Bayesian Inference with INLA

by
Virgilio Gómez-Rubio

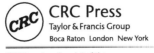

CRC Press
Taylor & Francis Group
Boca Raton London New York

CRC Press is an imprint of the
Taylor & Francis Group, an **informa** business

CRC Press
Taylor & Francis Group
6000 Broken Sound Parkway NW, Suite 300
Boca Raton, FL 33487-2742

© 2020 by Taylor & Francis Group, LLC
CRC Press is an imprint of Taylor & Francis Group, an Informa business

No claim to original U.S. Government works

Printed on acid-free paper
International Standard Book Number-13: 978-1-1380-3987-2 (Hardback)

Visit the Taylor & Francis Web site at
http://www.taylorandfrancis.com

and the CRC Press Web site at
http://www.crcpress.com

A mis padres, Victorina y Virgilio Benigno.

A Nerpio y sus gentes.

Contents

Preface   **xi**

1   Introduction to Bayesian Inference   1
1.1   Introduction 1
1.2   Bayesian inference 1
1.3   Conjugate priors 2
1.4   Computational methods 3
1.5   Markov chain Monte Carlo 3
1.6   The integrated nested Laplace approximation 4
1.7   An introductory example: U's in Game of Thrones books 5
1.8   Final remarks 11

2   The Integrated Nested Laplace Approximation   13
2.1   Introduction 13
2.2   The Integrated Nested Laplace Approximation 13
2.3   The R-INLA package 17
2.4   Model assessment and model choice 24
2.5   Control options 28
2.6   Working with posterior marginals 30
2.7   Sampling from the posterior 35

3   Mixed-effects Models   39
3.1   Introduction 39
3.2   Fixed-effects models 39
3.3   Types of mixed-effects models 42
3.4   Information on the latent effects 63
3.5   Additional arguments 63
3.6   Final remarks 73

4   Multilevel Models   75
4.1   Introduction 75
4.2   Multilevel models with random effects 75
4.3   Multilevel models with nested effects 82
4.4   Multilevel models with complex structure 87
4.5   Multilevel models for longitudinal data 90
4.6   Multilevel models for binary data 93
4.7   Multilevel models for count data 97

5   Priors in R-INLA   103
5.1   Introduction 103
5.2   Selection of priors 103
5.3   Implementing new priors 107

5.4	Penalized Complexity priors	111
5.5	Sensitivity analysis with R-INLA	113
5.6	Scaling effects and priors	114
5.7	Final remarks	116

6 Advanced Features   **119**

6.1	Introduction	119
6.2	Predictor Matrix	119
6.3	Linear combinations	121
6.4	Several likelihoods	128
6.5	Shared terms	131
6.6	Linear constraints	138
6.7	Final remarks	140

7 Spatial Models   **141**

7.1	Introduction	141
7.2	Areal data	141
7.3	Geostatistics	155
7.4	Point patterns	166

8 Temporal Models   **177**

8.1	Introduction	177
8.2	Autoregressive models	177
8.3	Non-Gaussian data	183
8.4	Forecasting	187
8.5	Space-state models	188
8.6	Spatio-temporal models	192
8.7	Final remarks	198

9 Smoothing   **201**

9.1	Introduction	201
9.2	Splines	201
9.3	Smooth terms with INLA	206
9.4	Smoothing with SPDE	212
9.5	Non-Gaussian models	214
9.6	Final remarks	218

10 Survival Models   **219**

10.1	Introduction	219
10.2	Non-parametric estimation of the survival curve	220
10.3	Parametric modeling of the survival function	222
10.4	Semi-parametric estimation: Cox proportional hazards	224
10.5	Accelerated failure time models	227
10.6	Frailty models	230
10.7	Joint modeling	233

11 Implementing New Latent Models   **243**

11.1	Introduction	243
11.2	Spatial latent effects	243
11.3	R implementation with `rgeneric`	245
11.4	Bayesian model averaging	251
11.5	INLA within MCMC	254

11.6 Comparison of results 257
11.7 Final remarks 257

12 Missing Values and Imputation **259**
12.1 Introduction 259
12.2 Missingness mechanism 259
12.3 Missing values in the response 260
12.4 Imputation of missing covariates 267
12.5 Multiple imputation of missing values 272
12.6 Final remarks 277

13 Mixture models **279**
13.1 Introduction 279
13.2 Bayesian analysis of mixture models 279
13.3 Fitting mixture models with INLA 283
13.4 Model selection for mixture models 289
13.5 Cure rate models 293
13.6 Final remarks 298

Packages used in the book **299**

Bibliography **303**

Index **313**

Preface

The integrated nested Laplace approximation (INLA) is a method for approximate Bayesian inference. In the last years it has established itself as an alternative to other methods such as Markov chain Monte Carlo because of its speed and ease of use via the R-INLA package. Although the INLA methodology focuses on models that can be expressed as latent Gaussian Markov random fields (GMRF), this encompasses a large family of models that are used in practice.

This book is aimed at providing an introduction to the INLA method and the associated `INLA` (or R-INLA) package. It starts with a short introduction to Bayesian inference in order to place INLA within context. Next, an introduction to the INLA method is given, and followed by two simple examples on using the `INLA` package for the R statistical software. Next, different types of widely used models are described in different chapters. To mention a few, these include mixed-effects models, multilevel models, spatial and spatio-temporal models, smoothing methods, survival analysis and others.

In addition to describing how to use the `INLA` package for model fitting, some advanced features available are covered as well. These are commonly employed to build different types of models, as well as to implement new latent effects and priors within the INLA framework. This is particularly important as it makes model fitting more flexible. Among the advanced features discussed, it is worth mentioning models with several likelihoods (to build joint models), shared effects between different likelihoods and the possibility to embed INLA within MCMC algorithms for flexible model fitting.

One idea that has been stressed in the book is that INLA can be used as a toolbox and that it can be combined with other methods for Bayesian inference. This is particular interesting when building models that do not fall within the class of latent GMRF. Two examples include mixture models and imputation mechanisms of missing observations in the latent GMRF.

Another important issue about this book is that a Gitbook version is available from the book website, and I can only thank my editor John Kimmel and the publisher for agreeing with this. This has also been possible thanks to the use of `rmarkdown` (Xie et al., 2018) and the `bookdown` (Xie, 2016) packages. Furthermore, all examples in the book are fully reproducible, with datasets and R code available from the book website.

Prerequisites

Although Chapter 1 provides a bit of context about Bayesian inference, the book assumes that the reader has a good understanding of Bayesian inference. In particular, a general course about Bayesian inference at the M.Sc. or Ph.D. level would be good starting point. Kruschke (2015) and McElreath (2016) are two recent books that can be used to learn about

Bayesian inference. Carlin and Louis (2008) and Gelman et al. (2013) provide a more in depth approach to Bayesian inference. Specific references to particular methods described in the book are mentioned wherever necessary.

This book does not assume any knowledge of the integrated nested Laplace approximation and the INLA package. However, the reader may want to check the nice introduction in Morrison (2017), as well as the examples provided in Bakka (2019) and Faraway (2019b).

Data and code sources

Most data and code sources are from R packages and they are cited in the appropriate chapters. However, some data have been obtained from different external sources and these are listed below. We have been as thorough as possible when acknowledging data and code sources and we hope that there are no omissions.

- In Chapter 4, the original data about the 1988 election in the United States of America have been obtained from Prof. Andrew Gelman's website, which can be downloaded from `http://www.stat.columbia.edu/~gelman/arm/examples/election88`.

- In Chapter 4, the original data about "stop-and-frisk" in New York have been obtained from Prof. Andrew Gelman's website at `http://www.stat.columbia.edu/~gelman/arm/examples/police`.

  Current precinct boundaries have been obtained from the web of the City of New York at `https://data.cityofnewyork.us/Public-Safety/Police-Precincts/78dh-3ptz/data`.

- In Chapter 8, the original New Mexico dataset health data has been obtained from the SaTScan™ website at `https://www.satscan.org` and completed with the county boundaries available from the US Census Bureau website (`https://www.census.gov`).

- In Chapter 9, the temperature dataset has been obtained from the associated website of Fahrmeir and Kneib (2011) at `http://www.smoothingbook.org/`.

- In Chapter 12, the code for the analysis of the nhanes2 dataset is available from GitHub at `https://github.com/becarioprecario/INLAMCMC_examples`.

- Some general on-line resources that I have found interesting include Bakka (2019), Faraway (2019b), Jovanovic (2015) and Morrison (2017).

- Finally, the book cover has been generated using several packages R packages, that include tmap (Tennekes, 2018) and leaflet (Cheng et al., 2019), and it uses data copyrighted OpenStreetMap contributors (available from `https://www.openstreetmap.org`).

Acknowledgements

First of all, I would like to thank Håvard Rue and coauthors for giving us INLA and all its derived works. I have had the chance to discuss many issues about INLA with them throughout the years and they have always been a source of inspiration and new ideas.

My friends and colleagues from the VALència Bayesian Research group (`http://vabar.es`) have also provided a nurturing environment for the development of this book. Furthermore, thanks to all my co-authors for coming with interesting research questions. Some of our joint work has been illustrated in this book. I am profoundly indebted to Susie Bayarri, Juan Ferrándiz and Antonio López, with whom I took my first steps in the Bayesian world.

And last but not least, I wanted to thank John Kimmel as the editor in charge of this book for his continuous support and patience every time I requested an extension to the previous deadline. He also made sure that early versions of the book where thoroughfully reviewed by a number of anonymous reviewers. Thanks to their comments the book has improved.

This work has also been partly supported by grants PPIC-2014-001-P and SB-PLY/17/180501/000491, funded by Consejería de Educación, Cultura y Deportes (Junta de Comunidades de Castilla-La Mancha, Spain) and FEDER, and grant MTM2016-77501-P, funded by Ministerio de Economía y Competitividad (Spain).

Virgilio Gómez-Rubio

La Noguera (Nerpio, Albacete, Spain)

1

Introduction to Bayesian Inference

1.1 Introduction

Bayesian inference has experienced a boost in recent years due to important advances in computational statistics. This book will focus on the integrated nested Laplace approximation (INLA, Rue et al., 2009) for approximate Bayesian inference. INLA is one of several recent computational breakthroughs in Bayesian statistics that allows fast and accurate model fitting.

The aim of this introduction is not to provide a thorough introduction to Bayesian inference but to introduce some notation and context for the other chapters of the book. For those readers that may require it, recent introductory texts to Bayesian inference include Kruschke (2015) and McElreath (2016). Both texts cover the basics and provide a good number of examples using a number of programming languages for Bayesian computation. More advanced texts include classics Gelman et al. (2013) and Carlin and Louis (2008), which provide more in depth details on a wide range of topics on Bayesian inference.

1.2 Bayesian inference

In the Bayesian paradigm all unknown quantities in the model are treated as random variables and the aim is to compute (or estimate) the joint *posterior* distribution. This is, the distribution of the parameters, $\boldsymbol{\theta}$, conditional on the observed data $\mathbf{y}$. The way that posterior distribution is obtained relies on Bayes' theorem:

$$\pi(\boldsymbol{\theta} \mid \mathbf{y}) = \frac{\pi(\mathbf{y} \mid \boldsymbol{\theta})\pi(\boldsymbol{\theta})}{\pi(\mathbf{y})}$$

Here, $\pi(\mathbf{y} \mid \boldsymbol{\theta})$ is the likelihood of the data $\mathbf{y}$ given parameters $\boldsymbol{\theta}$ (that take values in a parametric space Θ), $\pi(\boldsymbol{\theta})$ is the prior distribution of the parameters and $\pi(\mathbf{y})$ is the marginal likelihood, which acts as a normalizing constant. The marginal likelihood is often difficult to compute as it is equal to

$$\int_{\Theta} \pi(\mathbf{y} \mid \boldsymbol{\theta})\pi(\boldsymbol{\theta})d\boldsymbol{\theta}$$

Note that the posterior distribution $\pi(\boldsymbol{\theta} \mid \mathbf{y})$ is often a highly multivariate distribution and that it is only available in closed form for a few models because the marginal likelihood $\pi(\mathbf{y})$ is often difficult to estimate. In practice, the posterior distribution is estimated without computing the marginal likelihood. This is why Bayes' theorem is often stated as

$$\pi(\boldsymbol{\theta} \mid \mathbf{y}) \propto \pi(\mathbf{y} \mid \boldsymbol{\theta})\pi(\boldsymbol{\theta})$$

This means that the posterior can be estimated by re-scaling the product of the likelihood and the prior so that it integrates up to one.

The likelihood of the model describes the data generating process given the parameters, and the prior usually reflects any previous knowledge about the model parameters. When this knowledge is scarce, vague priors are assumed so that the posterior distribution is driven by the observed data.

Summary statistics on the model parameters $\boldsymbol{\theta}$ can be obtained from the joint posterior distribution $\pi(\boldsymbol{\theta} \mid \mathbf{y})$. In addition, the posterior *marginal* distribution of each element of $\boldsymbol{\theta}$ can be obtained by integrating the remainder of the parameters out:

$$\pi(\theta_i \mid \mathbf{y}) = \int \pi(\boldsymbol{\theta} \mid \mathbf{y})d\boldsymbol{\theta}_{-i}, \ i = 1, \ldots, \dim(\boldsymbol{\theta})$$

Here, θ_{-i} represents the set of elements in $\boldsymbol{\theta}$ minus θ_i. Posterior marginal distributions are very useful to summarize individual parameters and to compute summary statistics. Important quantities are the posterior mean, standard deviation, mode and quantiles.

1.3   Conjugate priors

As mentioned above, the posterior distribution is only available in closed form for a few models. Models with *conjugate* priors are those in which the prior is of the same form as the likelihood. For example, if the likelihood is a Gaussian distribution with known precision, the conjugate prior on the mean is a Gaussian distribution. This will ensure that the posterior distribution of the mean is also a Gaussian distribution.

For example, let it be a set of observations $\{y_i\}_{i=1}^{n}$ that follow a Gaussian distribution

$$y_i \mid \mu, \tau \sim N(\mu, \tau), \ i = 1, \ldots, n$$

with μ the unknown mean and τ a known precision. The prior on μ can be a Normal distribution with mean μ_0 and precision τ_0:

$$\mu \sim N(\mu_0, \tau_0)$$

The posterior distribution of μ (i.e., the distribution of μ given data $\mathbf{y}$) is $N(\mu_1, \tau_1)$ with

$$\mu_1 = \mu_0 \frac{\tau_0}{\tau_0 + \tau n} + \overline{y}\frac{\tau n}{\tau_0 + \tau n}$$

$$\tau_1 = \tau_0 + n\tau$$

This illustrates Bayesian learning quite well. First of all, the posterior mean is a compromise between the prior mean μ_0 and the mean of the observed data $\overline{y}$. When the number of observations is large, then the posterior mean is close to that of the data. If n is small, more weight is given to our prior belief about the mean. Similarly, the posterior precision is a function of the prior precision and the likelihood precision and it tends to infinity with n, which means that the variance of μ tends to zero as the number of data increases.

Other well known conjugate models include the Beta-Binomial model and the Poisson-Gamma model (Gelman et al., 2013).

1.4 Computational methods

When the posterior distribution is not available in a closed form it is necessary to resort to other methods to estimate it or, alternatively, to draw samples from it. Given a sample from the posterior, the Ergodic theorem ensures that moments and other quantities of interest can be estimated (Brooks et al., 2011).

In general, computational methods aim at estimating the integrals that appear in Bayesian inference. For example, the posterior mean of parameter θ_i (with values in the parameter space Θ_i) is computed as

$$\int_{\Theta_i} \theta_i \pi(\theta_i \mid \mathbf{y}) d\theta_i$$

Distribution $\pi(\theta_i \mid \mathbf{y})$ is the marginal posterior distribution of univariate parameter θ_i. Similarly, the posterior variance or any other moment can be computed as well. Integrals of this type can be conveniently approximated using numerical integration methods and the Laplace approximation (Tierney and Kadane, 1986).

Furthermore, typical Monte Carlo methods to sample from densities known up to a constant can be used to obtain samples from the posterior distribution. These methods include rejection sampling and other methods (Carlin and Louis, 2008). However, most of these methods will not work well in high dimensional spaces.

Point estimates of the model parameters can be obtained by maximizing the the product of the likelihood and the prior. This is denoted by Maximum A Posteriori (MAP) estimation. Maximization of the posterior distribution is usually performed in the log scaled and it can be effectively achieved using different methods, such as the Newton-Raphson algorithm or the Expectation-Maximization algorithm (Gelman et al., 2013).

1.5 Markov chain Monte Carlo

Markov chain Monte Carlo (MCMC) methods (Gilks et al., 1996; Brooks et al., 2011) are a class of computational methods to draw samples from the joint posterior distribution. These methods are based on constructing a Markov Chain with stationary distribution the posterior distribution. Hence, by sampling from this Markov chain repeatedly, samples from the joint posterior distribution are obtained after a number of iterations.

Several algorithms have been proposed (see Brooks et al., 2011, for a recent summary) but two of them provide a toolbox for Bayesian inference: the Metropolis-Hastings algorithm and Gibbs sampling.

The Metropolis-Hastings algorithm uses a proposal distribution to obtain new values for the ensemble of parameters. This is, given current value $\boldsymbol{\theta}$ a new value $\boldsymbol{\theta}'$ is drawn from density $q(\cdot \mid \boldsymbol{\theta})$. The proposal distribution can be chosen in many different ways. However, not all proposals will be accepted. When a new proposal is drawn it is accepted with probability

$$\min\left\{1, \frac{q(\boldsymbol{\theta} \mid \boldsymbol{\theta}')\pi(\boldsymbol{\theta}' \mid \mathbf{y})}{q(\boldsymbol{\theta}' \mid \boldsymbol{\theta})\pi(\boldsymbol{\theta} \mid \mathbf{y})}\right\}$$

Here, $q(\boldsymbol{\theta} \mid \boldsymbol{\theta}')$ represents the density of the proposal distribution $q(\cdot \mid \boldsymbol{\theta}')$ evaluated at $\boldsymbol{\theta}$. Note also that the acceptance probability contains the posterior distributions to be estimated (and that are unknown). However, the previous acceptance probability can be rewritten as

$$\min\left\{1, \frac{q(\boldsymbol{\theta} \mid \boldsymbol{\theta}')\pi(\mathbf{y} \mid \boldsymbol{\theta}')\pi(\boldsymbol{\theta}')}{q(\boldsymbol{\theta}' \mid \boldsymbol{\theta})\pi(\mathbf{y} \mid \boldsymbol{\theta})\pi(\boldsymbol{\theta})}\right\}$$

by using Bayes' rule. Note that now the scaling constant $\pi(\mathbf{y})$ is not needed to compute the ratio, which is why the Metropolis-Hastings algorithm is so popular.

The ratio essentially ensures that newly proposed values are accepted in the right proportion to be samples from the posterior distribution. In addition, the ratio also will favor moving to new values when there is a high chance of coming back to the current value. This makes sense because this will avoid getting trapped in areas of low posterior probability.

Gibbs sampling (Geman and Geman, 1984) can be regarded as a particular case of the Metropolis-Hastings algorithm in which the proposal distributions are the full conditional distribution of the model parameters, i.e., $\pi(\theta_i \mid \mathbf{y}, \boldsymbol{\theta}_{-i})$. This ensures that the acceptance probability in the Metropolis-Hastings algorithm is always one, which means that all proposals are automatically accepted.

In practice, convergence to the posterior distribution will take a number of iterations, and the first batch of simulations (or *burn-in*) is discarded for inference. Furthermore, given that samples are often correlated, a thinning is applied to the remaining samples, and many of them will be discarded as well (see, for example, Link and Eaton, 2012, and the references therein). Several criteria can be used to assess that the simulation have converged to the stationary state (Gelman and Rubin, 1992; Brooks and Gelman, 1998).

1.6 The integrated nested Laplace approximation

Rue et al. (2009) have developed a novel computational method for Bayesian inference. In particular, they focus on estimating the posterior marginals of the model parameters. Hence, instead of estimating a highly multivariate joint posterior distribution $\pi(\boldsymbol{\theta} \mid \mathbf{y})$ they focus on obtaining approximations to univariate posterior distributions $\pi(\theta_i \mid \mathbf{y})$. They have termed this approximation the *integrated nested Laplace approximation* (INLA).

Although the models that INLA can fit are restricted to the class of models that can be expressed as a latent Gaussian Markov random field (Rue and Held, 2005), this includes a myriad of commonly used models. In addition, the authors have developed an R package, INLA, for easy model fitting.

1.7 An introductory example: U's in Game of Thrones books

In order to introduce the different approaches to Bayesian inference outlined above, an introductory example is developed here. Note that the aim is to show where the INLA methodology fits into the Bayesian ecosystem and that some knowledge of Bayesian inference is required to follow the example.

We will consider the average number of u's on a page of any of the books in the Game of Thrones series. For data collection, only pages from the *Preface* of each of the five books published by Bantam Books in 2001 were considered. Pages with headers or that were not complete (i.e., had missing lines) were not considered. Data were collected by participants in the 2nd Valencia International Bayesian Summer School (VIBASS2, `http://vabar.es`) held in Valencia (Spain) in July 2018.

Data is provided in a CSV file that can be loaded and summarized as follows:

```
GoT <- read.csv2(file = "data/GoT.csv")
summary(GoT)
```

```
##        Us
##  Min.   :15.0
##  1st Qu.:27.5
##  Median :31.0
##  Mean   :33.0
##  3rd Qu.:36.5
##  Max.   :62.0
```

Altogether, there are 31 observations. Because this is a counting process, a Poisson likelihood seems a reasonable choice:

$$U_i \sim Po(\lambda), \ i = 1, \ldots, 31$$

Parameter λ is the mean of the Poisson distribution and the parameter that we are interested in. Remember that the probability distribution of a Poisson is

$$P(X = x \mid \lambda) = \frac{\exp(-\lambda)\lambda^x}{x!}$$

Note that letter *u* is not the most common vowel in English, and this fact can be used to make a choice about the prior distribution. Each page has about 20 lines and, say that we are certain that there will be about one or two u's per line. This prior guess can be used to set a prior on the parameter λ.

A Gamma distribution is the conjugate prior for a Poisson likelihood (Gelman et al., 2013). This is defined by two parameters, a and b, that define the mean, a/b, and variance, a/b^2. The probability density of the Gamma distribution is

$$f_X(x \mid a, b) = b \exp(-b \cdot x) \frac{(b \cdot x)^{a-1}}{\Gamma(a)}$$

Given our prior guess, we can take a Gamma with mean 30 and variance 5, which gives a high prior probability to λ being between 20 and 40. Hence, the parameters of the prior Gamma distribution are $a = 180$ and $b = 6$.

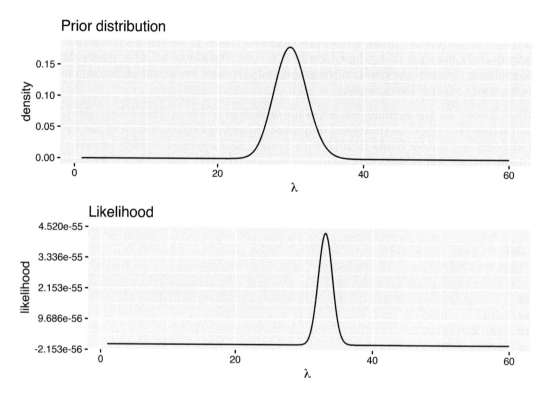

FIGURE 1.1 Likelihood and prior of the number of u's on a page of Game of Thrones.

A common way to visualize the likelihood and the prior is to plot them together. Figure 1.1 shows the prior and the likelihood. Note how they are in different scales but the modes are close, which means that our prior guess was not that bad after all. The posterior distribution will be obtained by combining the prior and the likelihood using Bayes' rule.

The maximum likelihood estimate is simply the mean of the data:

```
mean(GoT$Us)
```

```
## [1] 33.03
```

The Maximum A Posteriori (MAP) estimate can be obtained by maximizing the sum of the log-prior and the log-likelihood:

```
got.logposterior <- function(lambda) {
  dgamma(lambda, 180, 6, log = TRUE) + sum(dpois(GoT$Us, lambda,
    log = TRUE))
}
```

```
#Maximize log-posterior
```

```
got.MAP <- optim(30, got.logposterior, control = list(fnscale = -1))
got.MAP$par
```

```
## [1] 32.51
```

Given that the Gamma distribution is conjugate for a Poisson likelihood, the posterior is available in a closed form, and it is a Gamma with parameters $a + \sum_{i=1}^{31} U_i$ and $b + n$. The posterior distribution has been plotted in Figure 1.2.

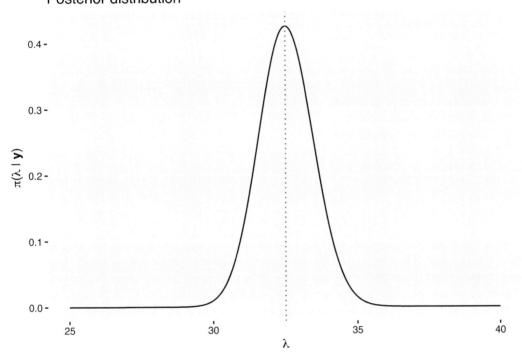

FIGURE 1.2 Posterior distribution of the number of u's in a book of Game of Thrones using a conjugate prior (black solid line) and MAP estimate (dotted red line).

A Metropolis-Hastings algorithm to estimate the posterior distribution of the parameter λ can be implemented in this case. As a proposal density we will consider a log-Normal distribution centered at the current value of the mean λ and with small standard deviation equal to 0.05.

The algorithm will obtain 2100 values of λ, starting at 20:

```
n.sim <- 2100
lambda <- rep(NA, n.sim)
lambda[1] <- 20
```

The implementation of the Metropolis-Hastings algorithm is the following:

```
set.seed(1)
for (i in 2:n.sim) {
  # Draw new value
  lambda.new <- rlnorm(1, log(lambda[i - 1]), 0.05)

  #Log-acceptance probability
  acc.prob <- dlnorm(lambda[i -1], log(lambda.new), 0.05, log = TRUE) +
    dgamma(lambda.new, 180, 6, log = TRUE) +
    sum(dpois(GoT$Us, lambda.new, log = TRUE)) -
    dlnorm(lambda.new, log(lambda[i - 1]), 0.05, log = TRUE) -
    dgamma(lambda[i - 1], 180, 6, log = TRUE) -
    sum(dpois(GoT$Us, lambda[i - 1], log = TRUE))

  acc.prob <- min(1, exp(acc.prob))

  # Accept/reject new value
  if(runif(1) < acc.prob) {
    lambda[i] <- lambda.new
  } else {
    lambda[i] <- lambda[i -1]
  }

}
```

Figure 1.3 shows the samples of λ obtained with the Metropolis-Hastings algorithm. The first iterations provide values that are too close to the initial value and these are often taken as a *burn-in* and discarded. The remaining values are used for inference. However, given that they seem a bit correlated it is usual to conduct a thinning on them. In this case, 100 iterations will be taken as burn-in, and thinning will be done on the remaining observations, so that only one in five is kept. As a result, there will be 400 values for inference.

Removing the burn-in iterations and thinning can be done as follows:

```
lambda2 <- lambda[seq(101, n.sim, by = 5)]
```

Summary statistics of the posterior distribution of λ can be obtained by taking summary statistics on the sampled values:

```
summary(lambda2)
```

```
##    Min. 1st Qu.  Median    Mean 3rd Qu.    Max.
##    30.0    32.0    32.7    32.6    33.2    36.2
```

Kernel density can be used to obtain an estimate of the posterior marginal distribution of λ from the final set of values. This is shown in the plot at the bottom in Figure 1.3. It is worth mentioning that the estimates obtained with the Metropolis-Hastings algorithm are very close to those obtained with the other methods computed so far because we are actually fitting the same model. Any differences are due to the Monte Carlo error inherent to MCMC methods, but this error can usually be reduced by increasing the number of samples drawn.

In any case, we provide a comparison and summary of the different estimates obtained at the end of this section.

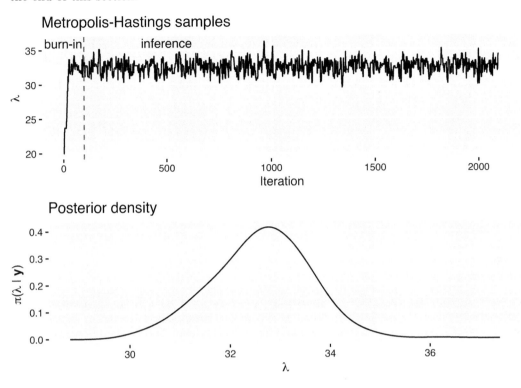

FIGURE 1.3 Samples of λ obtained with the Metropolis-Hastings algorithm (top) and kernel density estimate of the posterior distribution using the samples (bottom).

Finally, we show how to fit these models using INLA. First of all, the model fit will be the following:

$$U_i \sim Po(\lambda), \ i = 1, \ldots, 31$$

$$\log(\lambda) = \alpha$$

$$\pi(\alpha) \propto 1$$

Parameter α is the intercept of the linear predictor and it is assigned a constant prior. This is an improper prior because it does not integrate to one but these are sometimes useful to provide a vague prior. Note that λ is not modeled directly but in the log-scale through the intercept of the linear predictor α. This model can be implemented with **INLA** using the following code (that will not be discussed here in detail):

```
GoT.inla <- inla(Us ~ 1, data = GoT, family = "poisson",
   control.predictor = list(compute = TRUE)
)
```

Summary statistics of the posterior distribution of α are:

```
GoT.inla$summary.fixed
```

```
##                  mean      sd 0.025quant 0.5quant 0.975quant   mode        kld
## (Intercept) 3.498 0.03127      3.436     3.498       3.558 3.498 4.926e-07
```

The posterior distribution of λ can be obtained by transforming the posterior distribution of α given that $\lambda = \exp(\alpha)$ (see Section 2.6):

```
marg.lambda <- inla.tmarginal(exp, GoT.inla$marginals.fixed[[1]])
inla.est <- inla.zmarginal(marg.lambda)
```

```
## Mean              33.049
## Stdev             1.02682
## Quantile  0.025   31.059
## Quantile  0.25    32.3464
## Quantile  0.5     33.0376
## Quantile  0.75    33.7378
## Quantile  0.975   35.0905
```

In order to compare the different approaches, we have produced Table 1.1 that includes estimates based on the methods described so far. In this case, point estimates of parameter λ are very similar. Note also that the maximum likelihood estimate is very close to the posterior modes obtained with all Bayesian methods. The point estimates of the posterior standard deviation are also very similar among the three Bayesian methods that computed them. The quantiles computed are also very close. It is worth mentioning that in this particular case the mode is simple and we have enough data to estimate the only parameter in the model. Hence, it would be expected that all results should be similar.

TABLE 1.1: Summary of estimates using different Bayesian estimation methods.

Method	Mean	Mode	St. dev.	0.025 quant.	0.975 quant.
Max. lik.	NA	33.03	NA	NA	NA
MAP	NA	32.51	NA	NA	NA
Conjugate	32.54	32.51	0.9378	30.73	34.40
M-H	32.47	32.77	1.2625	30.55	34.33
INLA	33.05	33.02	1.0268	31.06	35.09

Figure 1.4 shows the different estimates of the posterior marginal and MAP estimate of parameter λ obtained with the different methods presented here. As we had seen previously, all methods provide very similar estimates of the posterior marginal. Note that for more complex models it may simply not be possible to obtain the marginals in a closed form and that estimation will most often rely on MCMC or INLA methods.

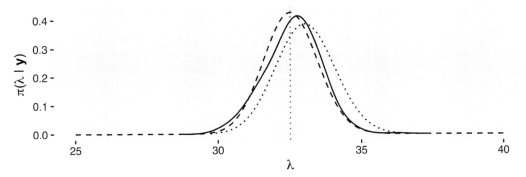

FIGURE 1.4 Comparison of the different estimates of the posterior marginal of λ provided by the methods described in this chapter: MCMC (solid line), conjugate prior (dashed line), INLA (dotted line) and MAP (vertical red dotted line).

1.8   Final remarks

As stated at the beginning of this chapter, the aim is to provide an introduction to Bayesian inference. In particular, to provide some context so that readers can place the integrated nested Laplace approximation within the Bayesian ecosystem. This is important for many reasons. First of all, INLA is one of many ways to make Bayesian inference. INLA may be the right approach in many occasions, but it might simply be the wrong approach on some other occasions. Secondly, this also means that having a deep knowledge of INLA is useful to identify models where it will work well and other where it will perform badly.

Chapter 2 introduces the integrated nested Laplace approximation methodology and the use of the INLA package for Bayesian model fitting. A number of latent effects for model building are described in Chapter 3. Next, multilevel models are tackled in Chapter 4. Prior distributions are summarized in Chapter 5. Additional features that can be used to fit more complex models are detailed in Chapter 6. Different types of models with spatial dependence are depicted in Chapter 7. The analysis of time series by means of temporally correlated models and spatio-temporal models are presented in Chapter 8. Splines and other smoothing methods are described in Chapter 9. The analysis of time-to-event data using survival and joint models is examined in Chapter 10. Different ways of fitting new models not implemented in the INLA package are illustrated in Chapter 11. Handling missing values in both the response and covariates is described in Chapter 12. Finally, the analysis of mixture models with INLA is explained in Chapter 13.

2

The Integrated Nested Laplace Approximation

2.1 Introduction

For many years, Bayesian inference has relied upon Markov chain Monte Carlo methods (Gilks et al., 1996; Brooks et al., 2011) to compute the joint posterior distribution of the model parameters. This is usually computationally very expensive as this distribution is often in a space of high dimension.

Rue et al. (2009) propose a novel approach that makes Bayesian inference faster. First of all, rather than aiming at estimating the joint posterior distribution of the model parameters, they suggest focusing on individual posterior marginals of the model parameters. In many cases, marginal inference is enough to make inference of the model parameters and latent effects, and there is no need to deal with multivariate posterior distributions that are difficult to obtain. Secondly, they focus on models that can be expressed as latent Gaussian Markov random fields (GMRF). This provides the computational advantages (see Rue and Held, 2005) that reduce computation time of model fitting. Furthermore, Rue et al. (2009) develop a new approximation to the posterior marginal distributions of the model parameters based on the Laplace approximation (see, for example, MacKay, 2003). A recent review on INLA can be found in Rue et al. (2017).

2.2 The Integrated Nested Laplace Approximation

In order to describe the models that INLA can fit, a vector of n observations $\mathbf{y} = (y_1, \ldots, y_n)$ will be considered. Note that some of them may be missing observations. Furthermore, these observations will have an associated likelihood (not necessarily from the exponential family). In general, mean μ_i of observation y_i can be linked to the linear predictor η_i via a convenient function.

Observations will be independent given its linear predictor, i.e.,

$$\eta_i = \alpha + \sum_{j=1}^{n_\beta} \beta_j z_{ji} + \sum_{k=1}^{n_f} f^{(k)}(u_{ki}) + \varepsilon_i; \; i = 1, \ldots, n$$

Here, α is the intercept, β_j, $j = 1, \ldots, n_\beta$, coefficients of some covariates $\{\mathbf{z}_j\}_{j=1}^{n_\beta}$, functions $f^{(k)}$ define n_f random effects on some vector of covariates $\{\mathbf{u}_k\}_{k=1}^{n_f}$. Finally, ε_i is an error term, that may be missing depending on the likelihood.

Within the INLA framework, the vector of latent effects $\mathbf{x}$ will be represented as follows:

$$\mathbf{x} = (\eta_1, \ldots, \eta_n, \alpha, \beta_1, \ldots)$$

Rue et al. (2009) make further assumptions about the model and consider that this latent structure is that of a GMRF (Rue and Held, 2005). Also, observations are considered to be independent given latent effects $\mathbf{x}$, whose distributions depend on a vector of hyperparameters $\boldsymbol{\theta}_1$.

The latent GRMF structure of the model will have zero mean and precision matrix $\mathbf{Q}(\boldsymbol{\theta}_2)$, which will depend on a vector of hyperparameters $\boldsymbol{\theta}_2$. To simplify notation we will consider $\boldsymbol{\theta} = (\boldsymbol{\theta}_1, \boldsymbol{\theta}_2)$ and will avoid referring to $\boldsymbol{\theta}_1$ or $\boldsymbol{\theta}_2$ individually. Given the structure of GMRF, precision matrix $\mathbf{Q}(\boldsymbol{\theta})$ will often be very sparse. INLA will take advantage of this sparse structure as well as conditional independence properties of GMRFs in order to speed up computations.

The posterior distribution of the latent effects $\mathbf{x}$ can then be written down as:

$$\pi(\mathbf{x}, \boldsymbol{\theta} \mid \mathbf{y}) = \frac{\pi(\mathbf{y} \mid \mathbf{x}, \boldsymbol{\theta})\pi(\mathbf{x}, \boldsymbol{\theta})}{\pi(\mathbf{y})} \propto \pi(\mathbf{y} \mid \mathbf{x}, \boldsymbol{\theta})\pi(\mathbf{x}, \boldsymbol{\theta})$$

In the previous equation, $\pi(\mathbf{y})$ represents the marginal likelihood of the model, which is a normalizing constant that is often ignored as it is usually difficult to compute. However, INLA provides an accurate approximation to this quantity (Hubin and Storvik, 2016), as described below.

Also, $\pi(\mathbf{y} \mid \mathbf{x}, \boldsymbol{\theta})$ represents the likelihood. Given that it is assumed that observations $(y_1, \ldots, y_n)$ are independent given the latent effects $\mathbf{x}$ and $\boldsymbol{\theta}$, the likelihood can be re-written as:

$$\pi(\mathbf{y} \mid \mathbf{x}, \boldsymbol{\theta}) = \prod_{i \in I} \pi(y_i \mid x_i, \boldsymbol{\theta})$$

Here, the set of indices I is a subset of all integers from 1 to n and only includes the indices of the observations y_i that have been actually observed. This is, if a value in the response is missing, then its corresponding index will not be included in I. For the observations with missing values, their predictive distribution can be easily computed by INLA (as described in Chapter 12).

The joint distribution of the random effects and the hyperparameters, $\pi(\mathbf{x}, \boldsymbol{\theta})$, can be rearranged as $\pi(\mathbf{x} \mid \boldsymbol{\theta})\pi(\boldsymbol{\theta})$, with $\pi(\boldsymbol{\theta})$ the prior distribution of the ensemble of hyperparameters $\boldsymbol{\theta}$. As many of the hyperparameters will be independent a priori, $\boldsymbol{\theta}$ is likely to be the product of several (univariate) priors.

Hence, because $\mathbf{x}$ is a GMRF, the posterior distribution of the latent effects is:

$$\pi(\mathbf{x} \mid \boldsymbol{\theta}) \propto |\mathbf{Q}(\boldsymbol{\theta})|^{1/2} \exp\{-\frac{1}{2}\mathbf{x}^T \mathbf{Q}(\boldsymbol{\theta})\mathbf{x}\}$$

Taking all these considerations, the joint posterior distribution of the latent effects and hyperparameters can be written down as:

$$\pi(\mathbf{x}, \boldsymbol{\theta} \mid \mathbf{y}) \propto \pi(\boldsymbol{\theta})|\mathbf{Q}(\boldsymbol{\theta})|^{1/2} \exp\{-\frac{1}{2}\mathbf{x}^T \mathbf{Q}(\boldsymbol{\theta})\mathbf{x}\} \prod_{i \in I} \pi(y_i \mid x_i, \boldsymbol{\theta}) =$$

$$\pi(\boldsymbol{\theta})|\mathbf{Q}(\boldsymbol{\theta})|^{1/2}\exp\{-\frac{1}{2}\mathbf{x}^T\mathbf{Q}(\boldsymbol{\theta})\mathbf{x}+\sum_{i\in I}\log(\pi(y_i\mid x_i,\boldsymbol{\theta}))\}$$

As mentioned earlier, INLA will not attempt to estimate the previous posterior distribution but the marginals of the latent effects and hyperparameters. For a latent parameter x_l, this is

$$\pi(x_l\mid\mathbf{y})=\int\pi(x_l,\boldsymbol{\theta}\mid\mathbf{y})\pi(\boldsymbol{\theta}\mid\mathbf{y})d\boldsymbol{\theta}$$

In a similar way, the posterior marginal for a hyperparameter θ_k is

$$\pi(\theta_k\mid\mathbf{y})=\int\pi(\boldsymbol{\theta}\mid\mathbf{y})d\boldsymbol{\theta}_{-k}$$

Here, $\boldsymbol{\theta}_{-k}$ is a vector of hyperparameters $\boldsymbol{\theta}$ without element θ_k.

The approximation to the joint posterior of $\boldsymbol{\theta}$, $\tilde{\pi}(\boldsymbol{\theta}\mid\mathbf{y})$ proposed by Rue et al. (2009) can be used to compute the marginals of the latent effects and hyperparameters as follows:

$$\tilde{\pi}(\boldsymbol{\theta}\mid\mathbf{y})\propto\frac{\pi(\mathbf{x},\boldsymbol{\theta},\mathbf{y})}{\tilde{\pi}_G(\mathbf{x}\mid\boldsymbol{\theta},\mathbf{y})}\Big|_{\mathbf{x}=\mathbf{x}^*(\boldsymbol{\theta})}$$

In the previous equation, $\tilde{\pi}_G(\mathbf{x}\mid\boldsymbol{\theta},\mathbf{y})$ is a Gaussian approximation to the full condition of the latent effects, and $\mathbf{x}^*(\boldsymbol{\theta})$ represents the mode of the full conditional for a given value of the vector of hyperparameters $\boldsymbol{\theta}$.

Posterior marginal $\pi(\theta_k\mid\mathbf{y})$ can be approximated by integrating $\boldsymbol{\theta}_{-k}$ out in the previous approximation $\tilde{\pi}(\boldsymbol{\theta}\mid\mathbf{y})$. Similarly, an approximation to posterior marginal $\pi(x_i\mid\mathbf{y})$ using numerical integration, but a good approximation to $\pi(x_i,\boldsymbol{\theta}\mid\mathbf{y})$ is required. A Gaussian approximation is possible, but Rue et al. (2009) obtain better approximations by resorting to other methods, such as the Laplace approximation.

2.2.1 Approximations to $\pi(x_i\mid\boldsymbol{\theta},\mathbf{y})$

The approximation to the marginals of the hyperparameters can be computed by marginalizing over $\tilde{\pi}(\boldsymbol{\theta}\mid\mathbf{y})$ above to obtain $\tilde{\pi}(\theta_i\mid\mathbf{y})$. The approximation to the marginals of the latent effects requires integrating the hyperparameters out and marginalizing over the latent effects. INLA uses the following approximation

$$\pi(x_i\mid\mathbf{y})\simeq\sum_{k=1}^{K}\tilde{\pi}(x_i\mid\boldsymbol{\theta}^{(k)},\mathbf{y})\tilde{\pi}(\boldsymbol{\theta}^{(k)}\mid\mathbf{y})\Delta_k$$

Here, $\{\boldsymbol{\theta}^{(k)}\}_{k=1}^{K}$ represent a set of values of $\boldsymbol{\theta}$ that are used for numerical integration and each one has an associated integration weight Δ_k. INLA will obtain these integration points by placing a regular grid about the posterior mode of $\boldsymbol{\theta}$ or by using a central composite design (CCD, Box and Draper, 1987) centered at the posterior mode (see Section 2.2.2 below).

Rue et al. (2009) describe three different approximations for $\pi(x_i\mid\boldsymbol{\theta},\mathbf{y})$. The first one is simply a Gaussian approximation, which estimates the mean $\mu_i(\boldsymbol{\theta})$ and variance $\sigma_i^2(\boldsymbol{\theta})$. This is computationally cheap because during the exploration of $\pi(\boldsymbol{\theta}\mid\mathbf{y})$ the distribution $\tilde{\pi}_G(\mathbf{x}\mid\boldsymbol{\theta},\mathbf{y})$ is computed, so $\tilde{\pi}_G(x_i\mid\boldsymbol{\theta},\mathbf{y})$ can be easily computed by marginalizing.

A second approach could be based on the Laplace approximation, so that the approximation to $\pi(x_i \mid \boldsymbol{\theta}, \mathbf{y})$ would be

$$\pi_{LA}(x_i \mid \boldsymbol{\theta}, \mathbf{y}) \propto \left. \frac{\pi(\mathbf{x}, \boldsymbol{\theta}, \mathbf{y})}{\tilde{\pi}_{GG}(\mathbf{x}_{-i} \mid x_i, \boldsymbol{\theta}, \mathbf{y})} \right|_{\mathbf{x}_{-i} = \mathbf{x}^*_{-i}(x_i, \boldsymbol{\theta})}$$

Distribution $\tilde{\pi}_{GG}(\mathbf{x}_{-i} \mid x_i, \boldsymbol{\theta}, \mathbf{y})$ represents the Gaussian approximation to $\mathbf{x}_{-i} \mid x_i, \boldsymbol{\theta}, \mathbf{y}$ and $\mathbf{x}_{-i} = \mathbf{x}^*_{-i}(x_i, \boldsymbol{\theta})$ is its mode. This is more computationally expensive than the Gaussian approximation because it must be computed for each value of x_i.

For this reason, Rue et al. (2009) propose a modified approximation that relies on

$$\pi_{LA}(x_i \mid \mathbf{x}, \boldsymbol{\theta}) \propto N(x_i \mid \mu_i(\boldsymbol{\theta}), \sigma_i^2(\boldsymbol{\theta})) \exp(spline(x_i))$$

Hence, the Laplace approximation relies on the product of the Gaussian approximation and a cubic spline $spline(x_i)$ on x_i. The spline is computed at selected values of x_i and its role is to correct the Gaussian approximation.

The third approximation, $\tilde{\pi}_{SLA}(x_i \mid \boldsymbol{\theta}, \mathbf{y})$, is termed the *simplified* Laplace approximation and it relies on a series expansion of $\tilde{\pi}_{LA}(x_i \mid \boldsymbol{\theta}, \mathbf{y})$ around $x_i = \mu_i(\boldsymbol{\theta})$. With this, the Gaussian approximation $\tilde{\pi}_G(x_i \mid \boldsymbol{\theta}, \mathbf{y})$ can be corrected for location and skewness and it is very fast computationally.

2.2.2   Estimation procedure

The whole estimation procedure in INLA is made of several steps. First of all, the mode of $\tilde{\pi}(\boldsymbol{\theta} \mid \mathbf{y})$ is obtained by maximizing $\log(\tilde{\pi}(\boldsymbol{\theta} \mid \mathbf{y}))$ on $\boldsymbol{\theta}$. This is done using a quasi-Newton method. Once the posterior mode $\boldsymbol{\theta}^*$ has been obtained, finite differences are used to compute minus the hessian, $\mathbf{H}$, at the mode. Note that $\mathbf{H}^{-1}$ would be the variance matrix if the posterior is a Gaussian distribution.

Next, $\mathbf{H}^{-1}$ is decomposed using a eigenvalue decomposition so that $\mathbf{H}^{-1} = \mathbf{V}\boldsymbol{\Lambda}\mathbf{V}^\top$. With this decomposition, for each value of the hyperparameter $\boldsymbol{\theta}$ we can obtain a re-scaled $\mathbf{z}$ so that $\boldsymbol{\theta}(\mathbf{z}) = \boldsymbol{\theta}^* + \mathbf{V}\boldsymbol{\Lambda}^{1/2}\mathbf{z}$. This re-scaling is useful to explore the space of $\boldsymbol{\theta}$ more efficiently as it corrects for scale and rotation.

Finally, $\log(\tilde{\pi}(\boldsymbol{\theta} \mid \mathbf{y}))$ is explored using the $\mathbf{z}$ parameterization in two different ways. The first one uses a regular grid of step h centered at the mode ($\mathbf{z} = \mathbf{0}$) and points in the grid are considered only if

$$|\log(\tilde{\pi}(\boldsymbol{\theta}(\mathbf{0}) \mid \mathbf{y})) - \log(\tilde{\pi}(\boldsymbol{\theta}(\mathbf{z}) \mid \mathbf{y}))| < \delta$$

with δ a given threshold. Exploration is done first along the axis in the $\mathbf{z}$ parameterization and then all intermediate points that fulfill the previous condition are added.

This will provide a set of configurations of the hyperparameters about the posterior mode that can be used in the numerical integration procedures required in INLA. This is often known as the *grid* strategy.

Alternatively, a central composite design (CCD, Box and Draper, 1987) centered at $\boldsymbol{\theta}(\mathbf{0})$ can be used so that a few strategically placed points are obtained instead of using points in a regular grid. This can be more efficient that the grid strategy as the dimension of the hyperparameter space increases.

Both integration strategies are exemplified in Figure 2.1 where the grid and CCD strategies are shown. For the grid strategy, the log-density is explored along the axes (black dots) first. Then, all combinations of their values are explored (gray dots) and only those with a difference up to a threshold δ with the log-density at the mode are considered in the integration strategy. For the CCD approach, a number of points that fill the space are chosen using a response surface approach. Rue et al. (2009) point out that this method worked well in many cases.

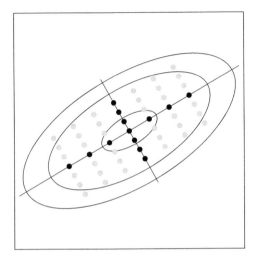 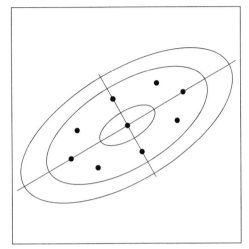

FIGURE 2.1 Exploration of $\log(\tilde{\pi}(\boldsymbol{\theta} \mid \mathbf{y}))$ using a grid (left) and CCD (right) strategy.

A cheaper option, which may work with a moderately large number of hyperparameters, is an empirical Bayes approach that will plug the posterior mode of $\boldsymbol{\theta} \mid \mathbf{y}$. This will work when the variability in the hyperparameters does not affect the posterior of the latent effects $\mathbf{x}$. This type of plug-in estimators may be useful to fit highly parameterized models and they can provide good approximations in a number of scenarios (Gómez-Rubio and Palmí-Perales, 2019).

Finally, recent reviews of INLA can be found in Martins et al. (2013) and Rue et al. (2017) as well. In addition to this review paper, several of the most important features of the implementation of INLA in a the `INLA` package will be discussed in the next sections and Chapter 6.

2.3 The R-INLA package

INLA is implemented as an R package called `INLA`, although this package is also called R-INLA. The package is not available from the main R repository CRAN, but from a specific repository at `http://www.r-inla.org`. The `INLA` package is available for Windows, Mac OS X and Linux, and there are a stable and a testing version.

A simple way to install the stable version is shown below. For the testing version, simply replace `stable` by `testing` when setting the repository.

```
# Set INLA repository
options(repos = c(getOption("repos"),
    INLA="https://inla.r-inla-download.org/R/stable"))

# Install INLA and dependencies (from CRAN)
install.packages("INLA", dep = TRUE)
```

The main function in the package is `inla()`, which is the one used to fit the Bayesian models using the INLA methodology. This function works in a similar way as function `glm()` (for generalized linear models) or `gam()` (for generalized additive models). A formula is used to specify the model to be fitted and it can include a mix of fixed and other effects conveniently specified.

Specific (random) effects are specified using the `f()` function. This includes an index to map the effect to the observations, the type of effect, additional parameters and the priors on the hyperparameters of the effect. When including a random effect in the model, not all of these options need to be specified.

2.3.1   Multiple linear regression

As a first example on the use of the `INLA` package we will show a simple example of multiple linear regression. The `cement` dataset in the `MASS` package contains measurements in an experiment on heat evolved (y, in cals/gm) depending on the proportions of 4 active components (x1, x2, x3 and x4). Data can be loaded and summarized as follows:

```
library("MASS")
summary(cement)
```

```
##       x1              x2              x3              x4
## Min.   : 1.00   Min.   :26.0   Min.   : 4.0   Min.   : 6
## 1st Qu.: 2.00   1st Qu.:31.0   1st Qu.: 8.0   1st Qu.:20
## Median : 7.00   Median :52.0   Median : 9.0   Median :26
## Mean   : 7.46   Mean   :48.1   Mean   :11.8   Mean   :30
## 3rd Qu.:11.00   3rd Qu.:56.0   3rd Qu.:17.0   3rd Qu.:44
## Max.   :21.00   Max.   :71.0   Max.   :23.0   Max.   :60
##       y
## Min.   : 72.5
## 1st Qu.: 83.8
## Median : 95.9
## Mean   : 95.4
## 3rd Qu.:109.2
## Max.   :115.9
```

The model to be fitted is the following:

$$y_i = \beta_0 + \sum_{j=1}^{4} \beta_j x_{j,i} + \varepsilon_i$$

Here, y_i represents the heat evolved of observation i, and $x_{j,i}$ is the proportion of component j in observation i. Parameter β_0 is an intercept and $\beta_j, j = 1, \ldots, 4$ are coefficients associated with the covariates. Finally, $\varepsilon_i, i = 1, \ldots, n$ is an error term with a Gaussian distribution with zero mean and precision τ.

By default, the intercept has a Gaussian prior with mean and precision equal to zero. Coefficients of the fixed effects also have a Gaussian prior by default with zero mean and precision equal to 0.001. The prior on the precision of the error term is, by default, a Gamma distribution with parameters 1 and 0.00005 (shape and rate, respectively).

The parameters of the priors on the fixed effects (i.e., intercept and coefficients) can be changed with option `control.fixed` in the call to `inla()`, which sets some of the options for the fixed effects. Table 2.1 displays a summary of the different options and their default values. A complete list of options and their default values can be obtained by running `inla.set.control.fixed.default()`. Control options are described below in Section 2.5.

TABLE 2.1: Summary of some options in `control.fixed` to set the priors on the fixed effects of the model.

Argument	Default	Description
`mean.intercept`	0	Mean of Gaussian prior on the intercept.
`prec.intercept`	0	Precision of Gaussian prior on the intercept.
`mean`	0	Mean of Gaussian prior on a coefficient.
`prec`	0.001	Precision of Gaussian prior on a coefficient.

The `inla()` function is the main function in the INLA package as it takes care of all model fitting. It works in a very similar way to the `glm()` function and, in its simplest form, it will take a formula with the model to fit and the data. It returns an object of class `inla` with all the results from model fitting. An `inla` object is essentially a named list and Table 2.2 shows some of its elements.

TABLE 2.2: Some of the elements in an `inla` object returned by a call to `inla()`. All summary statistics are computed using the posterior marginals.

Name	Description
`summary.fitted.values`	Summary statistics of fitted values.
`summary.fixed`	Summary statistics of fixed effects.
`summary.random`	Summary statistics of random effects.
`summary.linear.predictor`	Summary statistics of linear predictors.
`marginals.fitted.values`	Posterior marginals of fitted values.
`marginals.fixed`	Posterior marginals of fixed effects.
`marginals.random`	Posterior marginals of random effects.
`marginals.linear.predictor`	Posterior marginals of linear predictors.
`mlik`	Estimate of marginal likelihood.

To illustrate the use of the `inla()` function, in the next example a model with four fixed effects is fit using the `cement` dataset:

```
library("INLA")
```

```
m1 <- inla(y ~ x1 + x2 + x3 + x4, data = cement)
summary(m1)
```

```
##
## Call:
##    "inla(formula = y ~ x1 + x2 + x3 + x4, data = cement)"
## Time used:
##      Pre = 1.11, Running = 0.0933, Post = 0.0678, Total = 1.27
## Fixed effects:
##               mean     sd 0.025quant 0.5quant 0.975quant    mode kld
## (Intercept) 62.508 70.321    -78.180   62.495    203.045  62.481   0
## x1           1.550  0.747      0.054    1.550      3.043   1.550   0
## x2           0.509  0.726     -0.945    0.509      1.960   0.509   0
## x3           0.101  0.757     -1.415    0.101      1.614   0.101   0
## x4          -0.145  0.712     -1.569   -0.145      1.276  -0.145   0
##
## Model hyperparameters:
##                                            mean     sd 0.025quant 0.5quant
## Precision for the Gaussian observations 0.209 0.093      0.068      0.195
##                                        0.975quant   mode
## Precision for the Gaussian observations     0.429 0.167
##
## Expected number of effective parameters(stdev): 5.00(0.001)
## Number of equivalent replicates : 2.60
##
## Marginal log-Likelihood:  -59.50
```

The summary of the model displays summary statistics on the posterior marginals of the model latent effects and hyperparameters and other quantities of interest.

Furthermore, INLA provides an estimate of the effective number of parameters (and its standard deviation), which can be used as a measure of the complexity of the model. In addition, the number of equivalent replicates is computed as well, which is the number of observations divided by the effective number of parameters. Hence, this can be regarded as the average number of observations available to estimate each parameter in the model and higher values are better (Rue, 2009).

By default, INLA also computes the marginal likelihood of the model in the logarithmic scale. This is an important (and often neglected) feature in INLA as it not only serves as a criterion for model choice but also can be used to build more complex models with INLA as explained in later chapters.

2.3.2 Generalized linear models

INLA can handle generalized linear models similar to the glm() function by setting a convenient likelihood via the family argument. In addition to families from the exponential family, INLA can work with many other types of likelihoods. Table 2.3 summarizes a few of these distributions, but at the time of this writing INLA can work with more than 60 different likelihoods. In addition to the typical likelihoods used in practice (Gaussian, Poisson, etc.), this includes likelihoods for censored and zero-inflated data and many others. A complete list of available likelihoods can be obtained by running inla.models() as follows:

```
names(inla.models()$likelihood)
```

TABLE 2.3: Some likelihoods available in INLA.

Value	Likelihood
poisson	Poisson
binomial	Binomial
t	Student's t
gamma	Gamma

Function `inla.models()` provides a summary of the different likelihoods, latent models, etc. implemented in the INLA package and it can be used to assess the internal parameterization used by INLA and the default priors of the hyperparameters, for example. Table 2.4 shows a summary of the different blocks of information provided by `inla.models()`.

TABLE 2.4: Summary of some of the elements returned by a call to `inla.models()`. Each element provides a description of the functions or effects available, as well as the internal parameterization of the hyperparameters and their default priors.

Value	Description
latent	Latent models available
group	Models available when grouping observations
link	Link function available
hazard	Models for the baseline hazard function in survival models
likelihood	List of likelihoods available
prior	List of priors available

In order to provide an example of fitting a GLM with INLA, please note the `nc.sids` dataset in the `spData` package (Bivand et al., 2019). It contains information about the number of deaths by sudden infant death syndrome (SIDS) in North Carolina in two time periods (1974-1978 and 1979-1984). Some of the variables in the dataset are summarized in Table 2.5.

TABLE 2.5: Summary of some variables in the `nc.sids` dataset.

Variable	Description
CNTY.ID	County id number
BIR74	Number of births in the period 1974-1978
SID74	Number of cases of SIDS in the period 1974-1978
NWBIR74	Number of non-white births in the period 1974-1978
BIR79	Number of births in the period 1979-1984
SID79	Number of cases of SIDS in the period 1979-1984
NWBIR79	Number of non-white births in the period 1979-1984

In addition to the number of births and the number of cases, the number of non-white births has also been recorded and it can be used as a proxy socio-economic indicator.

These data can be modeled using a Poisson regression to explain the number of cases of SIDS in the available covariates. The period 1974-1978 will be considered, and the model to be fit is

$$O_i \sim Po(\mu_i), \ i = 1, \ldots, 100$$

$$\log(\mu_i) = \log(E_i) + \beta_0 + \beta_1 nw_i, \ i = 1, \ldots, 100$$

Here, O_i is the number of cases of SIDS in a time period 1974-1978 in county i, E_i the expected number of cases and nw_i the proportion of non-white births in the same period.

The expected number of cases is included as an offset in the model to account for the uneven distribution of the population across the counties in North Carolina. In this case, it is computed by multiplying the overall mortality rate of SIDS by the number of births in each county P_i (which is the population at risk), i.e.,

$$E_i = P_i \frac{\sum_{i=1}^{100} O_i}{\sum_{i=1}^{100} P_i}$$

Hence, the `nc.sids` dataset can be loaded and the overall rate for the first time period available (1974-1978) computed to obtain the expected number of SIDS cases per county:

```
library("spdep")
data(nc.sids)

# Overall rate
r <- sum(nc.sids$SID74) / sum(nc.sids$BIR74)

# Expected SIDS per county
nc.sids$EXP74 <- r * nc.sids$BIR74
```

The proportion of non-white births in each county can be easily computed by dividing the number of non-white births by the total number of births:

```
# Proportion of non-white births
nc.sids$NWPROP74 <- nc.sids$NWBIR74 / nc.sids$BIR74
```

The expected number of cases can be passed using an offset or using option E in the call to inla. Hence, the model can be fit as:

```
m.pois <- inla(SID74 ~ NWPROP74, data = nc.sids, family = "poisson",
  E = EXP74)
summary(m.pois)

##
## Call:
##    c("inla(formula = SID74 ~ NWPROP74, family = \"poisson\", data =
##    nc.sids, ", " E = EXP74)")
## Time used:
```

```
##      Pre = 0.905, Running = 0.0858, Post = 0.0567, Total = 1.05
## Fixed effects:
##                 mean    sd 0.025quant 0.5quant 0.975quant    mode kld
## (Intercept) -0.646 0.090     -0.824   -0.645     -0.470 -0.644   0
## NWPROP74     1.869 0.217      1.440    1.869      2.294  1.870   0
##
## Expected number of effective parameters(stdev): 2.00(0.00)
## Number of equivalent replicates : 49.90
##
## Marginal log-Likelihood:  -226.12
```

The results point to an increase of cases of SIDS in counties with a high proportion of non-white births.

This dataset has been studied by several authors (Cressie and Read, 1985; Cressie and Chan, 1989). In particular, Cressie and Read (1985) note the strong spatial pattern in the cases of SIDS, which produces overdispersion in the data. The inclusion of the proportion of non-white births has a similar spatial pattern and it accounts for some of the over-dispersion, but including a term to account for the extra variation can help to model overdispersion in the data.

A simple way to include a term to account for overdispersion is to include i.i.d Gaussian random effects in the model, i.e., now the log-mean is modeled as

$$\log(\mu_i) = \log(E_i) + \beta_0 + \beta_1 nw_i + u_i, \ i = 1, \ldots, 100$$

Effect u_i is Gaussian distributed with zero mean and precision τ_u. By default, **INLA** will assign this precision a Gamma prior with parameters 1 and 0.00005. The random effect is included in the model by using the f() function as follows:

```
m.poisover <- inla(SID74 ~ NWPROP74 + f(CNTY.ID, model = "iid"),
  data = nc.sids, family = "poisson", E = EXP74)
```

The first argument in the definition of the random effect (CNTY.ID) is an index that assigns a random effect to each observation. This index can be the same for different observations if they should share the same effect. This will happen, for example, when the observations are clustered in groups and the random effects are used to model the cluster effects.

In this case, each county has a different value but indices could have been repeated if two areas share the same random effect. If an index had not been available in the data we could have simply computed one and used it to fit the model:

```
# Add index for latent effect
nc.sids$idx <- 1:nrow(nc.sids)
# Model fitting
m.poisover <- inla(SID74 ~ NWPROP74 + f(idx, model = "iid"),
  data = nc.sids, family = "poisson", E = EXP74)
```

The summary of the model fit is obtained with:

```
summary(m.poisover)
```

```
##
## Call:
##    c("inla(formula = SID74 ~ NWPROP74 + f(CNTY.ID, model = \"iid\"),
##    ", " family = \"poisson\", data = nc.sids, E = EXP74)")
## Time used:
##     Pre = 1.18, Running = 0.129, Post = 0.0608, Total = 1.37
## Fixed effects:
##                 mean    sd 0.025quant 0.5quant 0.975quant    mode kld
## (Intercept) -0.646 0.093     -0.829   -0.645     -0.466 -0.644   0
## NWPROP74     1.871 0.224      1.431    1.871      2.310  1.872   0
##
## Random effects:
##   Name      Model
##     CNTY.ID IID model
##
## Model hyperparameters:
##                             mean        sd 0.025quant 0.5quant 0.975quant
## Precision for CNTY.ID 15986.29 19485.83      14.01  9360.20   69109.76
##                             mode
## Precision for CNTY.ID 15.70
##
## Expected number of effective parameters(stdev): 5.04(7.11)
## Number of equivalent replicates : 19.83
##
## Marginal log-Likelihood:  -227.84
```

Note the large posterior mean and median of the precision of the Gaussian random effects. This probably indicates that the covariate explains the overdispersion in the data well (as discussed in Bivand et al., 2013). Furthermore, the marginal likelihood of the latest model is smaller than that of the previous one, and it cannot be considered as a model with a better fit. The new model is also more complex in terms of its structure and the estimated effective number of parameters. Hence, the model with no random effects should be preferred for this analysis.

2.4   Model assessment and model choice

INLA computes a number of Bayesian criteria for model assessment (Held et al., 2010) and model choice. Model assessment criteria are useful to check whether a given model is doing a good job at representing the data, while model choice criteria will be of help when selecting among different models.

All the criteria presented here can be computed by setting the respective option in control.compute when calling inla(). Table 2.6 shows the different criteria for model assessment and model selection available, the corresponding option in control.compute and whether it is computed by default. All but the marginal likelihood are not computed by default.

TABLE 2.6: Options to compute model assessment and model choice
criteria with `control.compute`.

Criterion	Option	Default
Marginal likelihood	`mlik`	Yes
Conditional predictive ordinate (CPO)	`cpo`	No
Predictive integral transform (PIT)	`cpo`	No
Deviance information criterion (DIC)	`dic`	No
Widely applicable Bayesian information criterion (WAIC)	`waic`	No

2.4.1 Marginal likelihood

The marginal likelihood of a model is the probability of the observed data under a given model, i.e., $\pi(\mathbf{y})$. When a set of M models $\{\mathcal{M}_m\}_{m=1}^M$ is considered, their respective marginal likelihoods can be represented as $\pi(\mathbf{y} \mid \mathcal{M}_m)$ to indicate that they are different for different models.

In general, the marginal likelihood is difficult to compute. Chib (1995), Chib and Jeliazkov (2001), for example, describe several methods to compute this quantity when using MCMC algorithms. The approximation provided by INLA is computed as

$$\tilde{\pi}(\mathbf{y}) = \int \left. \frac{\pi(\boldsymbol{\theta}, \mathbf{x}, \mathbf{y})}{\tilde{\pi}_{\mathrm{G}}(\mathbf{x} \mid \boldsymbol{\theta}, \mathbf{y})} \right|_{\mathbf{x} = \mathbf{x}^*(\boldsymbol{\theta})} d\boldsymbol{\theta}.$$

Hubin and Storvik (2016) investigated the accuracy of this approximation by comparing to the methods described in Chib (1995), Chib and Jeliazkov (2001) and others, and they found out that, in general, this approximation is quite accurate. Gómez-Rubio and Rue (2018) use this approximation to implement the Metropolis-Hastings algorithm with INLA and their results also suggest that this approximation is quite good. Hence, INLA can easily compute an important quantity for model choice that would be difficult to compute otherwise.

Furthermore, the marginal likelihood can be used to compute the posterior probabilities of the model fitted as

$$\pi(\mathcal{M}_m \mid \mathbf{y}) \propto \pi(\mathbf{y} \mid \mathcal{M}_m)\pi(\mathcal{M}_m)$$

The prior probability of each model is set by $\pi(\mathcal{M}_m)$.

Gómez-Rubio et al. (2017) use posterior model probabilities to select among different models in the context of spatial econometrics. They use a flat prior, which assigns the same prior probability to each model, and an informative prior, which penalizes for the *complexity* of the model (in this case, the number of nearest neighbors used to build the adjacency matrix for the spatial models).

Finally, the marginal likelihood can be use to compute Bayes factors (Gelman et al., 2013) to compare two given models. The Bayes factor for models $\mathcal{M}_1$ and model $\mathcal{M}_2$ is given by

$$\frac{\pi(\mathcal{M}_1 \mid \mathbf{y})}{\pi(\mathcal{M}_2 \mid \mathbf{y})} = \frac{\pi(\mathbf{y} \mid \mathcal{M}_1)\pi(\mathcal{M}_1)}{\pi(\mathbf{y} \mid \mathcal{M}_2)\pi(\mathcal{M}_2)}$$

2.4.2   Conditional predictive ordinates (CPO)

Conditional predictive ordinates (CPO, Pettit, 1990) are a cross-validatory criterion for model assessment that is computed for each observation as

$$CPO_i = \pi(y_i \mid y_{-i})$$

Hence, for each observation its CPO is the posterior probability of observing that observation when the model is fit using all data but y_i. Large values indicate a better fit of the model to the data, while small values indicate a bad fitting of the model to that observation and, perhaps, that it is an outlier.

A measure that summarizes the CPO is

$$-\sum_{i=1}^{n} \log(CPO_i)$$

with smaller values pointing to a better model fit.

2.4.3   Predictive integral transform (PIT)

The next criterion to be considered in the predictive integral transform (PIT, Marshall and Spiegelhalter, 2003) which measures, for each observation, the probability of a new value to be lower than the actual observed value:

$$PIT_i = \pi(y_i^{new} \leq y_i \mid y_{-i})$$

For discrete data, the adjusted PIT is computed as

$$PIT_i^{adjusted} = PIT_i - 0.5 * CPO_i$$

In this case, the case $y_i^{new} = y_i$ is only counted as half.

If the model represents the observation well, the distribution of the different values should be close to a uniform distribution between 0 and 1. See Gelman et al. (1996) and Marshall and Spiegelhalter (2003), for example, for a detailed description and use of this criterion for model assessment. Held et al. (2010) provide a description on how the CPO and PIT are computed in INLA and provide a comparison with MCMC.

2.4.4   Information-based criteria (DIC and WAIC)

The deviance information criterion (DIC) proposed by Spiegelhalter et al. (2002) is a popular criterion for model choice similar to the AIC. It takes into account goodness-of-fit and a penalty term that is based on the complexity of the model via the estimated effective number of parameters. The DIC is defined as

$$DIC = D(\hat{\mathbf{x}}, \hat{\boldsymbol{\theta}}) + 2p_D$$

Here, $D(\cdot)$ is the deviance, $\hat{\mathbf{x}}$ and $\hat{\boldsymbol{\theta}}$ the posterior expectations of the latent effects and hyperparameters, respectively, and p_D is the effective number of parameters. This can be computed in several ways. Spiegelhalter et al. (2002) use the following:

TABLE 2.7 Summary of values of DIC, WAIC, CPO and marginal likelihood for different models fit to the North Carolina SIDS data.

Model	DIC	WAIC	CPO	MLIK
Poisson	441.6	442.7	221.4	-226.1
Poisson + r. eff.	439.6	439.8	221.3	-226.9

$$p_D = E[D(\cdot)] - D(\hat{\mathbf{x}}, \hat{\boldsymbol{\theta}})$$

Posterior estimates $\hat{\mathbf{x}}$ and $\hat{\boldsymbol{\theta}}$ are the posterior means of $\mathbf{x}$ and $\boldsymbol{\theta}$, respectively. INLA uses the posterior means of the latent field $\mathbf{x}$ but the posterior mode of the hyperparameters because these may be very skewed. The DIC favors models with lower values, and this should be preferred.

The Watanabe-Akaike information criterion, also known as widely applicable Bayesian information criterion, is similar to the DIC but the effective number of parameters is computed in a different way. See Watanabe (2013) and Gelman et al. (2014) for details.

2.4.5   North Carolina SIDS data revisited

In order to compare all these different criteria and see them in action, the models for the SIDS dataset will be refit and these criteria computed. As stated before, some options need to be passed to `inla` within the `control.compute` options:

```
# Poisson model
m.pois <- inla(SID74 ~ NWPROP74, data = nc.sids, family = "poisson",
  E = EXP74, control.compute = list(cpo = TRUE, dic = TRUE, waic = TRUE))


# Poisson model with iid random effects
m.poisover <- inla(SID74 ~ NWPROP74 + f(CNTY.ID, model = "iid"),
  data = nc.sids, family = "poisson", E = EXP74,
  control.compute = list(cpo = TRUE, dic = TRUE, waic = TRUE))
```

Table 2.7 displays a summary of the DIC, WAIC, CPO (i.e., minus the sum of the log-values of CPO) and the marginal likelihood computed for the model fit to the North Carolina SIDS data. All criteria (but the marginal likelihood) slightly favor the most complex model with `iid` random effects. Note that because this difference is small, we may still prefer the model that does not include random effects.

Similarly, Figure 2.2 compares the values of the CPOs and PITs for these two models. In general, values are pretty similar, which means that both models fit the data in a very similar way. Hence, given that these two models give very similar results we may prefer to choose the simplest one following the law of parsimony.

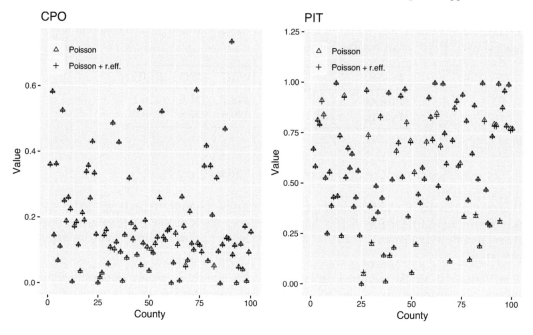

FIGURE 2.2 Values of CPOs and PITs computed for the models fit to the North Carolina SIDS data.

2.5   Control options

INLA has a number of arguments in the `inla()` function that allow us to control several options about how the estimation process is carried and the output is reported. Table 2.8 shows a summary of the different control options available in INLA. All these arguments have a manual page that can be accessed in the usual way (e.g., `?control.compute`) with detailed information about the different options. In addition, the list of options for each control argument and their default values can be obtained with functions `inla.set.CONTROL.default()`, where CONTROL refers to the control argument. For example, for argument `control.compute` the list of options and default values can be obtained with `inla.set.control.compute.default()`.

TABLE 2.8: Summary of control options available in INLA.

Argument	Description
`control.compute`	Options on what is actually computed during model fitting.
`control.expert`	Options on several internal issues.
`control.family`	Options on the likelihood of the model.
`control.fixed`	Options on the fixed effects of the model.
`control.hazard`	Options on how the hazard function is computed in survival models.
`control.inla`	Options on how the INLA method is used in model fitting.
`control.lincomb`	Options on how to compute linear combinations.
`control.mode`	Options on the initial values of the hyperparameters for model fitting.

Argument	Description
`control.predictor`	Options on how the linear predictor is computed.
`control.results`	Options on the marginals to be computed.
`control.update`	Options on how the posterior is updated.

The different values that all these arguments can take will not be discussed here, but only wherever they are used in the book. The index at the end of the book can help to find where the different control options are used. As stated above, the documentation in the INLA package can provide full details about the different options.

It is worth mentioning that `control.inla` options allow the user to set the approximation used by the INLA method for model fitting described in Section 2.2. For this reason, these are covered next.

2.5.1 Model fitting strategies

Control options in `control.inla` can be used to set how the model is fit using the different methods described in Section 2.2. Some of the options provided by `control.inla` are summarized in Table 2.9.

TABLE 2.9: Some options in `control.inla`.

Option	Default	Description
`strategy`	`'simplified.laplace'`	Strategy used for the approximations ('gaussian', 'simplified.laplace', 'laplace' or 'adaptive').
`int.strategy`	`'auto'`	Integration strategy ('auto', 'ccd', 'grid', 'eb' (empirical Bayes), 'user' or 'user.std').
`adaptive.max`	10	Maximum length of latent effect to use the user defined strategy.
`int.design`	NULL	Matrix (by row) of hyperparameters values and associated weights.

Regarding the strategy used for the approximations, the options cover all the methods described before in Section 2.2. The 'adaptive' strategy refers to a method in which the chosen strategy is used for all fixed effects and all latent effects with a length equal or less to option `adaptive.max`, while all the other effects are estimated using the Gaussian approximation.

The integration strategy also covers the methods described in Section 2.2 and, in particular, Section 2.2.2. Note strategies `user` and `user.std` for user defined integration points and weights, which are provided with option `int.design`.

To illustrate the different approaches, the Poisson model with random effects will be fit using three different strategies as well as three different integration strategies:

```
m.strategy <- lapply(c("gaussian", "simplified.laplace", "laplace"),
  function(st) {
    return(lapply(c("ccd", "grid", "eb"), function(int.st) {
```

```
inla(SID74 ~ NWPROP74 + f(CNTY.ID, model = "iid"),
  data = nc.sids, family = "poisson", E = EXP74,
  control.inla = list(strategy = st, int.strategy = int.st),
  control.compute = list(cpo = TRUE, dic = TRUE, waic = TRUE))
}))
})
```

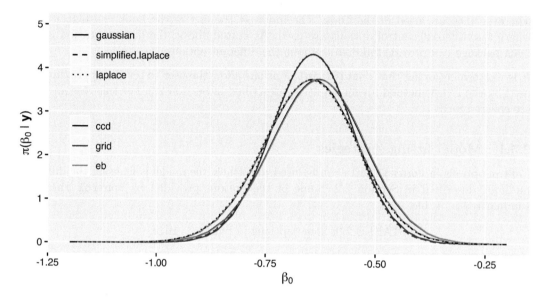

FIGURE 2.3 Posterior marginal of the intercept β_0 estimated with INLA.

Figure 2.3 and Figure 2.4 show the estimates of the posterior marginal of the intercept β_0 and the coefficient β_1, respectively. In general, all combinations of strategy and integration strategy produce very similar results.

Figure 2.5 shows the posterior marginal of the precision of the random effects. As can be seen, the main differences are with respect to the integration strategy. The grid strategy produces results that are different to the CCD and empirical Bayes strategies. In this case, the main differences are probably due to the long tails of the grid strategy. The estimates of the posterior modes are very close for all the methods considered.

As a final comment, function `inla.hyperpar()` can take an `inla` object and improve the estimates of the posterior marginals of the hyperparameters of the model.

2.6   Working with posterior marginals

As INLA focuses on the posterior marginal distributions of the latent effects and the hyperparameters it is important to be able to exploit these for inference. INLA provides a number of functions to make computations on the posterior marginals. These are summarized in Table 2.10.

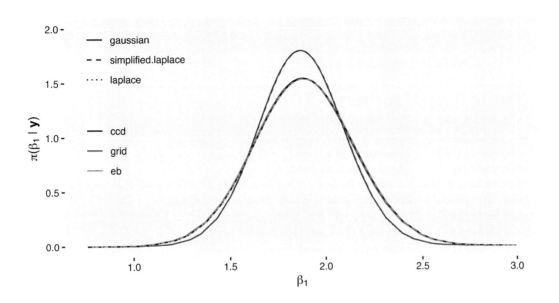

FIGURE 2.4 Posterior marginal of the intercept β_1 estimated with INLA.

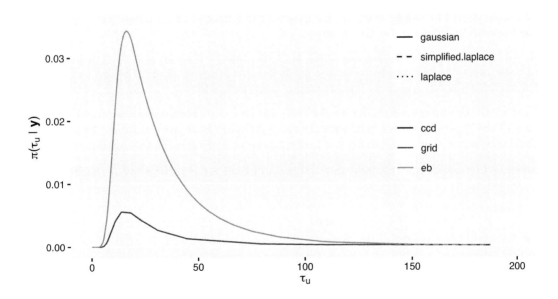

FIGURE 2.5 Posterior marginal of the precision of the random effects τ_u.

All these functions are properly documented in the INLA package manual pages. Note that a posterior marginal is a density function, and four functions to compute its density, cumulative probability, quantiles and draw random samples using the typical notation in R.

TABLE 2.10: Summary of functions to manipulate marginal distribution in the INLA package.

Function	Description
inla.dmarginal	Compute density function.
inla.pmarginal	Compute cumulative probability function.
inla.qmarginal	Compute a quantile.
inla.rmarginal	Draw a random sample.
inla.hpdmarginal	Compute highest posterior density (HPD) credible interval.
inla.smarginal	Spline smoothing of the posterior marginal.
inla.emarginal	Compute expected value of a function.
inla.mmarginal	Compute the posterior mode.
inla.tmarginal	Transform marginal using a function.
inla.zmarginal	Compute summary statistics.

Given a marginal $\pi(x)$, function inla.emarginal() computes the expected value of a function $f(x)$, i.e., $\int f(x)\pi(x)dx$. This is useful to compute summary statistics and other quantities of interest. Typical summary statistics can be directly obtained with function inla.zmarginal(), that computes the posterior mean, standard deviation and some quantiles.

When the posterior marginal of a transformation of a latent effect or hyperparameter is required, function inla.tmarginal() can be used to transform the original posterior marginal. A typical case is to obtain the posterior marginal of the standard deviation using the posterior marginal of the precision.

As an example, we will revisit the analysis of the cement data to show how to use some of these functions. We will focus on the coefficient of covariate x1 and the precision of the Gaussian likelihood, which is a hyperparameter in the model.

First of all, the marginals of the fixed effects are stored in m1$marginals.fixed and the ones of the hyperparameters in m1$marginals.hyperpar. Both are named list identified by the corresponding name of the effect or hyperparameter. For example, the posterior marginal of the coefficient of x1 and the precision have been plotted in Figure 2.6 using

```
library("ggplot2")
library("gridExtra")

# Posterior of coefficient of x1
plot1 <- ggplot(as.data.frame(m1$marginals.fixed$x1)) +
  geom_line(aes(x = x, y = y)) +
  ylab (expression(paste(pi, "(", "x", " | ", bold(y), ")")))

# Posterior of precision
plot2 <- ggplot(as.data.frame(m1$marginals.hyperpar[[1]])) +
  geom_line(aes(x = x, y = y)) +
```

```
ylab (expression(paste(pi, "(", tau, " | ", bold(y), ")")))
```

```
grid.arrange(plot1, plot2, nrow = 2)
```

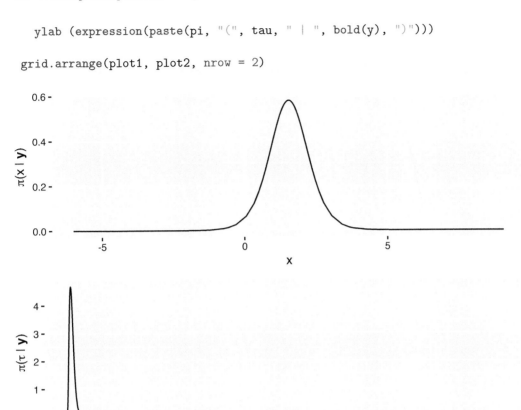

FIGURE 2.6 Posterior marginals of the coefficient of covariate x1 (top) and the precision of the Gaussian likelihood (bottom).

In order to know whether covariate x1 has a (positive) association with the response, the probability of its coefficient being higher than one can be computed:

```
1 - inla.pmarginal(0, m1$marginals.fixed$x1)
```

```
## [1] 0.9781
```

For the precision, an 95% highest posterior density (HPD) credible interval could be computed:

```
inla.hpdmarginal(0.95, m1$marginals.hyperpar[[1]])
```

```
##                low    high
## level:0.95 0.04999 0.3939
```

The posterior marginal of the standard deviation of the Gaussian likelihood σ_u can be computed by noting that the standard deviation is $\tau_u^{-1/2}$, where τ_u is the precision. Hence, function `inla.tmarginal()` can be used to transform the posterior marginal of the precision as follows:

```
marg.stdev <- inla.tmarginal(function(tau) tau^(-1/2),
  m1$marginals.hyperpar[[1]])
```

This marginal is plotted in Figure 2.7.

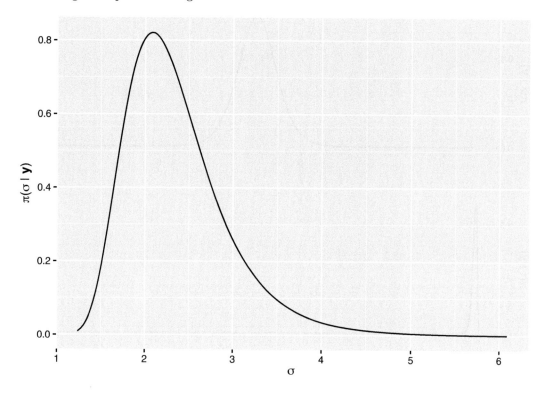

FIGURE 2.7 Posterior marginal of the standard deviation of the Gaussian likelihood in the linear model fit to the `cement` dataset.

Summary statistics from the posterior marginal of the standard deviation can be obtained with `inla.zmarginal()`:

```
inla.zmarginal(marg.stdev)
```

```
## Mean                2.36885
## Stdev               0.591117
## Quantile  0.025 1.5284
## Quantile  0.25  1.95211
## Quantile  0.5   2.2626
## Quantile  0.75  2.66346
## Quantile  0.975 3.82448
```

Note that the posterior mean is $\int \sigma \pi(\sigma \mid \mathbf{y}) d\sigma$, which could have also been computed with function `inla.emarginal()` as

```
inla.emarginal(function(sigma) sigma, marg.stdev)
```

```
## [1] 2.369
```

The posterior mode of the standard deviation is computed with function `inla.mmarginal()`:

```
inla.mmarginal(marg.stdev)
```

```
## [1] 2.084
```

2.7 Sampling from the posterior

INLA can draw samples from the approximate posterior distribution of the latent effects and the hyperparameters. Function `inla.posterior.sample()` draws samples from the (approximate) joint posterior distribution of the latent effects and the hyperparameters. In order to use this option, the model needs to be fit with options `config` equal to `TRUE` in `control.compute`. This will make INLA keep the internal representation of the latent GMRF in the object returned by `inla()`. Furthermore, function `inla.posterior.sample.eval()` can be used to evaluate a function on the samples drawn.

Table 2.11 shows the different arguments that inla.posterior.sample()' can take.

TABLE 2.11: Arguments that can be passed to function `inla.posterior.sample()`.

Argument	Default	Description
n	1L	Number of samples to draw.
result		An `inla` object.
selection		A named list with the components of the model to return.
intern	FALSE	Whether samples are in the internal scale of the hyperparameters.
use.improved.mean	TRUE	Whether to use the posterior marginal means when sampling.
add.names	TRUE	Add names of elements in each sample.
seed	0L	Seed for random number generator.
num.threads	NULL	Number of threads to be used.
verbose	FALSE	Verbose mode.

Sampling from the posterior may be useful when inference requires computing a function on the latent effects and the hyperparameters that INLA cannot handle. Non-linear functions or functions that depend on several hyperparameters that require multivariate inference for several parameters are a typical example (sse, for example, Gómez-Rubio et al., 2017).

For example, we might be interested in the posterior distribution of the product of the coefficients of variables x1 and x2 in the analysis of the cement dataset. First of all, the model needs to be fit again with `config` equal to `TRUE`:

```
# Fit model with config = TRUE
m1 <- inla(y ~ x1 + x2 + x3 + x4, data = cement,
   control.compute = list(config = TRUE))
```

Next, the random sample is obtained. We will draw 100 samples from the posterior:

```
m1.samp <- inla.posterior.sample(100, m1, selection = list(x1 = 1, x2 = 1))
```

Note that here we have used the **selection** argument to keep just the sampled values of the coefficients of x1 and x2. Note that the expression x1 = 1 means that we want to keep the first element in effect x1. Note that in this case there is only a single value associated with x1 (i.e., the coefficient) but this can be extended to other latent random effects with possibly more values.

The object returned by inla.posterior.sample() is a list of length 100, where each element contains the samples of the different effects in the model in a name list. For example, the names for the first element of m1.samp are

```
names(m1.samp[[1]])
```

```
## [1] "hyperpar" "latent"    "logdens"
```

which correspond to the first sample of the simulated values of the hyperparameters, latent effects and the log-density of the posterior at those values. We can inspect the simulated values:

```
m1.samp[[1]]
```

```
## $hyperpar
## Precision for the Gaussian observations
##                                  0.1503
##
## $latent
##        sample1
## x1:1    1.733
## x2:1    0.561
##
## $logdens
## $logdens$hyperpar
## [1] 1.522
##
## $logdens$latent
## [1] 62.37
##
## $logdens$joint
## [1] 63.89
```

Note that because we have used option **select** above there are no samples from the coefficients of covariates x3 and x4. This can be used to speed up simulations and reduce memory requirements.

Finally, function `inla.posterior.sample.eval()` is used to compute the product of the two coefficients:

```
x1x2.samp <- inla.posterior.sample.eval(function(...) {x1 * x2},
    m1.samp)
```

Note that the first argument is the function to be computed (using the names of the effects) and the second one the output from `inla.posterior.sample`. `x1x2.samp` is a matrix with 1 row and 100 columns so that summary statistics can be computed from the posterior as usual:

```
summary(as.vector(x1x2.samp))
```

```
##    Min. 1st Qu. Median   Mean 3rd Qu.   Max.
## -0.513   0.158  0.642  1.151   1.653  8.670
```

When the interest is on the hyperparameters alone, function `inla.hyperpar.sample()` can be used to draw samples from the approximate joint posterior distribution of the hyperparameters. Table 2.12 shows the arguments that can be passed to this function.

TABLE 2.12: List of arguments that can be passed to function `inla.hyperpar.sample()`.

Argument	Default	Description
n		Number of samples to be drawn.
result		An `inla` object.
intern	FALSE	Whether samples are in the internal scale of the hyperparameters.
improve.marginals	FALSE	Improve samples by using better estimates of the marginals in `results`.

In this case the model has only one hyperparameter (i.e., the precision of the Gaussian likelihood) and its posterior marginal could be used for inference. However, we will illustrate the use of `inla.hyperpar.sample()` by using it to obtain a random sample and compare its distribution of values to the posterior marginal. They should be very close.

```
# Sample hyperpars from joint posterior
set.seed(123)
prec.samp <- inla.hyperpar.sample(1000, m1)
```

Note that the returned object (`prec.samp`) is a matrix with as many columns as hyperparameters and a number of rows equal to the number of simulated samples. Figure 2.8 shows a histogram of the sampled values and the posterior marginal has been added for comparison purposes. Both distributions are very close. However, note that in order to validate the approximation provided by INLA it would be required to compare to other exact approaches such as MCMC. This is particularly important when the posterior marginal is very skewed. Furthermore, the samples drawn by `inla.posterior.sample()` rely on the approximation provided by INLA, and they should be considered as sampled from an approximation to the posterior. At the time of this writing members of the INLA team are working on providing a skewness correction for the `inla.posterior.sample()` function.

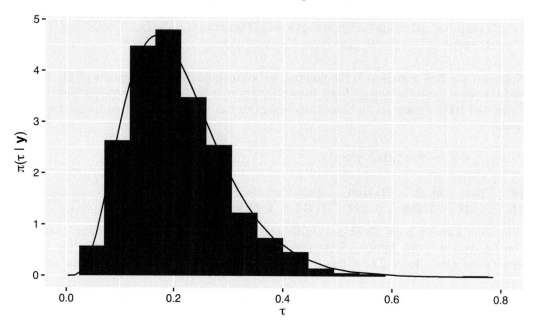

FIGURE 2.8 Sample from the posterior of the precision hyperparameter τ using `inla.hyperpar.sample()` (histogram) and posterior marginal (solid line).

3

Mixed-effects Models

3.1 Introduction

In Chapter 2 we have already introduced how to fit models with fixed and random effects. In this chapter a more detailed description of the different types of fixed and random effects available in INLA will be provided.

First of all, let's recall that a covariate should enter the model as a linear fixed effect when it is thought that it affects all observations in the same way (in a linear way, in fact) and that this effect is of primary interest in the study.

Random effects, on the other hand, are often adopted to take into account variation produced by variables in the model that are not our primary object of study. For example, in a study to investigate the effect of different irrigation systems on plant growth, measurement may include the type of irrigation, type of soil and variables associated with the trees, such as a numerical identifier of the tree, age, etc. Trees themselves in the study are not the primary object of study as they are a (random) sample of the population of trees. However, depending on the actual tree being measured, growth may be faster or slower and it will affect the growth measurement. In this case, because the trees in the study are taken as a random sample from the total population of trees, their effect is included as a random effect.

In a Bayesian context, a fixed effect will have an associated coefficient which is often assigned a vague prior, such as a Gaussian with zero mean and large variance. On the other hand, random effects will have a common Gaussian prior with a zero mean and a precision, to which a prior will be assigned.

3.2 Fixed-effects models

As explained in Section 2.3, fixed effects can be easily included in the model formula. The default prior assigned to the associated coefficients (and the intercept) is a Gaussian distribution, and its parameters can be set through option `control.fixed` in the call to `inla()`.

Fixed effects can also be included in the model by including one or more terms in the model formula using the the `f()` function. Table 3.1 summarizes the two types of fixed effects implemented in INLA, which will be described in more detail below.

TABLE 3.1: Summary of types of fixed effects implemented in `INLA`.

Name	Description
`linear`	Linear fixed effect.
`clinear`	Linear fixed effect with constrained coefficient.

3.2.1   `linear` fixed effect

The `linear` effect is similar to including a covariate in the formula in the usual way and it implements the effect βx_i, where x_i is the value of the covariate for observation i and β the associated coefficient. The prior on β is a Gaussian distribution with mean and precision that can be specified in the call to the `f()` function when the model is defined in the formula. Table 3.2 summarizes the specific options available for this effect. Alternatively, parameter `control.fixed` can be used to set the prior on the coefficient.

TABLE 3.2: Summary of options of the `linear` effect.

Argument	Default	Description
`mean.linear`	0	Mean of Gaussian prior on a coefficient.
`prec.linear`	0.001	Precision of Gaussian prior on a coefficient.

3.2.2   `clinear` fixed effect

Sometimes it is necessary to fit a model in which the covariate coefficients are constrained in some way, e.g., we want to force the coefficient to be non-negative. This can be achieved by means of the `clinear` effect. Table 3.3 shows the different options available to specify this effect. Note that `precision` is the precision of a (tiny) error that is added to the actual value of βx_i required by how this latent effect is implemented.

TABLE 3.3: Summary of options of the `clinear` effect.

Argument	Default	Description
`range`	`c(-Inf, Inf)`	Vector of length two with the range of the linear coefficient.
`precision`	`exp(14)`	Tiny precision to implement this latent effect.

The implementation of this effect distinguishes three different possibilities depending on how `range` is defined:

- `range = c(-Inf, Inf)`

  In this case there are not constraints and the model is equivalent to the `linear` effect. The parameterization is $\beta = \theta$, where θ is the parameter in the internal scale used by `INLA` to estimate the model.

- `range = c(a, Inf)`

  In this case `a` is the lower bound of the parameter and there is no upper limit, so the internal parameterization is

$$\beta = a + \exp(\theta)$$

- range = c(a, b)

  This is the model general case in which both limits, lower bound a and upper bound b, are real numbers. The internal parameterization is now:

$$\beta = a + (b - a)\frac{\exp(\theta)}{1 + \exp(\theta)}$$

In all cases the prior of this model is set on the internal parameter θ and it is a Gaussian distribution with default mean equal to 1 and precision equal to 10.

In order to illustrate the use of the two models for fixed effects we will revisit the example on the SIDS dataset. A model will be fitted to constrain to a positive coefficient on the covariate that represents the proportion of non-white births in a county.

First of all, the dataset will be loaded and the required variables computed (see Chapter 2 for details):

```
library("spdep")
data(nc.sids)

# Overall rate
r <- sum(nc.sids$SID74) / sum(nc.sids$BIR74)
nc.sids$EXP74 <- r * nc.sids$BIR74

# Proportion of non-white births
nc.sids$NWPROP74 <- nc.sids$NWBIR74 / nc.sids$BIR74
```

Next, the two models will be fitted. First of all, the model using the linear effect:

```
m.pois.lin1 <- inla(SID74 ~ f(NWPROP74, model = "linear"),
  data = nc.sids, family = "poisson", E = EXP74)

summary(m.pois.lin1)
```

```
##
## Call:
##    c("inla(formula = SID74 ~ f(NWPROP74, model = \"linear\"), family
##    = \"poisson\", ", " data = nc.sids, E = EXP74)")
## Time used:
##     Pre = 0.989, Running = 0.0827, Post = 0.061, Total = 1.13
## Fixed effects:
##                 mean    sd 0.025quant 0.5quant 0.975quant    mode kld
## (Intercept) -0.646 0.090     -0.824   -0.645     -0.470  -0.644   0
## NWPROP74     1.869 0.217      1.440    1.869      2.294   1.870   0
##
## Expected number of effective parameters(stdev): 2.00(0.00)
## Number of equivalent replicates : 49.90
##
## Marginal log-Likelihood:  -226.12
```

Note how the posterior marginal of the coefficient of covariate `NWPROP74` has a 95% credible interval which is above zero. In case we wanted this coefficient to be positive, this is how the model with a constraint on the coefficient using the `clinear` effect is fitted:

```
library("INLA")
m.pois.clin1 <- inla(SID74 ~ f(NWPROP74, model = "clinear",
  range = c(0, Inf)), data = nc.sids, family = "poisson",
  E = EXP74)

summary(m.pois.clin1)
```

```
##
## Call:
##    c("inla(formula = SID74 ~ f(NWPROP74, model = \"clinear\", range =
##    c(0, ", " Inf)), family = \"poisson\", data = nc.sids, E = EXP74)"
##    )
## Time used:
##     Pre = 1.09, Running = 0.121, Post = 0.0614, Total = 1.27
## Fixed effects:
##              mean    sd 0.025quant 0.5quant 0.975quant   mode   kld
## (Intercept) -0.672 0.084     -0.843    -0.67     -0.514 -0.666 0.002
##
## Random effects:
##   Name      Model
##     NWPROP74 Constrained linear
##
## Model hyperparameters:
##                   mean    sd 0.025quant 0.5quant 0.975quant mode
## Beta for NWPROP74 1.93 0.201       1.54     1.93       2.33 1.93
##
## Expected number of effective parameters(stdev): 1.00(0.00)
## Number of equivalent replicates : 99.55
##
## Marginal log-Likelihood:  -222.89
```

It can be seen how the estimates of the intercept and the coefficient of the proportion of non-white births are very similar between the unconstrained and the constrained model.

3.3   Types of mixed-effects models

The list of random effects implemented in INLA is quite rich. Random effects in INLA are defined using a multivariate Gaussian distribution with zero mean and precision matrix $\tau\Sigma$, where τ is a generic precision parameter and Σ is a matrix that defines the dependence structure of the random effects and that may depend on further parameters. When the random effects are a latent Gaussian Markov random field the structure of Σ is quite sparse and this can be exploited for computational purposes (Rue and Held, 2005). Given a vector **u** of random effects, this will be represented as:

$$\mathbf{u} \sim N(0, \tau\Sigma).$$

Table 3.4 summarizes the ones described in this chapter, but other types of random effects are discussed in different chapters.

TABLE 3.4: Summary of some of the random effects implemented in INLA.

Name	Description
iid	Independent and identically distributed Gaussian random effect.
z	"Classical" specification of random effects.
generic0	Generic specification (type 0).
generic1	Generic specification (type 1).
generic2	Generic specification (type 2).
generic3	Generic specification (type 3).
rw1	Random walk of order 1.
rw2	Random walk of order 2.
crw2	Continuous random walk of order 2.
seasonal	Seasonal variation with a given periodicity.
ar1	Autoregressive model of order 1.
ar	Autoregressive model of arbitrary order.
iid1d	Correlated random effects of dimension 1.
iid2d	Correlated random effects of dimension 2.
iid3d	Correlated random effects of dimension 3.
iid4d	Correlated random effects of dimension 4.
iid5d	Correlated random effects of dimension 5.

3.3.1 Independent random effects (iid model)

Independent and identically distributed random effects have already been introduced in Chapter 2 and they are probably the simplest way to account for unstructured variability in the data.

The precision matrix of iid random effects is $\tau\Sigma$ with Σ a diagonal matrix of scaling factors $\{s_1, \ldots, s_n\}$ (which are all equal to 1 by default). Scaling factors are defined by means of parameter scale within the f() function used to define the latent effect in the formula.

The internal parameterization of the hyperparameter of this model is $\theta = \log(\tau)$, which by default is assigned a log-Gamma distribution with parameters 1 and 0.00005. In other words, the prior of τ is a Gamma distribution.

The first argument passed to the f() function should be an index of values that define the grouping of the observations in order to define the number of random effects. The length of parameter scale, if used, must be equal to the number of groups defined. Scaling may be used, for example, to account for different sample sizes in the groups defined by the data (see Section 5.6).

This type of random effects is often used to account for overdispersion in Poisson models. For this reason, the example will be again based on the SIDS dataset. The first step is to create an index for the random effects:

```
nc.sids$ID <- 1:100
```

Here, the index goes from 1 to 100 because we want a different value of the random effect for each county. If different counties must share the same random effect then the index variable should assign the same value to these counties.

The `iid` is then added to the model formula, using the `f()` function:

```
m.pois.iid <- inla(SID74 ~ f(ID, model = "iid"),
  data = nc.sids, family = "poisson",
  E = EXP74)

summary(m.pois.iid)
```

```
##
## Call:
##    c("inla(formula = SID74 ~ f(ID, model = \"iid\"), family =
##    \"poisson\", ", " data = nc.sids, E = EXP74)")
## Time used:
##     Pre = 1.14, Running = 0.164, Post = 0.0596, Total = 1.37
## Fixed effects:
##                 mean    sd 0.025quant 0.5quant 0.975quant    mode kld
## (Intercept) -0.027 0.063     -0.154   -0.026      0.092  -0.023   0
##
## Random effects:
##   Name     Model
##     ID IID model
##
## Model hyperparameters:
##                    mean    sd 0.025quant 0.5quant 0.975quant mode
## Precision for ID 7.26 2.57       3.79     6.77      13.61    6.02
##
## Expected number of effective parameters(stdev): 40.44(6.52)
## Number of equivalent replicates : 2.47
##
## Marginal log-Likelihood:  -245.54
```

The posterior mean of the precision of the random effects is 7.2609, which is a clear sign of overdispersion.

The same model can now include the covariate on the proportion of non-white births:

```
m.pois.iid2 <- inla(SID74 ~ NWPROP74 + f(ID, model = "iid"),
  data = nc.sids, family = "poisson",
  E = EXP74)

summary(m.pois.iid2)
```

```
##
## Call:
```

```
##    c("inla(formula = SID74 ~ NWPROP74 + f(ID, model = \"iid\"),
##    family = \"poisson\", ", " data = nc.sids, E = EXP74)")
## Time used:
##     Pre = 1.04, Running = 0.135, Post = 0.061, Total = 1.24
## Fixed effects:
##               mean    sd 0.025quant 0.5quant 0.975quant    mode kld
## (Intercept) -0.646 0.093     -0.829   -0.645     -0.466 -0.644   0
## NWPROP74     1.871 0.224      1.431    1.871      2.310  1.872   0
##
## Random effects:
##    Name       Model
##      ID IID model
##
## Model hyperparameters:
##                     mean       sd 0.025quant 0.5quant 0.975quant  mode
## Precision for ID 15986.29 19485.83      14.01  9360.20   69109.76 15.70
##
## Expected number of effective parameters(stdev): 5.04(7.11)
## Number of equivalent replicates : 19.83
##
## Marginal log-Likelihood:  -227.84
```

Now, the posterior mean of the precision of the random effects is 1.5986×10^4. This means that the covariate explains most of the overdispersion in the data.

3.3.2 Generic specification

In general, `iid` random effects are not suitable to model complex covariate structures that often appear in experimental design. For this reason, `INLA` provides a number of generic specifications for random effects, in addition to some specific ones (that are described later in this chapter).

3.3.3 Mixed-effects design matrix (z model)

The **z** latent model can be used to define a term $Z\mathbf{u}$ in the linear predictor where Z is a defined matrix and $\mathbf{u}$ is a vector of iid random effects with zero mean and precision τC. C is a known matrix, and it is taken to be a diagonal matrix of the appropriate dimension if it is not specified.

This random effect allows for the following representation of the linear predictor:

$$\eta = X\beta + Z\mathbf{u}$$

which is a standard and generic representation of mixed-effects models (Pinheiro and Bates, 2000). Hence, Z can be regarded as a "design matrix" for the random effects and it will allow one observation to depend on more than one random effect. Note that Z will have as many rows as observations and as many columns as elements in the vector of random effects $\mathbf{u}$.

Because of the way this latent effect is implemented in `INLA`, the actual model is:

$$\eta = Z\mathbf{u} + \varepsilon$$

Here, η is the contribution of the **z** random effect to the linear predictor and ε a tiny random error added. The precision of this tiny error can be set when the random effect is defined. All the specific options of this random effect that can be passed to the f() function are shown in Table 3.5.

TABLE 3.5: Summary of options of the z random effect.

Argument	Default	Description
z	—	Mixed-effects design matrix Z.
Cmatrix	Diagonal matrix	Structure of precision of random effects (C matrix).
precision	exp(14)	Precision of tiny noise ε.

The next example shows how to fit the model with random effects on the SIDS dataset using the z random effect:

```
m.pois.z <- inla(SID74 ~ f(ID, model = "z", Z = Diagonal(nrow(nc.sids), 1)),
  data = nc.sids, family = "poisson", E = EXP74)

summary(m.pois.z)
```

```
##
## Call:
##    c("inla(formula = SID74 ~ f(ID, model = \"z\", Z =
##    Diagonal(nrow(nc.sids), ", " 1)), family = \"poisson\", data =
##    nc.sids, E = EXP74)")
## Time used:
##     Pre = 1.03, Running = 0.196, Post = 0.0627, Total = 1.29
## Fixed effects:
##               mean    sd 0.025quant 0.5quant 0.975quant    mode kld
## (Intercept) -0.027 0.063     -0.154   -0.026      0.092  -0.023   0
##
## Random effects:
##   Name      Model
##     ID Z model
##
## Model hyperparameters:
##                  mean    sd 0.025quant 0.5quant 0.975quant mode
## Precision for ID 7.26 2.57       3.79     6.77      13.61 6.02
##
## Expected number of effective parameters(stdev): 40.44(6.52)
## Number of equivalent replicates : 2.47
##
## Marginal log-Likelihood:  -245.54
```

Note how the estimates of the intercept and the precision of the random effects are very similar to the model fit before using the iid latent effects.

3.3.4 Type 0 generic specification (generic0 model)

In this latent effect the value of matrix Σ is a fixed matrix C that is completely known and does not depend on any other hyperparameter. This is specified via the Cmatrix argument in the f() function and it must be a non-singular symmetric matrix, so that a proper precision matrix is defined.

This latent effect has a single hyperparameter precision τ, and the prior is set on $\theta = \log(\tau)$ and it is, by default, a log-Gamma with parameters 1 (shape) and 0.00005 (rate).

We go back to the model with random effects using the SIDS dataset. In this case, we set matrix C to be diagonal as this defines the same model used in previous examples:

```
m.pois.g0 <- inla(SID74 ~ f(ID, model = "generic0",
  Cmatrix = Diagonal(nrow(nc.sids), 1)),
  data = nc.sids, family = "poisson", E = EXP74)

summary(m.pois.g0)
```

```
##
## Call:
##    c("inla(formula = SID74 ~ f(ID, model = \"generic0\", Cmatrix =
##    Diagonal(nrow(nc.sids), ", " 1)), family = \"poisson\", data =
##    nc.sids, E = EXP74)")
## Time used:
##      Pre = 0.996, Running = 0.162, Post = 0.0611, Total = 1.22
## Fixed effects:
##                 mean    sd 0.025quant 0.5quant 0.975quant    mode kld
## (Intercept) -0.027 0.063     -0.154   -0.026      0.092 -0.023   0
##
## Random effects:
##    Name      Model
##      ID Generic0 model
##
## Model hyperparameters:
##                   mean    sd 0.025quant 0.5quant 0.975quant mode
## Precision for ID 7.26 2.57       3.79     6.77      13.61 6.02
##
## Expected number of effective parameters(stdev): 40.44(6.52)
## Number of equivalent replicates : 2.47
##
## Marginal log-Likelihood:  -245.54
```

Given than the fit model is the same one as in previous examples, the estimates of the intercept and the precision are very similar to those obtained above.

3.3.5 Type 1 generic specification (generic1 model)

This latent effect has a structure of the precision matrix which is $(I - \frac{\beta}{\lambda_{max}}C)$, where I is the diagonal matrix, C a known matrix, λ_{max} its maximum eigenvalue and β a parameter in the $[0, 1)$ interval. Matrix C is passed to the f() function using the Cmatrix argument.

The internal parameterization of this latent effect is $\theta_1 = \log(\tau)$ and $\theta_2 = \text{logit}(\beta)$. For θ_1 the default prior is a log-Gamma with parameters 1 and 0.00005, while for θ_2 is a Gaussian with zero mean and precision 0.01.

The generic1 latent effect has been used to implement some spatial models (Bivand et al.,

2014, 2015) not included in the `INLA` package. An example on the use of the `generic1` latent effect is provided in Section 7.2 to fit the spatial model proposed in Leroux et al. (1999).

3.3.6   Type 2 generic specification (`generic2` model)

This latent effect is used to represent the following hierarchical model:

$$v \sim N(0, \tau_v C)$$

$$u \mid v \sim N(v, \tau_u I)$$

and results in the following structure for the precision matrix:

$$Q = \begin{bmatrix} \tau_u I & -\tau_u I \\ -\tau_u I & \tau_u I + \tau_v C \end{bmatrix}$$

Hence, the resulting vector of random effects is (u, v). Matrix C is passed to the `f()` function using the `Cmatrix` argument.

The priors are set on internal parameters $\theta_1 = \log(\tau_v)$ and $\theta_2 = \log(\tau_u)$ By default, they are both a log-Gamma with parameters 1 and 0.00005, and 1 and 0.001, respectively.

3.3.7   Type 3 generic specification (`generic3` model)

The last form of generic random effect has a precision matrix that is a linear combination of K different terms:

$$Q = \tau \sum_{i=1}^{K} \tau_i C_i$$

Here, τ is a common precision parameter, τ_i a term-specific precision parameter associated with matrix C_i. K is the number of terms in the sum, and it must be an integer value from 1 to 10. Matrices C_i are passed using a list with argument `Cmatrix` in the definition of the latent effect in the model formula.

Priors are set on parameters $\theta_1, \ldots, \theta_{11}$, with $\theta_i = \log(\tau_i), i = 1, \ldots, 10$ and $\theta_{11} = \log(\tau)$. By default, priors on θ_i, $i = 1, \ldots, 10$ are log-Gamma with parameters 1 and 0.00005. Parameter θ_{11} is fixed to zero by default (i.e., $\tau = 1$ by default).

Note that in order to make this model identifiable only K precision parameters can be free out of the $K + 1$ in the model. For this reason, τ is fixed by default to a fixed value of 1 (0 in the log-scale). This parameter could be set to a different fixed value to rescale all other precision parameters, which sometimes help to identify the model parameters better. See also Section 5.6 for a general discussion on scaling of hyperparameters in `INLA`.

In the following example we consider the SIDS dataset again and fit a Poisson model with a random effect for overdispersion using the `generic3` latent effect. First, a diagonal matrix `K1` is defined and then a list with this matrix is used to define the latent effect:

```
K1 <- Diagonal(nrow(nc.sids), 1)

m.pois.g2 <- inla(SID74 ~ f(ID, model = "generic3", Cmatrix = list(K1)),
  data = nc.sids, family = "poisson", E = EXP74)

summary(m.pois.g2)
```

```
##
## Call:
##    c("inla(formula = SID74 ~ f(ID, model = \"generic3\", Cmatrix =
##    list(K1)), ", " family = \"poisson\", data = nc.sids, E = EXP74)")
## Time used:
##     Pre = 1.02, Running = 0.156, Post = 0.0601, Total = 1.24
## Fixed effects:
##               mean    sd 0.025quant 0.5quant 0.975quant    mode kld
## (Intercept) -0.027 0.063     -0.154   -0.026      0.092 -0.023   0
##
## Random effects:
##   Name      Model
##     ID Generic3 model
##
## Model hyperparameters:
##                                  mean    sd 0.025quant 0.5quant 0.975quant
## Precision for Cmatrix[[1]] for ID 7.26 2.57       3.79     6.77      13.61
##                                  mode
## Precision for Cmatrix[[1]] for ID 6.02
##
## Expected number of effective parameters(stdev): 40.44(6.52)
## Number of equivalent replicates : 2.47
##
## Marginal log-Likelihood: -245.54
```

As expected, the estimates of the intercept and precision are equal to the ones obtained when the same model was fitted using other random effects.

3.3.8 Correlated effects (iid?d models)

So far, we have discussed latent effects defined on a single vector of random effects $\mathbf{u}$ but INLA implements a number of random effects to introduce correlation among the random effects. These latent effects are particularly useful when defining joint models, as seen in Chapter 10. The models for correlated random effects are iid1d, iid2d, iid3d, iid4d and iid5d. They are named after the dimension of the vector of correlated random effects. For example, if a vector of three correlated random effects $\mathbf{u}$, $\mathbf{v}$ and $\mathbf{w}$ is needed, namely (u_i, v_i, w_i) then latent effect iid3d should be used.

Following the description of these effects in the manual page of the INLA package, we will describe the case for dimension 2, and we will consider two vectors of random effects, $\mathbf{u}$ and $\mathbf{v}$, so that (u_i, v_i) are correlated. A bivariate Gaussian distribution with zero mean and precision W will be considered. Furthermore, the prior on precision matrix W is a Wishart with r degrees of freedom and scale matrix R^{-1}.

The covariance of the correlated random effects is parameterized as:

$$W^{-1} = \begin{bmatrix} \tau_a & \rho/\sqrt{\tau_a \tau_b} \\ \rho/\sqrt{\tau_a \tau_b} & \tau_b \end{bmatrix}$$

Note that τ_a and τ_b are the marginal precisions and ρ is the correlation coefficient. These parameters are represented internally in INLA as $\boldsymbol{\theta} = (\theta_1, \theta_2, \theta_3)$, with $\theta_1 = \log(\tau_a)$, $\theta_2 = \log(\tau_b)$ and θ_3 defined as

$$\rho = 2\frac{\exp(\theta_3)}{1 + \exp(\theta_3)} - 1$$

Given that the prior is a Wishart, the prior parameters are $(r, R_{11}, R_{22}, R_{12})$, where r are the degrees of freedom and R_{ij} the corresponding elements in the inverse scale matrix R. By default, $r = 4$ and R is the diagonal matrix of dimension 2.

If each vector of the correlated random effects is of dimension m, then the resulting vector handled by INLA with both random effects will be of length $2 \cdot m$. This total length must be passed to the f() function through parameter n. See Table 3.6.

TABLE 3.6: Summary of options of the iid?d random effect.

Argument	Default	Description
n	—	Total length of vector of correlated random effects.

Correlated random effects up to 5 dimensions can be defined. These are analogously defined as the two-dimension case. More information is provided in the INLA documentation, which can be accessed with inla.doc("iid2d").

In the next example we will fit a model to the North Carolina SIDS data that considers data from both periods of time (1974-78 and 1979-84). The reason is that we might expect the overdispersion in the first period to be similar to the second.

First of all, the expected number of cases for the second time period will be computed and added to nc.sids:

```
#Overall rate
r79 <- sum(nc.sids$SID79) / sum(nc.sids$BIR79)
nc.sids$EXP79 <- r79 * nc.sids$BIR79
```

A new data.frame with data for both periods of time must be created. Here, we have included a factor PERIOD to identify each period of time (so that a different intercept for each period is considered). Furthermore, an index from 1 to 200 will be created (names ID) to define the iid2d latent effect:

```
#New data.frame
nc.new <- data.frame(SID = c(nc.sids$SID74, nc.sids$SID79),
   EXP = c(nc.sids$EXP74, nc.sids$EXP79),
   PERIOD = as.factor(c(rep("74", 100), rep("79", 100))),
   ID = 1:200)
```

The vector of random effects will be of length 200, but in practice it can be regarded as a vector $(\mathbf{u}, \mathbf{v})$, where both $\mathbf{u}$ and $\mathbf{v}$ are of length 100. Hence, the iid2d will make each pair (u_i, v_i), $i = 1, \ldots, 100$ to be correlated. Because we have two vectors of length 100, the value of n used to define the random effect must be 200, and this is passed to the f() as n = 2 * 100 in the code to fit the model:

```
m.pois.iid2d <- inla(SID ~ 0 + PERIOD + f(ID, model = "iid2d", n = 2 * 100),
  data = nc.new, family = "poisson", E = EXP)
```

```
summary(m.pois.iid2d)
```

```
##
## Call:
##    c("inla(formula = SID ~ 0 + PERIOD + f(ID, model = \"iid2d\", n =
##    2 * ", " 100), family = \"poisson\", data = nc.new, E = EXP)")
## Time used:
##     Pre = 1.05, Running = 0.362, Post = 0.0639, Total = 1.48
## Fixed effects:
##             mean    sd 0.025quant 0.5quant 0.975quant    mode kld
## PERIOD74 -0.041 0.066     -0.174   -0.039      0.087 -0.037   0
## PERIOD79 -0.007 0.055     -0.117   -0.007      0.098 -0.005   0
##
## Random effects:
##    Name       Model
##      ID IID2D model
##
## Model hyperparameters:
##                                 mean      sd 0.025quant 0.5quant 0.975quant
## Precision for ID (component 1) 5.557 1.459      3.234    5.375       8.93
## Precision for ID (component 2) 9.057 2.398      5.235    8.759      14.60
## Rho1:2 for ID                  0.398 0.156      0.065    0.409       0.67
##                                 mode
## Precision for ID (component 1) 5.030
## Precision for ID (component 2) 8.195
## Rho1:2 for ID                  0.432
##
## Expected number of effective parameters(stdev): 82.13(6.86)
## Number of equivalent replicates : 2.44
##
## Marginal log-Likelihood:  -489.90
```

Figure 3.1 shows the posterior means of the correlated random effects (u_i, v_i). The positive correlation between both random effects is evident. Also, variability in $\mathbf{v}$ is smaller than the variability of $\mathbf{u}$ and this is also shown in the model estimates of the precisions of the random effects.

This type of correlated effects is commonly used in joint models, where different coefficients in the model need to be correlated. For example, in Chapter 12 a joint model is built to estimate height and weight. Because these two variables are usually highly correlated, their coefficients in regression models can sometimes be assumed to be similar.

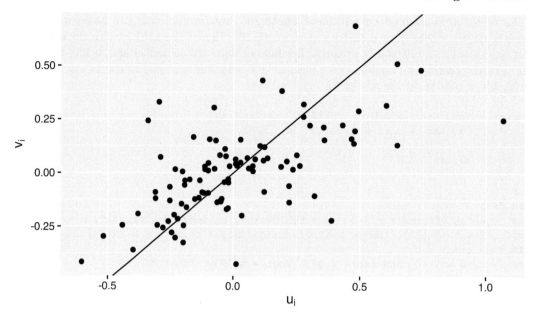

FIGURE 3.1 Posterior means of correlated random effects using a `iid2d` model. The solid line represents the identity line.

3.3.9   Random walks (`rw1` and `rw2` models)

Random walks of order one and two are also available as latent effects in **INLA**. Given a vector of Gaussian observations $u = (u_1, \ldots, u_n)$, the random walk of order one is defined assuming that increments $\Delta u_i = u_i - u_{i-1}$ follow a Gaussian distribution with zero mean and precision τ. This is equivalent to assuming that the distribution of vector u is Gaussian with zero mean and precision matrix τQ, where Q contains the neighborhood structure of the model.

Similarly, the random walk of order two is defined by assuming that second order increments $\Delta^2 u_i = u_i - 2u_{i-1} + u_{i-2}$ follow a Gaussian distribution with zero mean and precision τ.

In both cases the random walk can be defined to be cyclic, and the model can be scaled to have an average variance (i.e., the diagonal of the generalized inverse of Q) equal to 1 (see Section 5.6). See Table 3.7 for options `cyclic` and `scale.model`, respectively.

Although this is a discrete latent effect, it can be used to model continuous variables by using the `values` argument. In particular, the values of the covariate can be binned so that they are associated with a particular value of the vector of random effects. This is particularly interesting to model non-linear dependence on covariates in the linear predictor.

A continuous random walk of order 2 is implemented as model `crw2` in **INLA**. See Chapter 3 in Rue and Held (2005) for details on how this model is defined as a latent Gaussian Markov random field. In particular, these models are consistent with respect to the choice of the locations and the resolution, and their precision matrix is sparse due to the fact that they fulfill a Markov property.

TABLE 3.7: Summary of options of the `rw1d` and `rw2d` random effects.

Argument	Default	Description
values	—	Values of the covariate for which the effect is estimated.
cyclic	FALSE	Cyclic adjacency.
scale.model	FALSE	Whether to scale variance matrix.

The `AirPassengers` dataset records the number of total monthly international airline passengers from 1949 to 1960 (Box et al., 1976). This data is an object of class `ts` (i.e., time-series) and the next lines of R code show how to load the data and create a `data.frame` with the number of passengers, year, month of the year and id to identify the row in the dataset:

```
data(AirPassengers)

airp.data <- data.frame(airp = as.vector(AirPassengers),
  month = as.factor(rep(1:12, 12)),
  year = as.factor(rep(1949:1960, each = 12)),
  ID = 1:length(AirPassengers))
```

Figure 3.2 shows the original times series and the log of the number of passengers. The original data show an increasing variance with time, which is not observed in the log-transformed time series. Given that the random walk assumes a common precision, it will be better to model the data in the log-scale.

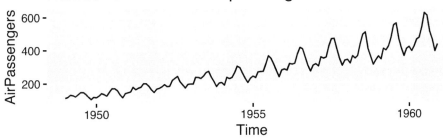

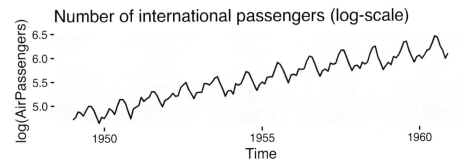

FIGURE 3.2 Monthly international airline passengers: original data (top) and log-scale (bottom).

The first model to be fit to the data is a linear model with a fixed effect on year and a `rw1` random effect:

```
airp.rw1 <- inla(log(AirPassengers) ~ 0 + year + f(ID, model = "rw1"),
  control.family = list(hyper = list(prec = list(param = c(1, 0.2)))),
  data = airp.data, control.predictor = list(compute = TRUE))
```

```
summary(airp.rw1)
```

```
##
## Call:
##    c("inla(formula = log(AirPassengers) ~ 0 + year + f(ID, model =
##    \"rw1\"), ", " data = airp.data, control.predictor = list(compute
##    = TRUE), ", " control.family = list(hyper = list(prec = list(param
##    = c(1, ", " 0.2)))))")
## Time used:
##     Pre = 1.58, Running = 0.458, Post = 0.0742, Total = 2.11
## Fixed effects:
##             mean    sd 0.025quant 0.5quant 0.975quant  mode kld
## year1949 5.157 0.252      4.664    5.156      5.654 5.154   0
## year1950 5.207 0.220      4.776    5.206      5.641 5.205   0
## year1951 5.332 0.190      4.959    5.332      5.707 5.331   0
## year1952 5.420 0.165      5.096    5.420      5.745 5.420   0
## year1953 5.490 0.146      5.203    5.490      5.776 5.490   0
## year1954 5.517 0.135      5.251    5.517      5.782 5.517   0
## year1955 5.602 0.135      5.335    5.602      5.867 5.603   0
## year1956 5.670 0.146      5.381    5.670      5.956 5.671   0
## year1957 5.727 0.165      5.401    5.728      6.051 5.729   0
## year1958 5.736 0.190      5.360    5.736      6.109 5.737   0
## year1959 5.806 0.219      5.374    5.807      6.237 5.807   0
## year1960 5.843 0.251      5.348    5.843      6.336 5.844   0
##
## Random effects:
##   Name      Model
##     ID RW1 model
##
## Model hyperparameters:
##                                          mean     sd 0.025quant 0.5quant
## Precision for the Gaussian observations 100.90 18.11      69.24    99.65
## Precision for ID                        157.65 42.64      93.81   150.85
##                                         0.975quant   mode
## Precision for the Gaussian observations    139.98  97.41
## Precision for ID                           259.69 137.91
##
## Expected number of effective parameters(stdev): 58.90(8.78)
## Number of equivalent replicates : 2.44
##
## Marginal log-Likelihood:  2.04
## Posterior marginals for the linear predictor and
##  the fitted values are computed
```

Next, a `rw2` model is fitted:

```
airp.rw2 <- inla(log(AirPassengers) ~ 0 + year + f(ID, model = "rw2"),
  control.family = list(hyper = list(prec = list(param = c(1, 0.2)))),
  data = airp.data, control.predictor = list(compute = TRUE))
summary(airp.rw2)
```

```
##
## Call:
##    c("inla(formula = log(AirPassengers) ~ 0 + year + f(ID, model =
##    \"rw2\"), ", " data = airp.data, control.predictor = list(compute
##    = TRUE), ", " control.family = list(hyper = list(prec = list(param
##    = c(1, ", " 0.2)))))")
## Time used:
##     Pre = 1.58, Running = 0.461, Post = 0.074, Total = 2.11
## Fixed effects:
##             mean    sd 0.025quant 0.5quant 0.975quant  mode kld
## year1949 5.148 0.278      4.602    5.148      5.694 5.148   0
## year1950 5.203 0.243      4.726    5.203      5.679 5.203   0
## year1951 5.323 0.210      4.909    5.323      5.736 5.323   0
## year1952 5.417 0.183      5.058    5.417      5.775 5.417   0
## year1953 5.467 0.162      5.149    5.467      5.784 5.467   0
## year1954 5.501 0.150      5.206    5.501      5.795 5.501   0
## year1955 5.585 0.149      5.291    5.585      5.879 5.585   0
## year1956 5.653 0.161      5.336    5.653      5.969 5.653   0
## year1957 5.715 0.182      5.357    5.715      6.073 5.715   0
## year1958 5.755 0.210      5.341    5.755      6.168 5.755   0
## year1959 5.847 0.243      5.369    5.847      6.325 5.847   0
## year1960 5.893 0.279      5.344    5.893      6.442 5.893   0
##
## Random effects:
##   Name      Model
##     ID RW2 model
##
## Model hyperparameters:
##                                             mean     sd 0.025quant 0.5quant
## Precision for the Gaussian observations 101.38  16.61      72.19   100.22
## Precision for ID                        410.28 138.07     208.57   387.16
##                                         0.975quant   mode
## Precision for the Gaussian observations    137.41  98.09
## Precision for ID                           744.86 345.43
##
## Expected number of effective parameters(stdev): 47.16(4.53)
## Number of equivalent replicates : 3.05
##
## Marginal log-Likelihood:  -12.71
## Posterior marginals for the linear predictor and
##   the fitted values are computed
```

Note that `control.family` has been used to set a prior on the precision of the Gaussian likelihood to prevent overfitting (Faraway, 2019b; Bakka, 2019). See also Chapter 5 on priors and Section 6.5.2.

In order to compare how these two models fit the data, the times series (in the log scale) and the fitted values from these two models have been plotted in Figure 3.3. In general, fitted values from both models are very close to the observed time series. However, the estimates obtained with the `rw2` model seem to be smoother than those obtained with the `rw1`. This is not surprising as the `rw2` is of a higher order.

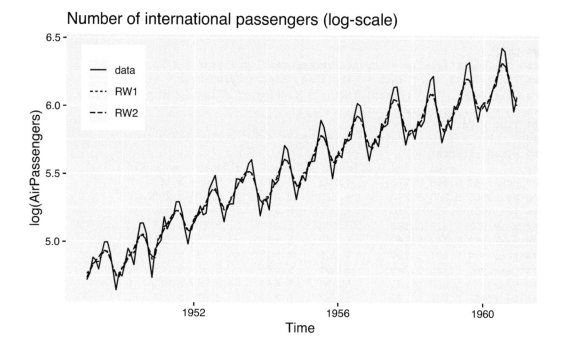

FIGURE 3.3 Fitted values (i.e., posterior means) of the number of international passengers.

Note that in this example, the latent effects are based on modeling the time series using values that are close in time, such as the one or two previous values. However, it is clear from Figure 3.2 that the time series has a strong season effect of period equal to one year. For this reason, it may be better to include a seasonal latent effect in the linear predictor.

3.3.10   Seasonal random effects

Seasonal effects can be modeled with the `seasonal` latent effect. In this case, the vector of random effects $\mathbf{u} = (u_1, \ldots, u_n)$ is assumed to have periodicity p (with $p < n$) and it is defined such as sums $x_i + x_{i+1} + \ldots + x_{i+m-1}$ are independent Gaussian observations with zero mean and precision τ.

Note that the precision matrix of the model is $Q = \tau R$, where R has the neighborhood structure of the model. This model can be scaled, similarly to the random walk models. See Table 3.8 for the different specific options of this model. Note how periodicity of the seasonal effect can be set with argument `season.length` when the model is defined within the `f()` function.

For seasonal latent effects, the internal parameter is $\theta = \log(\tau)$, and the default prior is a log-Gamma with parameters 1 and 0.00005. This prior can be modified as usual. See Section 3.5.1 and Chapter 5.

A `seasonal` model can be fit to the air passengers dataset as seen below. Note that we have set the periodicity to 12 so that the latent effect assumes that the seasonal effect covers one year. This is reasonable because the time series shows a clear seasonal effect of period equal to one year.

TABLE 3.8: Summary of options of the `seasonal` random effect.

Argument	Default	Description
season.length	—	Periodicity of the seasonal effect.
scale.model	FALSE	Whether to scale variance matrix.

Hence, the model is fit and summarized as follows:

```
airp.seasonal <- inla(log(AirPassengers) ~ 0 + year +
    f(ID, model = "seasonal", season.length = 12),
  control.family = list(hyper = list(prec = list(param = c(1, 0.2)))),
  data = airp.data)
summary(airp.seasonal)
```

```
##
## Call:
##    c("inla(formula = log(AirPassengers) ~ 0 + year + f(ID, model =
##    \"seasonal\", ", " season.length = 12), data = airp.data,
##    control.family = list(hyper = list(prec = list(param = c(1, ", "
##    0.2)))))")
## Time used:
##    Pre = 1.6, Running = 0.345, Post = 0.0682, Total = 2.01
## Fixed effects:
##             mean   sd 0.025quant 0.5quant 0.975quant  mode kld
## year1949  4.836 0.02      4.797    4.836      4.875 4.836   0
## year1950  4.931 0.02      4.891    4.931      4.970 4.931   0
## year1951  5.131 0.02      5.092    5.131      5.171 5.131   0
## year1952  5.277 0.02      5.238    5.277      5.317 5.277   0
## year1953  5.409 0.02      5.369    5.409      5.448 5.409   0
## year1954  5.467 0.02      5.427    5.467      5.506 5.467   0
## year1955  5.639 0.02      5.600    5.639      5.679 5.639   0
## year1956  5.784 0.02      5.745    5.784      5.824 5.784   0
## year1957  5.898 0.02      5.859    5.898      5.938 5.898   0
## year1958  5.931 0.02      5.891    5.931      5.970 5.931   0
## year1959  6.048 0.02      6.009    6.048      6.088 6.048   0
## year1960  6.154 0.02      6.115    6.154      6.194 6.154   0
##
## Random effects:
##    Name      Model
##      ID Seasonal model
##
## Model hyperparameters:
```

```
##                                              mean         sd 0.025quant
## Precision for the Gaussian observations    212.38      27.36     162.78
## Precision for ID                          40490.46  24851.53   10356.31
##                                           0.5quant 0.975quant      mode
## Precision for the Gaussian observations    211.01     270.20    208.66
## Precision for ID                          34835.03  104303.22  24772.46
##
## Expected number of effective parameters(stdev): 26.53(1.86)
## Number of equivalent replicates : 5.43
##
## Marginal log-Likelihood:   70.16
```

3.3.11 Autoregressive random effects

Autoregressive models of order p, denoted by $AR(p)$, are also available in INLA. In particular, an autoregressive model of order 1 (ar1) and a generic order p (ar) are implemented.

The $AR(1)$ model on a vector $\mathbf{u}$ can be defined as u_1 coming from a Gaussian distribution with zero mean and precision $\tau(1 - \rho^2)$, where τ is a precision parameter and ρ a correlation coefficient so that $|\rho| < 1$. The other elements in $\mathbf{u}$ are defined as $u_i = \rho x_{i-1} + \varepsilon_i, i = 2, \ldots, n$ with ε Gaussian observation with zero mean and precision τ.

Similarly as for the random walk models, autoregressive models can take the values argument when defined to set the values of the covariates for which the effects are being estimated. For the ar1 model, covariates can be included using argument control.ar1c when defining the model. Table 3.9 summarizes the specific options of the autoregressive latent effects.

TABLE 3.9: Summary of options of the ar1, ar1c and ar random effects.

Argument	Default	Description
values	—	Values of the covariate for which the effect is estimated.
order	—	Order of autoregressive model (for ar only).
control.ar1c	—	List with two objects: Z and Q.beta.
control.ar1c$Z	—	Matrix of covariates of dimension $n \times m$.
control.ar1c$Q.beta	—	$m \times m$ precision matrix of Gaussian prior on the coefficients of the covariates.

This model is parameterized using $\boldsymbol{\theta} = (\theta_1, \theta_2)$. The first internal hyperparameter is defined as $\theta_1 = \log(\kappa)$, where κ is the *marginal* precision:

$$\kappa = \tau(1 - \rho^2)$$

The second hyperparameter is defined as

$$\theta_2 = \log(\frac{1 + \rho}{1 - \rho})$$

The prior is defined on θ. The default is a log-Gamma with parameters 1 and 0.00005 for θ_1 and a Gaussian with zero mean and precision 1 for θ_2.

The AR(1) model can be extended to include covariates as follows:

$$u_i = \rho u_{i-1} + \sum_{j=1}^{m} \beta_j z_{i-1}^{(j)} + \varepsilon_i, i = 2, \ldots, n$$

This model is known as `ar1c`. Here, m covariates are used in the model, and $z_i^{(j)}$ is the value of the covariate j of observation i. The covariates have associated coefficients $\beta_j, j = 1, \ldots, m$.

Coefficients are assigned a multivariate Gaussian prior with known precision matrix. The matrix of covariates (by column) and the precision of the prior on the coefficients are defined in the `f()` function via parameter `control.ar1c`, and they are passed as a list with names `Z` and `Q.beta`, respectively. See Table 3.9 for details.

The AR(p) model is defined in a similar way, but it can now include a lag of order p on the vector of random effects:

$$u_i = \varphi_1 x_{i-1} + \ldots + \varphi_p u_{i-p} + \varepsilon_i, i = p, \ldots, n$$

Note that this model can handle values of p up to 10 (inclusive). The internal parameterization of this model is more complex and we refer the reader to the manual page, which can be accessed with `inla.doc("^ar$")`. The argument of `inla.doc` is due to the fact that this function used regular expressions to look up in the documentation files.

To illustrate the use of autoregressive models with `INLA` we will fit a number of models to the `AirPassengers` dataset. We will start with an AR(1) model:

```
airp.ar1 <- inla(log(AirPassengers) ~ 0 + year + f(ID, model = "ar1"),
  control.family = list(hyper = list(prec = list(param = c(1, 0.2)))),
  data = airp.data, control.predictor = list(compute = TRUE))
summary(airp.ar1)
```

```
## 
## Call:
##    c("inla(formula = log(AirPassengers) ~ 0 + year + f(ID, model =
##    \"ar1\"), ", " data = airp.data, control.predictor = list(compute
##    = TRUE), ", " control.family = list(hyper = list(prec = list(param
##    = c(1, ", " 0.2)))))")
## Time used:
##     Pre = 1.57, Running = 0.224, Post = 0.0744, Total = 1.87
## Fixed effects:
##            mean    sd 0.025quant 0.5quant 0.975quant  mode kld
## year1949 4.843 0.085      4.679    4.842      5.016 4.840   0
## year1950 4.940 0.081      4.781    4.939      5.104 4.938   0
## year1951 5.129 0.081      4.969    5.129      5.289 5.129   0
## year1952 5.277 0.080      5.117    5.277      5.437 5.277   0
## year1953 5.403 0.080      5.242    5.403      5.562 5.403   0
## year1954 5.478 0.081      5.320    5.477      5.640 5.476   0
## year1955 5.638 0.080      5.477    5.638      5.797 5.638   0
## year1956 5.776 0.081      5.613    5.777      5.934 5.778   0
## year1957 5.888 0.081      5.724    5.888      6.045 5.890   0
## year1958 5.932 0.081      5.771    5.933      6.091 5.933   0
```

```
## year1959 6.046 0.081        5.882     6.047     6.205 6.048   0
## year1960 6.124 0.085        5.947     6.127     6.287 6.130   0
##
## Random effects:
##   Name      Model
##      ID AR1 model
##
## Model hyperparameters:
##                                              mean      sd 0.025quant 0.5quant
## Precision for the Gaussian observations 102.135 17.968      70.66  100.908
## Precision for ID                         63.795 21.156      30.00   61.419
## Rho for ID                                0.753  0.075       0.59    0.759
##                                         0.975quant  mode
## Precision for the Gaussian observations    140.91 98.70
## Precision for ID                           111.82 56.50
## Rho for ID                                   0.88  0.77
##
## Expected number of effective parameters(stdev): 62.18(8.35)
## Number of equivalent replicates : 2.32
##
## Marginal log-Likelihood:  4.67
## Posterior marginals for the linear predictor and
##   the fitted values are computed
```

Next, an AR(3) is fitted:

```
airp.ar3 <- inla(log(AirPassengers) ~ 0 + year + f(ID, model = "ar",
    order = 3),
  control.family = list(hyper = list(prec = list(param = c(1, 0.2)))),
  data = airp.data, control.predictor = list(compute = TRUE))
summary(airp.ar3)
```

```
##
## Call:
##    c("inla(formula = log(AirPassengers) ~ 0 + year + f(ID, model =
##    \"ar\", ", " order = 3), data = airp.data, control.predictor =
##    list(compute = TRUE), ", " control.family = list(hyper = list(prec
##    = list(param = c(1, ", " 0.2)))))")
## Time used:
##     Pre = 1.6, Running = 0.484, Post = 0.086, Total = 2.17
## Fixed effects:
##          mean    sd 0.025quant 0.5quant 0.975quant  mode kld
## year1949 4.835 0.027      4.783    4.835      4.888 4.835   0
## year1950 4.930 0.027      4.877    4.930      4.983 4.930   0
## year1951 5.131 0.027      5.078    5.131      5.184 5.131   0
## year1952 5.277 0.027      5.224    5.277      5.330 5.277   0
## year1953 5.408 0.027      5.355    5.408      5.461 5.408   0
## year1954 5.465 0.027      5.413    5.465      5.518 5.465   0
## year1955 5.639 0.027      5.586    5.639      5.691 5.639   0
## year1956 5.784 0.027      5.731    5.784      5.837 5.784   0
## year1957 5.898 0.027      5.845    5.898      5.950 5.898   0
## year1958 5.930 0.027      5.877    5.930      5.983 5.930   0
## year1959 6.048 0.027      5.995    6.048      6.101 6.048   0
## year1960 6.154 0.027      6.101    6.154      6.207 6.154   0
```

```
##
## Random effects:
##    Name     Model
##      ID AR(p) model
##
## Model hyperparameters:
##                                          mean      sd 0.025quant 0.5quant
## Precision for the Gaussian observations 119.528 15.817     88.654  119.755
## Precision for ID                        115.377 89.603     17.752   92.407
## PACF1 for ID                              0.860  0.002      0.857    0.860
## PACF2 for ID                             -0.917  0.035     -0.971   -0.922
## PACF3 for ID                             -0.958  0.054     -0.999   -0.976
##                                        0.975quant    mode
## Precision for the Gaussian observations   150.303 121.477
## Precision for ID                          349.316  49.617
## PACF1 for ID                                0.864   0.860
## PACF2 for ID                               -0.835  -0.933
## PACF3 for ID                               -0.810  -0.997
##
## Expected number of effective parameters(stdev): 17.99(1.99)
## Number of equivalent replicates : 8.00
##
## Marginal log-Likelihood:  41.27
## Posterior marginals for the linear predictor and
##  the fitted values are computed
```

In previous models covariate `year` has been included as part of the linear predictor. In the next model this covariate is included as part of an AR(1) model with covariates (i.e., a `ar1c` model):

```
Z <- model.matrix (~ 0 + year, data = airp.data)
Q.beta <- Diagonal(12, 0.001)

airp.ar1c <- inla(log(AirPassengers) ~ 1 + f(ID, model = "ar1c",
  args.ar1c = list(Z = Z, Q.beta = Q.beta)),
  control.family = list(hyper = list(prec = list(param = c(1, 0.2)))),
  data = airp.data, control.predictor = list(compute = TRUE))
summary(airp.ar1c)
```

```
##
## Call:
##    c("inla(formula = log(AirPassengers) ~ 1 + f(ID, model = \"ar1c\",
##    ", " args.ar1c = list(Z = Z, Q.beta = Q.beta)), data = airp.data,
##    ", " control.predictor = list(compute = TRUE), control.family =
##    list(hyper = list(prec = list(param = c(1, ", " 0.2)))))")
## Time used:
##    Pre = 1, Running = 0.247, Post = 0.0682, Total = 1.32
## Fixed effects:
##              mean    sd 0.025quant 0.5quant 0.975quant  mode kld
## (Intercept) 4.724 0.135      4.458    4.724       4.99 4.724   0
##
## Random effects:
##    Name     Model
```

```
##       ID AR1C model
##
## Model hyperparameters:
##                                        mean      sd 0.025quant 0.5quant
## Precision for the Gaussian observations 99.117 18.770    66.763   97.632
## Precision for ID                       118.749 36.461    64.469  112.902
## Rho for ID                               0.522  0.089     0.331    0.529
##                                       0.975quant    mode
## Precision for the Gaussian observations   140.318  94.875
## Precision for ID                          206.108 102.174
## Rho for ID                                  0.678   0.543
##
## Expected number of effective parameters(stdev): 60.35(9.94)
## Number of equivalent replicates : 2.39
##
## Marginal log-Likelihood:  3.65
## Posterior marginals for the linear predictor and
##  the fitted values are computed
```

In all three models, the autoregressive effect seems to capture the high temporal autocorrelation in the data given the estimates of the autocorrelation parameter. Figure 3.4 shows the original time series (in the log scale) together with the posterior means of the fitted values.

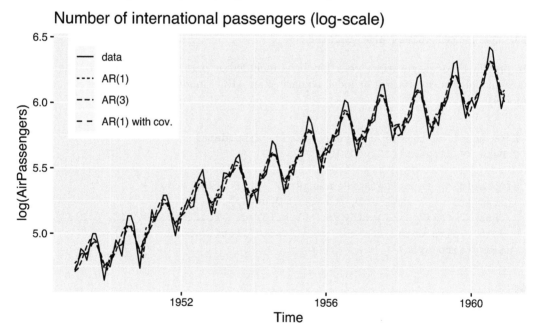

FIGURE 3.4 Fitted values (i.e., posterior means) of the number of international passengers using autoregressive models.

3.4 Information on the latent effects

The names of the hyperparameters in a given model, their internal parameterization and the default prior on the internal scale can be checked in the manual page (i.e., calling `inla.doc()`) or using function `inla.models()`. For example, the information about the `idd` model can be displayed with `inla.models()$latent$iid`, and similarly for any other random effects model.

This is particularly useful when in doubt about how a particular part of the model is defined, such as the internal representation of the parameters and their default priors. The full list of the elements that define the latent effect can be seen here:

```
names(inla.models()$latent$iid)
```

```
##  [1] "doc"              "hyper"          "constr"
##  [4] "nrow.ncol"        "augmented"      "aug.factor"
##  [7] "aug.constr"       "n.div.by"       "n.required"
## [10] "set.default.values" "pdf"
```

Although particular random effects may require the use of specific parameters, there are a number of common parameters to all models that are worth knowing. These are described in the next section.

3.5 Additional arguments

In addition to the specific parameters required by each one of the random effects previously described, there are a number of other arguments that can be used to tune specific parts of the model. Some of these are summarized in Table 3.10. All of them must be passed to the `f()` function when defining the latent effect in the model formula.

TABLE 3.10: Summary of additional arguments that can be passed when defining a random effect.

Argument	Default	Description
hyper	Default priors	Definition of priors for hyperparameters.
constr	FALSE	Sum-to-zero constraint on the random effects.
extraconstr	FALSE	Additional constraint on the random effects.
scale.model	FALSE	Scale variance matrix of random effects.
group	—	Variable to define the groups of random effect.
control.group	—	Control options for `group` parameter.

3.5.1 Priors of hyperparameters

Priors in `INLA` are described in detail in Chapter 5 but we include here a short introduction to how priors are set. Priors on the model hyperparameters are set with parameter `hyper`, which takes a named list using the names of the hyperparameters. Each element in the named list must be one of the variables shown in Table 3.11.

For example, the default parameters for the prior on the log-precision of the random effects of a `iid` random effects are:

```
prec.prior <- inla.models()$latent$iid$hyper$theta
prec.prior
```

```
## $hyperid
## [1] 1001
## attr(,"inla.read.only")
## [1] FALSE
##
## $name
## [1] "log precision"
## attr(,"inla.read.only")
## [1] FALSE
##
## $short.name
## [1] "prec"
## attr(,"inla.read.only")
## [1] FALSE
##
## $prior
## [1] "loggamma"
## attr(,"inla.read.only")
## [1] FALSE
##
## $param
## [1] 1e+00 5e-05
## attr(,"inla.read.only")
## [1] FALSE
##
## $initial
## [1] 4
## attr(,"inla.read.only")
## [1] FALSE
##
## $fixed
## [1] FALSE
## attr(,"inla.read.only")
## [1] FALSE
##
## $to.theta
## function (x)
## log(x)
## <bytecode: 0x7fcd8047b140>
## <environment: 0x7fcd804867c8>
## attr(,"inla.read.only")
## [1] TRUE
```

```
##
## $from.theta
## function (x)
## exp(x)
## <bytecode: 0x7fcd8047b028>
## <environment: 0x7fcd804867c8>
## attr(,"inla.read.only")
## [1] TRUE
```

Note that in this case there is a single hyperparameter θ and hence the `$theta` after `hyper`. Other random effects with more than one hyperparameter will name them `theta1`, etc.

In this example, the internal parameterization is $\theta = \log(\tau)$ (`prec.prior$to.theta` above), with τ the precision of the `iid` random effects. The default prior, on θ, is a log-Gamma (`prec.prior$prior`) with parameters 1 and 0.00005 (`prec.prior$param`), as seen in parameters `prior` and `param`. The starting value of θ is 4, as seen in parameter `prec.prior$initial` and it is not fixed by default (i.e., a posterior marginal will be estimated) because `prec.prior$fixed` is `FALSE`. When `fixed` is set to `TRUE`, the hyperparameter will be kept constant at the value in `initial`. In this particular case, as `initial` is 4 this will make the log-precision to be 4, i.e., $4 = \theta = \log(\tau)$, which implies that the precision would be fixed to $\tau = \exp(4)$. This will represent a very large precision or, equivalently, a very small variance which will make the random effects very close to zero.

Furthermore, functions set in `to.theta` and `from.theta` are used to convert the values of τ to and from θ (i.e., from the *model* scale to and from the *internal* scale). In this case, given that $\theta = \log(\tau)$, `to.theta` is the `log()` function while `from.theta` is the `exp()` function, because $\tau = \exp(\theta)$.

TABLE 3.11: Summary of parameters that are used to define a prior on a hyperparameter with INLA.

Argument	Description
hyperid	Internal id of prior.
name	Name of hyperparameter in internal scale.
short.name	Short name of hyperparameter to be used inside `hyper`.
prior	Name of prior distribution.
param	Parameter values of prior distributions.
initial	Initial value of hyperparameter in the internal scale.
fixed	Whether to keep the hyperparameter fixed (default is `FALSE`).
to.theta	Function to convert parameter into the internal scale.
from.theta	Function to convert the value in the internal scale to the model scale.

In general, not all arguments in the prior definition will be given a value when setting a non-default prior. For example, in the `iid` model the prior on the log-precision could be replaced by a Gaussian with zero mean and small precision. This could be easily done as follows:

```
hyper = list(prec = list(prior = "gaussian", param = c(0, 0.001)))
```

The former R code sets a Gaussian prior with zero mean and precision 0.001 on θ, i.e., a log-Gaussian prior on τ.

A full example on the North Carolina SIDS data using this prior would be:

```
m.pois.iid.gp <- inla(SID74 ~ f(ID, model = "iid",
    hyper = list(theta = list(prior = "gaussian", param = c(0, 0.001)))),
  data = nc.sids, family = "poisson",
  E = EXP74)
summary(m.pois.iid.gp)
```

```
##
## Call:
##    c("inla(formula = SID74 ~ f(ID, model = \"iid\", hyper =
##    list(theta = list(prior = \"gaussian\", ", " param = c(0,
##    0.001)))), family = \"poisson\", data = nc.sids, ", " E = EXP74)")
## Time used:
##     Pre = 1.02, Running = 0.115, Post = 0.0597, Total = 1.19
## Fixed effects:
##                mean    sd 0.025quant 0.5quant 0.975quant    mode kld
## (Intercept) -0.032 0.064     -0.162   -0.031      0.091 -0.028   0
##
## Random effects:
##    Name      Model
##      ID IID model
##
## Model hyperparameters:
##                   mean    sd 0.025quant 0.5quant 0.975quant mode
## Precision for ID 6.53 2.15       3.49     6.14      11.82 5.52
##
## Expected number of effective parameters(stdev): 42.44(6.26)
## Number of equivalent replicates : 2.36
##
## Marginal log-Likelihood:  -241.88
```

The estimates of the parameters are very similar to the previous examples but not equal and this is due to the choice of the priors. Note that in the named list passed to hyper we have used prec to set the prior for the hyperparameter. An alternative name could have been theta. i.e.,

```
hyper = list(theta = list(prior = "gaussian", param = c(0, 0.001)))
```

However, using prec makes the code easier to read and avoids possible errors when setting the priors for models with several hyperparameters. In this case, the list passed to hyper can have length higher than one. For example, for a model with two hyperparameters this would be:

```
hyper = list(theta1 = list(...), theta2 = list(...))
```

Detailed information on how priors can be set in INLA (including implementing new priors and other features) is given in Chapter 5.

3.5.2   Sum-to-zero constraint

Some of the models described above are *intrinsic*, i.e., their precision matrices are singular. Hence, the distribution is improper and may lead to an improper posterior. In other words, the precision matrix is not full-rank and additional constraints on the random effects are often imposed (see also Section 6.3).

A common one is a sum-to-zero constraint which will make the values of the random effects $\mathbf{u} = (u_1, \ldots, u_n)$ to be such as $\sum_{i=1}^{n} u_i = 0$. This can be achieved by setting parameter constr to TRUE when the model is defined. This sum-to-zero constraint is added by default to all intrinsic models implemented in INLA.

For example, for a rw1 model the constr parameter is set to TRUE by default:

```
inla.models()$latent$rw1$constr
```

```
## [1] TRUE
```

On the other hand, iid latent effects are not intrinsic and the parameter is set to FALSE by default:

```
inla.models()$latent$iid$constr
```

```
## [1] FALSE
```

Note that setting constraints on the random effects will likely affect the estimates of other parameters in the model as these constraints will shift the estimates of the random effects. In the previous example on the North Carolina SIDS data, the way to add a sum-to-zero constraint on the iid random effects (using the default prior) would be:

```
m.pois.iid.gp0 <- inla(SID74 ~ f(ID, model = "iid", constr = TRUE),
  data = nc.sids, family = "poisson", E = EXP74)

summary(m.pois.iid.gp0)
```

```
##
## Call:
##    c("inla(formula = SID74 ~ f(ID, model = \"iid\", constr = TRUE),
##    family = \"poisson\", ", " data = nc.sids, E = EXP74)")
## Time used:
##     Pre = 0.998, Running = 0.152, Post = 0.0592, Total = 1.21
## Fixed effects:
##                 mean    sd 0.025quant 0.5quant 0.975quant    mode kld
## (Intercept) -0.027 0.049     -0.125   -0.026      0.067 -0.025   0
##
## Random effects:
##    Name      Model
##       ID IID model
##
## Model hyperparameters:
##                   mean    sd 0.025quant 0.5quant 0.975quant mode
## Precision for ID 7.26 2.57       3.79     6.77      13.61 6.02
```

```
##
## Expected number of effective parameters(stdev): 40.44(6.52)
## Number of equivalent replicates : 2.47
##
## Marginal log-Likelihood:   -245.54
```

In this particular case, the parameter estimates are quite similar.

3.5.3   Additional constraints on the random effects

In addition to the sum-to-zero constraint there is also the possibility of setting additional constraints on the random effects. See Section 6.3 for a general discussion on how to set linear constraints on the latent effects in INLA.

Linear constraints are set with argument `extraconstr`. This will take a list with two elements, A and e, to define the constraint $Au = e$. Hence, A must be a matrix with the same number of columns as the length of the vector of random effects, and e must be a vector of the appropriate length, i.e., with the same number of rows as matrix A.

For example, a sum-to-zero constraint for a vector of random effects of length n could be added as follows:

```
A <- matrix(1, ncol = n, nrow = 1)
e <- rep(0, 1)

inla( ... ~ ... + f(..., extraconstr = list(A, e), ...), ...)
```

Hence, the previous example could be reproduced as follows using `extraconstr`:

```
n <- nrow(nc.sids)
A <- matrix(1, ncol = n, nrow = 1)
e <- rep(0, 1)
m.pois.iid.extrac <- inla(SID74 ~
    f(ID, model = "iid", extraconstr = list(A = A, e = e)),
  data = nc.sids, family = "poisson", E = EXP74)

summary(m.pois.iid.extrac)
```

```
##
## Call:
##    c("inla(formula = SID74 ~ f(ID, model = \"iid\", extraconstr =
##    list(A = A, ", " e = e)), family = \"poisson\", data = nc.sids, E
##    = EXP74)" )
## Time used:
##     Pre = 1.04, Running = 0.147, Post = 0.0594, Total = 1.25
## Fixed effects:
##               mean    sd 0.025quant 0.5quant 0.975quant    mode kld
## (Intercept) -0.027 0.049     -0.125   -0.026      0.067 -0.025   0
##
## Random effects:
##   Name      Model
```

```
##      ID IID model
##
## Model hyperparameters:
##                  mean   sd 0.025quant 0.5quant 0.975quant mode
## Precision for ID 7.26 2.57       3.79     6.77      13.61 6.02
##
## Expected number of effective parameters(stdev): 40.44(6.52)
## Number of equivalent replicates : 2.47
##
## Marginal log-Likelihood:  -245.54
```

Note how the fit model is the same as the previous one.

The main purpose to add additional constraint is for identifiability purposes. See, for example, Rue and Held (2005) for more details on this topic. Goicoa et al. (2018) show how additional constraints on the random effect can change the model estimates in spatio-temporal disease mapping models. However, this behavior is likely to be reproduced by models where the random effects are highly constrained for identifiability reasons.

3.5.4   Model scaling

Another feature that is particularly interesting when dealing with intrinsic models is the possibility to *scale* the model to make the diagonal of the structure variance (i.e., excluding the precision parameter) of the random effects to be re-scaled so that the generalized variance is equal to 1. This is fully described in Sørbye and Rue (2014), with a more practical example available in Sørbye (2013). Scaling in the context of prior setting is discussed later in Section 5.6.

The generalized variance is the geometric mean of the diagonal values of the covariance matrix (see Sørbye, 2013, for details). By setting this to one the precision parameter is re-scaled as well. As a result of this scaling, the precision parameters of different models will have a similar interpretation. Hence, imposing the same priors on them (e.g., the default prior) will make sense as they are in the same scale. Furthermore, scaled models will be less sensible to the scale of the data used to estimate the effects (as shown in Sørbye, 2013).

Scaling is set with parameter `scale.model`, which is `FALSE` by default. The `rw1` model fit to the air passengers data can be modified to scale the latent random effect:

```
airp.rw1.scale <- inla(log(AirPassengers) ~ 0 + year +
    f(ID, model = "rw1", scale.model = TRUE),
  control.family = list(hyper = list(prec = list(param = c(1, 0.2)))),
  data = airp.data)

summary(airp.rw1.scale)
```

```
##
## Call:
##    c("inla(formula = log(AirPassengers) ~ 0 + year + f(ID, model =
##    \"rw1\", ", " scale.model = TRUE), data = airp.data,
##    control.family = list(hyper = list(prec = list(param = c(1, ", "
##    0.2))))))")
## Time used:
```

```
##      Pre = 1.55, Running = 0.346, Post = 0.0682, Total = 1.96
## Fixed effects:
##              mean    sd 0.025quant 0.5quant 0.975quant  mode kld
## year1949 5.157 0.252      4.664    5.156       5.654 5.154   0
## year1950 5.207 0.220      4.777    5.206       5.641 5.205   0
## year1951 5.332 0.190      4.959    5.332       5.707 5.331   0
## year1952 5.420 0.165      5.096    5.420       5.745 5.420   0
## year1953 5.490 0.146      5.203    5.490       5.776 5.490   0
## year1954 5.517 0.135      5.251    5.517       5.782 5.517   0
## year1955 5.602 0.135      5.335    5.602       5.867 5.603   0
## year1956 5.670 0.146      5.382    5.670       5.955 5.671   0
## year1957 5.727 0.165      5.401    5.728       6.050 5.729   0
## year1958 5.736 0.190      5.360    5.736       6.109 5.737   0
## year1959 5.806 0.219      5.374    5.807       6.237 5.807   0
## year1960 5.843 0.251      5.348    5.843       6.335 5.844   0
##
## Random effects:
##   Name      Model
##      ID RW1 model
##
## Model hyperparameters:
##                                           mean     sd 0.025quant 0.5quant
## Precision for the Gaussian observations 100.86 18.11      69.21    99.61
## Precision for ID                          7.30  1.98       4.34     6.99
##                                        0.975quant  mode
## Precision for the Gaussian observations    139.96 97.36
## Precision for ID                            12.02  6.39
##
## Expected number of effective parameters(stdev): 58.87(8.81)
## Number of equivalent replicates : 2.45
##
## Marginal log-Likelihood:  -220.77
```

Figure 3.5 shows the effect of scaling a `rw1` model. The point estimates of the random effects do not seem to change but the posterior marginals of the precision are clearly in different scales. Note that this also means that the linear predictor is not affected by re-scaling and the fitted values will be the same. For the scaled model, the posterior marginal show smaller values than the one obtained with the non-scaled model.

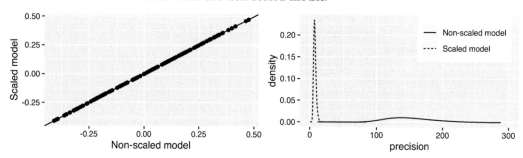

FIGURE 3.5 Non-scaled versus scaled models. Point estimates (i.e., posterior means) of the random effects (left) and posterior marginal of the precision of the random effect (right).

3.5.5   Grouped effects

Random effects can be grouped so that additional group-level correlation can be included using an appropriate latent effect. The variable that sets the group must be passed with parameter `group` and the actual model and other parameters are passed through the `control.group` parameter. This adds a new model to account for between group correlation, i.e., observations are already correlated using the primary random effects but also according to the grouped effect. In practice, the variance structure of the resulting model is the Kronecker product of the main and grouped random effects. This is further discussed in Section 8.6, where spatio-temporal models are discussed.

TABLE 3.12: Summary of options to be set with `control.group` when defining grouped random effects.

Argument	Description
adjust.for.con.comp	Adjust for connected components when the model is scaled (default is TRUE).
cyclic	Make the group model cyclic (only for ar1, rw1 and rw2 models)
graph	Graph specification (for besag model).
hyper	Definition of priors in the hyperparameters.
model	Group model (exchangable, exchangablepos, ar1, ar, rw1, rw2, besag or iid).
order	Order of the model (only available for ar models).
scale.model	Scale the grouped model (default is TRUE; only for rw1, rw2 or besag models).

Table 3.12 shows a summary of the options that can be passed to `control.group`. In general, these are the same that apply to the random effect when it is used.

In the next example we will analyze the air passengers data by using `iid` random effects on the year but correlated random effects using an `ar1` model for the months. This implies that the observations for the same month of consecutive years are correlated. First of all, two integer indices from 1 to 12 are created for the month (particularly important as this is passed to `group`) and year, and then the model is fitted:

```
airp.data$month.num <- as.numeric(airp.data$month)
airp.data$year.num <- as.numeric(airp.data$year)
airp.iid.ar1 <- inla(log(airp) ~ 0 + f(year.num, model = "iid",
    group = month.num, control.group = list(model = "ar1",
    scale.model = TRUE)),
  data = airp.data)
summary(airp.iid.ar1)
```

```
##
## Call:
##    c("inla(formula = log(airp) ~ 0 + f(year.num, model = \"iid\",
##    group = month.num, ", " control.group = list(model = \"ar1\",
##    scale.model = TRUE)), ", " data = airp.data)")
## Time used:
```

```
##       Pre = 0.955, Running = 0.336, Post = 0.0623, Total = 1.35
## Random effects:
##   Name      Model
##     year.num IID model
##
## Model hyperparameters:
##                                            mean        sd 0.025quant
## Precision for the Gaussian observations 2.24e+04 1.99e+04    2413.571
## Precision for year.num                  4.60e-02 1.60e-02       0.022
## GroupRho for year.num                   1.00e+00 0.00e+00       0.999
##                                         0.5quant 0.975quant    mode
## Precision for the Gaussian observations 1.69e+04    7.51e+04 6953.07
## Precision for year.num                  4.40e-02    8.40e-02    0.04
## GroupRho for year.num                   1.00e+00    1.00e+00    1.00
##
## Expected number of effective parameters(stdev): 142.44(1.66)
## Number of equivalent replicates : 1.01
##
## Marginal log-Likelihood:  43.39
```

Figure 3.6 shows the posterior estimates of the grouped random effects. Each plot represents a given month, and the increasing trend is clearly visible. In the model summary this can be appreciated by looking at the high correlation of the grouped effect, which has a posterior mean of 0.9997. Note also how summer months, for example, have higher estimates of the number of passengers.

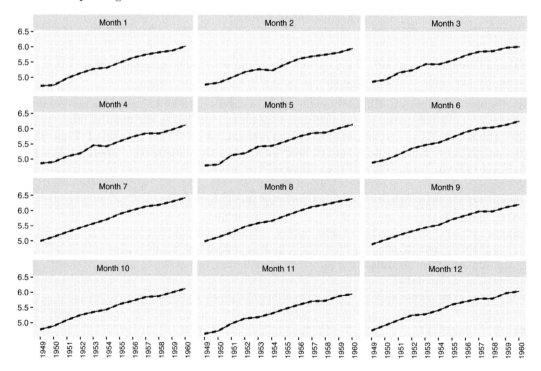

FIGURE 3.6 Grouped effects for the air passengers dataset. Solid lines represent the posterior means and the dashed lines 95% credible intervals.

3.6 Final remarks

In this chapter we have described some of the random effects implemented in the INLA package. However, this list is far from exhaustive. Table 3.13 shows a list of other random effects not discussed in this chapter. As INLA keeps growing, the list of available latent effects is likely to increase too, so the list below may miss some recent developments. Spatial random effects are described in detail in Chapter 7. In general, detailed information about the random effects can be obtained from the manual page that can be accessed with function inla.doc(). This function takes the name of the latent effect to be searched, e.g., inla.doc("ou").

TABLE 3.13: Summary of other random effects not described in this chapter.

Model	Description
ou	Ornstein-Uhlenbeck process.
sigm	Sigmoidal effect of a covariate.
revsigm	Reverse-sigmoidal effect of a covariate.
mec	Classical measurement error model.
meb	Berkson Measurement Error model.
matern2d	Gaussian field with Matérn correlation in a 2D lattice.
rw2d	2-dimensional random walk.
besag	Besag spatial model.
besag2	Weighted spatial effects model.
besagproper	Convolution spatial model.
besagproper2	Convolution spatial model.
bym	Convolution spatial model.
bym2	Reparameterized convolution spatial model.
slm	Spatial lag model.
spde	Spatial model based on Stochastic Partial Differential Equations.
rgeneric	Generic random effect.
fgn	Fractional Gaussian noise.
fgn2	Reparameterized fractional Gaussian noise.
copy	Copy a random effect.
log1exp	Non-linear effect of a positive covariate.
logdist	Non-linear effect of a positive covariate.

4

Multilevel Models

4.1 Introduction

Multilevel models (Goldstein, 2003) tackle the analysis of data that have been collected from experiments with a complex design. For example, multilevel models are typically used to analyze data from the students' performance at different tests. Performance is supposed to depend on a number of variables measured at different levels, such as the student, class, school, etc. Nesting occurs because some students will belong to the same class, several classes will belong to the same school and so on. Although the effect of the class or the school is seldom the primary object of study, its effect should be taken into account as it often has an impact on the students' performance. Hence, class, school, etc. are often modeled using random effects with a complex structure.

A typical problem in multilevel modeling is assessing the variances of the different group effects. For example, is performance among the students in the same class uniform? This can be determined by inspecting the variance estimates of the students' error terms in a linear mixed-effects model. In addition to the grouped or nested random effects, multilevel data may contain values of the covariates (usually introduced as fixed effects in the model) at different levels. For example, in the case of measuring students' performance, socio-economic information about the students is available at the individual level, as well as information about the class (size, course, etc.), school, region, etc. These additional data have also an implicit nested or hierarchical structure in different levels that will be included in the model.

Packages `nlme` (Pinheiro et al., 2018) and `lme4` (Bates et al., 2015) provide functions to fit mixed-effects models with complex structure, as well as numerous datasets and examples. Gelman and Hill (2006) provide an introduction to modeling multilevel data and hierarchical models, and provide a wealth of examples in R. The `multilevel` package (Bliese, 2016) provides a number of datasets with examples and a manual on how to fit multilevel models with R. Faraway (2006) also provides an excellent description of mixed-effects models and provides a good number of examples with R. Some of the examples in this chapter have also been discussed in Faraway (2019b) and Faraway (2019a).

4.2 Multilevel models with random effects

The first example will tackle the analysis of the `penicillin` dataset (Box et al., 1978), which is available in the `faraway` package (Faraway, 2016). This dataset measures the production of penicillin depending on the process for production and the blend used. These variables in the data are described in Table 4.1. The `penicillin` dataset can be loaded and summarized as follows:

```
library("faraway")
data(penicillin)
summary(penicillin)
```

```
## treat      blend        yield
## A:5    Blend1:4    Min.   :77
## B:5    Blend2:4    1st Qu.:81
## C:5    Blend3:4    Median :87
## D:5    Blend4:4    Mean   :86
##        Blend5:4    3rd Qu.:89
##                    Max.   :97
```

TABLE 4.1: Summary of variables in the `penicillin` dataset in the `faraway` package.

Variable	Description
yield	Production of penicillin.
treat	Production type (factor with 4 levels).
blend	Blend used for production (factor with 5 levels).

Figure 4.1 displays the data and shows the effect of the different production methods and blend.

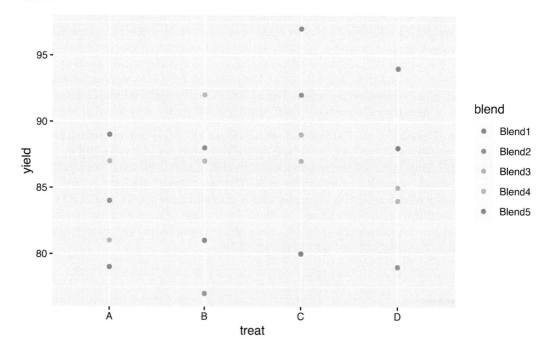

FIGURE 4.1 Penicillin production on production method (`treat`) and blend (`blend`).

In this analysis, the interest is on how the production method (`treat`) affects the production of penicillin. However, production methods use a raw material (corn steep liquor) which is quite variable and may affect the production. Furthermore, this is produced in blends that are only enough for four runs of the production of penicillin. Hence, there is the risk that an observed increment in the production may be due to the actual blend used and not the production method and it is required to account for the blend in the model even if it is not of interest.

Hence, `treat` will be introduced in the model as a fixed effect and `blend` will be introduced in the model as a random effect. Note that the four runs coming from the same blend will share the same value of the random effect. Hence, each observation of production of penicillin can be regarded as being in a level of the model, with each one of the four production types in level 2 of the model.

The model can be written down as:

$$\text{yield}_{ij} = \beta_i \text{treat}_i + u_j + e_{ij}; \; i = 1, \ldots, 4, \; j = 1 \ldots, 5$$

$$u_j \sim N(0, \tau_u); \; j = 1 \ldots, 5$$

Altogether, there are 20 observations. Note that we have not included an intercept in the model because we aim at estimating the different effects of the treatments directly.

Note that the term u_j is sometimes referred to as a *random intercept* as it is a random effect and it is the same for the same level of the `blend` variable, acting similarly as an intercept for the observations in that group alone. Also, the prior on the precision of the random effects τ_u is set to a Gamma distribution with parameters 0.001 and 0.001 as this is a commonly used vague prior. However, see Chapter 5 and, in particular, Gelman (2006) and Gelman and Hill (2006), Chapter 19, for a general discussion on priors for the precisions of the random effects and alternatives to the prior Gamma distribution.

The Gamma prior with parameters 0.001 and 0.001 can be set beforehand and used later in the definition of the latent random effects:

```
# Set prior on precision
prec.prior <- list(prec = list(param = c(0.001, 0.001)))
```

Before the analysis, the reference level of the production type will be set to D so that our results can be compared to those in Faraway (2006):

```
penicillin$treat <- relevel(penicillin$treat, "D")
```

The mixed-effects model can be fit with `INLA` as follows:

```
library("INLA")
inla.pen <- inla(yield ~ 1 + treat + f(blend, model = "iid",
    hyper = prec.prior),
  data = penicillin, control.predictor = list(compute = TRUE))
summary(inla.pen)

##
## Call:
##    c("inla(formula = yield ~ 1 + treat + f(blend, model = \"iid\",
##    hyper = prec.prior), ", " data = penicillin, control.predictor =
```

```
##     list(compute = TRUE))" )
## Time used:
##     Pre = 1.53, Running = 0.168, Post = 0.0728, Total = 1.78
## Fixed effects:
##              mean    sd 0.025quant 0.5quant 0.975quant   mode   kld
## (Intercept) 86.000 2.697     80.652   86.000     91.351 86.000 0.001
## treatA      -1.991 2.940     -7.857   -1.992      3.868 -1.993 0.000
## treatB      -0.996 2.940     -6.862   -0.996      4.863 -0.997 0.000
## treatC       2.987 2.940     -2.884    2.988      8.842  2.990 0.000
##
## Random effects:
##   Name      Model
##     blend IID model
##
## Model hyperparameters:
##
##                                            mean    sd 0.025quant 0.5quant
## Precision for the Gaussian observations 0.062 0.024      0.026    0.058
## Precision for blend                     0.169 0.268      0.012    0.091
##                                          0.975quant  mode
## Precision for the Gaussian observations      0.118 0.052
## Precision for blend                          0.810 0.030
##
## Expected number of effective parameters(stdev): 6.00(1.38)
## Number of equivalent replicates : 3.33
##
## Marginal log-Likelihood:  -83.99
## Posterior marginals for the linear predictor and
##   the fitted values are computed
```

In addition to the summary of the model fit above, Figure 4.2 shows the posterior marginals of the latent effects and hyperparameters in the model.

For comparison purposes, the same model has been fitted with function lmer() from package lme4 using restricted maximum likelihood:

```
library("lme4")
lmer.pen <- lmer(yield ~ 1 + treat + (1|blend), data = penicillin)
summary(lmer.pen)
```

```
## Linear mixed model fit by REML ['lmerMod']
## Formula: yield ~ 1 + treat + (1 | blend)
##    Data: penicillin
##
## REML criterion at convergence: 103.8
##
## Scaled residuals:
##    Min     1Q Median     3Q    Max
## -1.415 -0.502 -0.164  0.683  1.284
##
## Random effects:
##  Groups   Name         Variance Std.Dev.
```

```
## blend      (Intercept) 11.8      3.43
## Residual                18.8      4.34
## Number of obs: 20, groups:  blend, 5
##
## Fixed effects:
##              Estimate Std. Error t value
## (Intercept)     86.00       2.48   34.75
## treatA          -2.00       2.75   -0.73
## treatB          -1.00       2.75   -0.36
## treatC           3.00       2.75    1.09
##
## Correlation of Fixed Effects:
##          (Intr) treatA treatB
## treatA -0.554
## treatB -0.554  0.500
## treatC -0.554  0.500  0.500
```

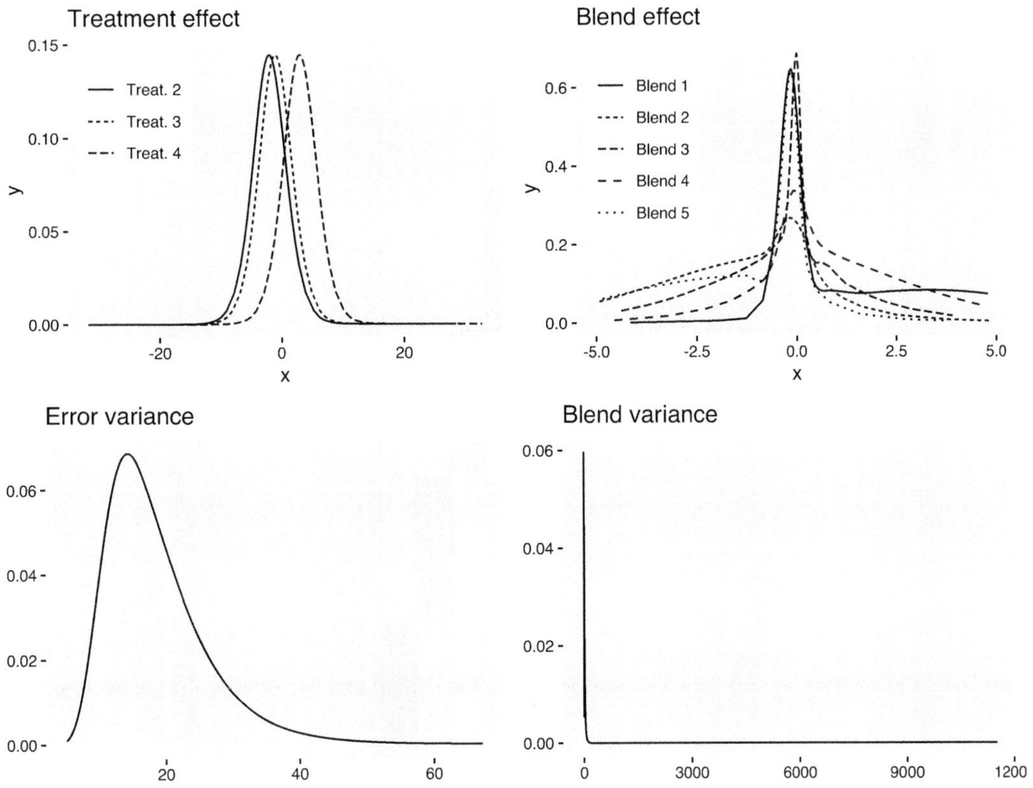

FIGURE 4.2 Marginals of fixed effects of the production method (top-left), blend random-effects (top-right), variance of the error term (bottom-left) and variance of the blend effect (bottom-right).

The main differences lie between the estimates of the variances of the random effects and the error term. As suggested in Faraway (2019b), a more informative prior on the precision of the blend random effects would be required here.

Alternatively, this model can be fit using the latent effect z, which requires a matrix of random effects. Although this is a rather simple model that can be easily fit with the `iid` latent effect, we will develop an example in order to show how the matrix of random effects can be obtained with function `model.matrix()`.

Function `model.matrix()` is usually employed to obtain the design matrix for linear models from a model formula and a dataset. It has the nice feature of expanding factors as dummy variables, which is what is needed to create a design matrix for the random effects. The resulting matrix is likely to be very sparse, so it makes sense to convert it into a `Matrix` (Bates and Maechler, 2019) to obtain a sparse representation.

The creation of the design matrix of the random effects can be as follows:

```
Z <- as(model.matrix(~ 0 + blend, data = penicillin), "Matrix")
```

Figure 4.3 shows the structure of the matrix created. Shaded elements are equal to 1 and all the other elements are zero. Note that this matrix is used to map the group-level random effects in the linear predictor of the observations.

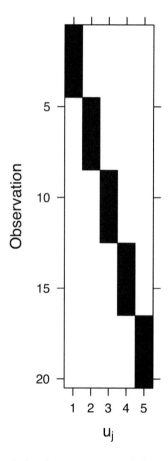

FIGURE 4.3 Representation of the design matrix of the random effects.

Once the matrix has been created, then a new index is needed (for random effect `z`) and the model can be fitted:

```
penicillin$ID <- 1:nrow(penicillin)

inla.pen.z <- inla(yield ~ 1 + treat +  f(ID, model = "z", Z = Z,
  hyper = list(prec = list(param = c(0.001, 0.001)))),
  data = penicillin, control.predictor = list(compute = TRUE))
summary(inla.pen.z)
```

```
##
## Call:
##    c("inla(formula = yield ~ 1 + treat + f(ID, model = \"z\", Z = Z,
##    ", " hyper = list(prec = list(param = c(0.001, 0.001)))), data =
##    penicillin, ", " control.predictor = list(compute = TRUE))")
## Time used:
##      Pre = 1.21, Running = 0.217, Post = 0.0651, Total = 1.49
## Fixed effects:
##                 mean    sd 0.025quant 0.5quant 0.975quant    mode kld
## (Intercept) 86.000 2.709     80.637   86.000     91.365  86.000   0
## treatA      -1.991 2.943     -7.862   -1.992      3.874  -1.993   0
## treatB      -0.996 2.943     -6.867   -0.996      4.868  -0.997   0
## treatC       2.987 2.943     -2.889    2.988      8.846   2.990   0
##
## Random effects:
##    Name       Model
##      ID Z model
##
## Model hyperparameters:
##                                             mean    sd 0.025quant 0.5quant
## Precision for the Gaussian observations 0.062 0.024      0.027    0.059
## Precision for ID                        0.172 0.286      0.011    0.090
##                                         0.975quant  mode
## Precision for the Gaussian observations     0.118 0.052
## Precision for ID                            0.841 0.029
##
## Expected number of effective parameters(stdev): 6.00(1.38)
## Number of equivalent replicates : 3.33
##
## Marginal log-Likelihood:  -83.91
## Posterior marginals for the linear predictor and
##   the fitted values are computed
```

The main difference between the iid and z latent effects is that the first one will produce exactly as many random effects as defined in the model. On the other hand, the z model will produce as many random effects as data, which are the random effects of the groups plus some tiny error. This is defined by the precision parameter when the latent effect is defined using the f() function. See Chapter 3 for details.

When the z model is used, INLA will report summary statistics on the subject-level random effects followed by the group-level random effects. As mentioned above, subject-level random effects are the corresponding group-level random effects plus some tiny noise that is required for model fitting. In this particular case, there are 20 observations, with 5 groups to define the random effects. Hence, the number of rows in inla.pen.z$summary.random$ID is 25.

Figure 4.4 shows the posterior means of the random effects obtained with the iid and the z model. In general, the agreement between the estimates from both models is quite good.

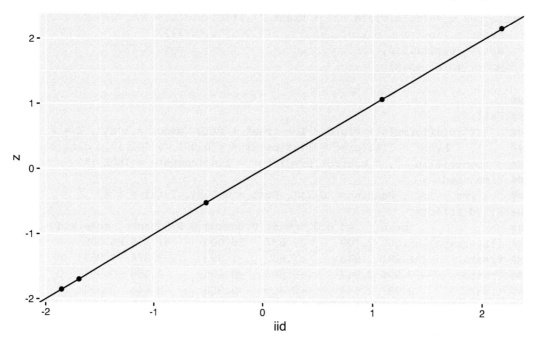

FIGURE 4.4 Multilevel models fitted with iid and z random effects.

4.3 Multilevel models with nested effects

The eggs dataset (Bliss, 1967) in the faraway package contains data on fat content in different samples of egg powder. The analyzes were carried out at different laboratories, by different technicians. Also, each sample was split into two parts that were analyzed separately by the same technician.

A summary of the variables in the dataset is in Table 4.2, which is loaded and summarized as follows:

```
data(eggs)

summary(eggs)
```

```
##       Fat           Lab      Technician Sample
##  Min.   :0.060   I  :8    one:24     G:24
##  1st Qu.:0.307   II :8    two:24     H:24
##  Median :0.370   III:8
##  Mean   :0.388   IV :8
##  3rd Qu.:0.430   V  :8
##  Max.   :0.800   VI :8
```

This is a typical example of *nested* random effects because the technicians are nested within laboratories, so their ids cannot be directly used when defining the random effects as this will consider technician one in laboratory I to be the same as technician one in laboratory II and so on. Hence, using the technician ids directly will make the effect of technician one in lab I to be the same as technician one in lab II, etc. Nesting of the random effects can be taken into account by simply creating a new index variable that accounts for the technician and the laboratory.

TABLE 4.2: Summary of the variables in the eggs dataset.

Variable	Description
Fat	Fat content.
Lab	Laboratory id (a factor from I to VI).
Technician	Technician id (a factor of one or two).
Sample	Sample id (a factor of G or H).

The model to be fitted now is:

$$\text{fat}_{ijkl} = \beta_0 + \text{lab}_i + \text{technician}_{j:i} + \text{sample}_{k:(j:i)} + \varepsilon_{ijkl}, i = 1, \ldots, 6; j = 1, 2; k = 1, 2; l = 1, 2$$

$$\varepsilon_{ijkl} \sim N(0, \tau)$$

$$\text{lab}_i \sim N(0, \tau_{lab}), i = 1, \ldots, 4$$

$$\text{technician}_{j:i} \sim N(0, \tau_{tec}), j : i = 1, \ldots, 12$$

$$\text{sample}_{k:(j:i)} \sim N(0, \tau_{sam}), k : (j : i) = 1, \ldots, 24$$

Indices are defined for laboratory (i), technician (j), samples (k) and half-sample (l). Index $j : i$ denotes that technician is nested within a laboratory and, similarly, index $k : (j : i)$ denotes nesting of samples within technicians (who are themselves nested within laboratories).

Similarly as in the previous example, function `model.matrix()` can be used with a formula that includes the nesting of the variable to create the matrices of the random effects:

```
Zlt <- as(model.matrix( ~ 0 + Lab:Technician, data = eggs), "Matrix")
Zlts <- as(model.matrix( ~ 0 + Lab:Technician:Sample, data = eggs), "Matrix")
```

Figure 4.5 shows the matrices created. Note how the non-zero elements appear in different ways in each matrix. For the nested random effect of the technician, the non-zero elements appear in groups of four, since each technician examined two samples (which were in turn split in two). For the nested random effect on `Sample`, these appear in groups of two as each sample was split in two and analyzed.

Note that now there are two nested random effects. The first one is the technician, which is nested within a laboratory, and the second one is the sample, which is analyzed by different technicians from different laboratories.

Before model fitting, two indices for the nested random effects must be created:

```
# Index for techinician
eggs$IDt <- 1:nrow(eggs)
# Index for technician:sample
eggs$IDts <- 1:nrow(eggs)
```

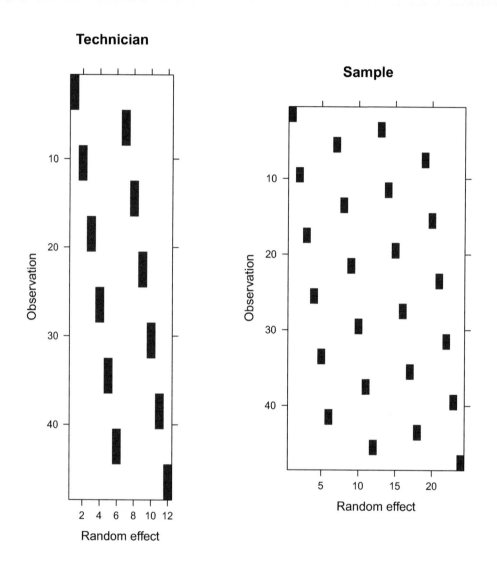

FIGURE 4.5 Representation of the design matrix of the random effects for the `eggs` dataset.

The final model contains a non-nested random effect for the laboratory (which is `iid`) plus the two nested random effects:

```
inla.eggs <- inla(Fat ~ 1 + f(Lab, model = "iid", hyper = prec.prior) +
    f(IDt, model = "z", Z = Z1t, hyper = prec.prior) +
```

```
        f(IDts, model = "z", Z = Zlts, hyper = prec.prior),
    data = eggs, control.predictor = list(compute = TRUE))

  summary(inla.eggs)
```

```
##
## Call:
##    c("inla(formula = Fat ~ 1 + f(Lab, model = \"iid\", hyper =
##    prec.prior) + ", " f(IDt, model = \"z\", Z = Zlt, hyper =
##    prec.prior) + f(IDts, ", " model = \"z\", Z = Zlts, hyper =
##    prec.prior), data = eggs, ", " control.predictor = list(compute =
##    TRUE))")
## Time used:
##     Pre = 1.45, Running = 0.272, Post = 0.0694, Total = 1.79
## Fixed effects:
##               mean    sd 0.025quant 0.5quant 0.975quant  mode kld
## (Intercept) 0.387 0.056      0.275    0.387      0.501 0.387   0
##
## Random effects:
##   Name      Model
##     Lab IID model
##     IDt Z model
##     IDts Z model
##
## Model hyperparameters:
##                                           mean      sd 0.025quant 0.5quant
## Precision for the Gaussian observations 154.23   41.91      86.27   149.63
## Precision for Lab                       364.90  698.40      22.60   173.33
## Precision for IDt                       207.63  213.88      28.15   144.53
## Precision for IDts                      342.48  293.44      60.81   259.96
##                                         0.975quant    mode
## Precision for the Gaussian observations    249.45  140.86
## Precision for Lab                         1890.53   55.77
## Precision for IDt                          769.82   71.97
## Precision for IDts                        1114.35  150.84
##
## Expected number of effective parameters(stdev): 16.84(2.58)
## Number of equivalent replicates : 2.85
##
## Marginal log-Likelihood:  7.70
## Posterior marginals for the linear predictor and
##   the fitted values are computed
```

Alternatively, an index variable can be created from the matrices of the random effects to be used with the iid random effect, as follows:

```
eggs$labtech <- as.factor(apply(Zlt, 1, function(x){names(x)[x == 1]}))
eggs$labtechsamp <- as.factor(apply(Zlts, 1, function(x){names(x)[x == 1]}))
```

Then, the model can be fit as follows:

```
inla.eggs.iid <- inla(Fat ~ 1 + f(Lab, model = "iid", hyper = prec.prior) +
    f(labtech, model = "iid", hyper = prec.prior) +
    f(labtechsamp, model = "iid", hyper = prec.prior),
  data = eggs, control.predictor = list(compute = TRUE))

summary(inla.eggs.iid)
```

```
##
## Call:
##    c("inla(formula = Fat ~ 1 + f(Lab, model = \"iid\", hyper =
##    prec.prior) + ", " f(labtech, model = \"iid\", hyper = prec.prior)
##    + f(labtechsamp, ", " model = \"iid\", hyper = prec.prior), data =
##    eggs, control.predictor = list(compute = TRUE))" )
## Time used:
##     Pre = 1.45, Running = 0.171, Post = 0.0683, Total = 1.69
## Fixed effects:
##              mean    sd 0.025quant 0.5quant 0.975quant  mode kld
## (Intercept) 0.387 0.056      0.275    0.387      0.501 0.388   0
##
## Random effects:
##   Name      Model
##     Lab IID model
##     labtech IID model
##     labtechsamp IID model
##
## Model hyperparameters:
##                                        mean      sd 0.025quant 0.5quant
## Precision for the Gaussian observations 154.18   41.88     86.26   149.59
## Precision for Lab                       364.90  698.40     22.60   173.33
## Precision for labtech                   207.63  213.88     28.15   144.53
## Precision for labtechsamp               342.49  293.44     60.81   259.96
##                                        0.975quant    mode
## Precision for the Gaussian observations    249.34  140.83
## Precision for Lab                         1890.52   55.77
## Precision for labtech                      769.80   71.97
## Precision for labtechsamp                 1114.37  150.84
##
## Expected number of effective parameters(stdev): 16.83(2.58)
## Number of equivalent replicates : 2.85
##
## Marginal log-Likelihood:  7.70
## Posterior marginals for the linear predictor and
##  the fitted values are computed
```

Note how both ways of fitting the model provide very similar estimates. The fact that some estimates of the precision are that high may indicate that these parameters are poorly identified in the model and may require the use of less vague priors.

It is important to mention that some of the estimates of the precisions are quite high and narrow, and it might be better to have a more informative prior on these precisions (Faraway, 2019b).

4.4   Multilevel models with complex structure

Multilevel models have traditionally been associated with education research on measuring students' performance. See, for example, Goldstein (2003) and the references therein. This type of research often creates rich datasets with data available at different levels: student, class, school, etc. Both covariates and a nesting structure are available for the design of mixed-effects models.

Carpenter et al. (2011) describe a multilevel model to analyze the performance of children using literacy and numeracy scores. This is a subset of the original dataset, which is fully described in Blatchford et al. (2002). The study aimed at measuring the effect of class size on children in their first full year of education. For this reason, literacy and numeracy scores are available at school entry and at the end of the first year of school for each student, in addition to the class size. Table 4.3 shows the variables included in this dataset.

TABLE 4.3: Summary of the variables in the analysis of school performance in children (Carpenter et al., 2011).

Variable	Description
clsnr	Class identifier.
pupil	Student identifier.
nlitpost	Standardized literacy score at the end of 1st school year
nmatpost	Standardized numeracy score at the end of 1st school year
nlitpre	Standardized literacy score at school entry
nmatpre	Standardized numeracy score at school entry
csize	Class size (as a factor with four levels)

The following code can be used to load the data into R. Note that the code includes some lines to handle missing values (coded as -9.9990e+029) and label the categories of class size into four groups.

```
#Read data
csize_data <- read.csv (file = "data/class_size_data.txt", header = FALSE,
  sep = "", dec = ".")

#Set names
names(csize_data) <- c("clsnr", "pupil", "nlitpre", "nmatpre", "nlitpost",
  "nmatpost", "csize")

#Set NA's
csize_data [csize_data < -1e+29 ] <- NA

#Set class size levels
csize_data$csize <- as.factor(csize_data$csize)
levels(csize_data$csize) <- c("<=19", "20-24", "25-29", ">=30")

summary(csize_data)
```

```
##        clsnr           pupil          nlitpre         nmatpre
## Min.   :  1     Min.   :   1    Min.   :-3.7    Min.   :-2.89
## 1st Qu.: 84     1st Qu.:1849    1st Qu.:-0.6    1st Qu.:-0.62
## Median :170     Median :3698    Median : 0.0    Median :-0.08
## Mean   :174     Mean   :3698    Mean   : 0.0    Mean   :-0.01
## 3rd Qu.:262     3rd Qu.:5546    3rd Qu.: 0.7    3rd Qu.: 0.68
## Max.   :400     Max.   :7394    Max.   : 3.4    Max.   : 1.88
##                                 NA's   :766     NA's   :302
##      nlitpost        nmatpost         csize
## Min.   :-2.8     Min.   :-3.1    <=19  : 301
## 1st Qu.:-0.7     1st Qu.:-0.7    20-24:1401
## Median : 0.0     Median : 0.0    25-29:3484
## Mean   : 0.0     Mean   : 0.0    >=30 :1520
## 3rd Qu.: 0.6     3rd Qu.: 0.7    NA's : 688
## Max.   : 2.7     Max.   : 2.8
## NA's   :1450     NA's   :1409
```

The dataset contains a number of missing values because the aim of Carpenter et al. (2011) was to deal with missing data in the study and impute them. However, we will consider here children with complete observations only, and focus on the numeracy score only, which is also discussed in the original paper.

Hence, the next step is to keep the rows with full observations in all variables (but `nlitpost`, which will be ignored for now):

```
csize_data2 <- na.omit(csize_data[, -5])
```

Note that this makes the dataset have 5033 rows instead of the original 7394. For now, we will forget about the observations with missing data but this is something that should be taken into account in the analysis at some point (see Chapter 12).

Carpenter et al. (2011) are interested in modeling the literacy and numeracy scores at the end of the first year of school on other variables, with particular interest in school size. Note that all the other variables have been measured at the student level and this makes this dataset multilevel. Note that now students are nested within classes. Furthermore, for this initial analysis the response variable will be `nmatpost`.

Following Carpenter et al. (2011), the multilevel model fitted now is:

$$\text{nmatpost}_{ij} = \beta_{0ij} + \beta_1 \text{nmatpre}_{ij} + \beta_2 \text{nlitpre}_{ij} + \beta_3 \text{csize}_{ij}^{20\text{-}24} + \beta_4 \text{csize}_{ij}^{25\text{-}29} + \beta_5 \text{csize}_{ij}^{\geq 30}$$

$$\beta_{0ij} = \beta_0 + u_j + \varepsilon_{ij}$$

$$u_j \sim N(0, \tau_u); \ \varepsilon_{ij} \sim N(0, \tau); i = 1, \dots, n_j; \ j = 1, \dots, n_c$$

Here, β_{0ij} represents a random term on the student, which comprises an overall intercept β_0, a class random effect u_j and a student random effect ε_{ij} (which is in fact modeled by the error of the Gaussian likelihood). Variable $\text{csize}_{ij}^{20\text{-}24}$ is a dummy variable that is 1 if the class size is "20-24" and 0 otherwise. $\text{csize}_{ij}^{25\text{-}29}$ and $\text{csize}_{ij}^{\geq 30}$ are defined analogously. The total number of classes is denoted by n_c and the number of students in class j by n_j.

The model can be summarized as students being in level 1 in the model, with student level numeracy and literacy scores and an associated error (or random effect) ε_{ij}. The next layer in the model, level 2, is about the class, for which covariate class size and a class-level random effect u_j is included. This multilevel model can be easily fitted with INLA:

```
inla.csize <- inla(nmatpost ~ 1 + nmatpre + nlitpre + csize +
  f(clsnr, model = "iid"), data = csize_data2)

summary(inla.csize)
```

```
##
## Call:
##    c("inla(formula = nmatpost ~ 1 + nmatpre + nlitpre + csize +
##    f(clsnr, ", " model = \"iid\"), data = csize_data2)")
## Time used:
##     Pre = 1.27, Running = 1.98, Post = 0.0744, Total = 3.32
## Fixed effects:
##                mean    sd 0.025quant 0.5quant 0.975quant    mode kld
## (Intercept)   0.270 0.141     -0.008    0.270      0.547   0.270   0
## nmatpre       0.367 0.015      0.337    0.367      0.397   0.367   0
## nlitpre       0.372 0.015      0.343    0.372      0.402   0.372   0
## csize20-24   -0.114 0.157     -0.422   -0.114      0.193  -0.115   0
## csize25-29   -0.319 0.149     -0.611   -0.319     -0.026  -0.319   0
## csize>=30    -0.340 0.160     -0.654   -0.340     -0.026  -0.340   0
##
## Random effects:
##   Name       Model
##     clsnr IID model
##
## Model hyperparameters:
##                                          mean    sd 0.025quant 0.5quant
## Precision for the Gaussian observations  2.67 0.055       2.56     2.67
## Precision for clsnr                      4.01 0.395       3.29     4.00
##                                         0.975quant mode
## Precision for the Gaussian observations       2.78 2.67
## Precision for clsnr                           4.84 3.97
##
## Expected number of effective parameters(stdev): 232.33(2.03)
## Number of equivalent replicates : 21.66
##
## Marginal log-Likelihood:  -5051.98
```

Point estimates of the model are very similar to those obtained using restricted maximum likelihood as reported in Carpenter et al. (2011).

Regarding the effect of class size on the numeracy score at the end of the first school year, it seems that this is reduced with the increase of the class size. Furthermore, variation between students is larger than between classes.

4.5   Multilevel models for longitudinal data

Belenky et al. (2003) describe a study of reaction time in patients under sleep deprivation up to 10 days. This dataset is available in package lme4 as dataset sleepstudy. See also Jovanovic (2015) for an analysis of this dataset with R using different methods.

TABLE 4.4: Summary of variables in the sleepstudy dataset in package lme4.

Variable	Description
Reaction	Average reaction time (in ms).
Days	Number of days in sleep deprivation.
Subject	Subject id in the study.

Table 4.4 shows the variables in the dataset, which can be loaded as follows:

```
library("lme4")
data(sleepstudy)
```

Reaction time will be rescaled by dividing by 1000 to have the reaction time in seconds as this makes estimation with INLA more stable:

```
#Scale Reaction
sleepstudy$Reaction <- sleepstudy$Reaction / 1000
```

Then, the resulting dataset can be summarized as:

```
summary(sleepstudy)
```

```
##     Reaction            Days         Subject
##  Min.   :0.194    Min.   :0.0    308    : 10
##  1st Qu.:0.255    1st Qu.:2.0    309    : 10
##  Median :0.289    Median :4.5    310    : 10
##  Mean   :0.298    Mean   :4.5    330    : 10
##  3rd Qu.:0.337    3rd Qu.:7.0    331    : 10
##  Max.   :0.466    Max.   :9.0    332    : 10
##                                  (Other):120
```

The analysis of this dataset is interesting because time deprivation seems to affect subjects' reaction time differently. This effect is shown in Figure 4.6. Hence, this is an interesting dataset for a longitudinal model.

In order to fit a reasonable model to the data we need to allow for different slopes for variable Days for different subjects in the study. This is often achieved by including a *random coefficient* in the model. This means that each subject will have an associated random effect that multiplies the value of the covariate and that will produce a different linear trend for each patient.

First of all, a mixed effects model with a fixed effect on Days and a random effect on Subject is fit. This model assumes the same slope of the effect of Days on the students.

```
inla.sleep <- inla(Reaction ~ 1 + Days + f(Subject, model = "iid"),
  data = sleepstudy)
```

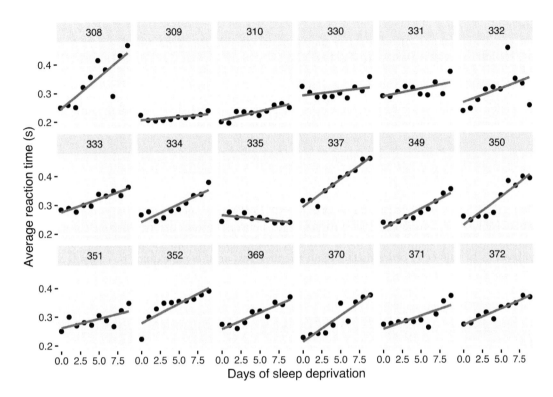

FIGURE 4.6 Effect of time (in days) of sleep deprivation on reaction time from the 'sleepstudy' dataset.

```
summary(inla.sleep)
```

```
##
## Call:
##    c("inla(formula = Reaction ~ 1 + Days + f(Subject, model =
##    \"iid\"), ", " data = sleepstudy)")
## Time used:
##    Pre = 1.05, Running = 0.179, Post = 0.0609, Total = 1.29
## Fixed effects:
##               mean    sd 0.025quant 0.5quant 0.975quant  mode kld
## (Intercept) 0.251 0.010      0.232    0.251      0.271 0.251   0
## Days        0.010 0.001      0.009    0.010      0.012 0.010   0
##
## Random effects:
##    Name      Model
##      Subject IID model
```

```
##
## Model hyperparameters:
##                                           mean      sd 0.025quant 0.5quant
## Precision for the Gaussian observations 1059.17 118.23     842.29  1054.03
## Precision for Subject                    833.27 296.04     383.51   791.37
##                                          0.975quant    mode
## Precision for the Gaussian observations    1306.94 1045.36
## Precision for Subject                      1532.04  709.98
##
## Expected number of effective parameters(stdev): 18.79(0.497)
## Number of equivalent replicates : 9.58
##
## Marginal log-Likelihood:  324.28
```

A model with subject-level random slopes on Days can be fitted by including a second term when defining the random effect with the values of the covariates:

```
inla.sleep.w <- inla(Reaction ~ 1 + f(Subject, Days, model = "iid"),
  data = sleepstudy, control.predictor = list(compute = TRUE))
```

Note that term f(Subject, Days, model = "iid") now includes two arguments before model. The first one defines the groups (and, hence, the number of random slopes) and the second one is the value of the covariate (which is, in principle, slightly different among subjects). In this case, order matters and the first two arguments cannot be exchanged. The summary of the model is:

```
summary(inla.sleep.w)
```

```
##
## Call:
##    c("inla(formula = Reaction ~ 1 + f(Subject, Days, model =
##    \"iid\"), ", " data = sleepstudy, control.predictor = list(compute
##    = TRUE))" )
## Time used:
##     Pre = 1.05, Running = 0.33, Post = 0.0664, Total = 1.45
## Fixed effects:
##               mean    sd 0.025quant 0.5quant 0.975quant  mode kld
## (Intercept) 0.255 0.004      0.247    0.255      0.263 0.255   0
##
## Random effects:
##   Name       Model
##     Subject IID model
##
## Model hyperparameters:
##                                           mean      sd 0.025quant
## Precision for the Gaussian observations 1205.63  135.09     957.89
## Precision for Subject                   7257.75 2440.40    3475.48
##                                          0.5quant 0.975quant    mode
## Precision for the Gaussian observations  1199.73    1488.80 1189.78
## Precision for Subject                    6936.32   12965.01 6306.55
```

```
##
## Expected number of effective parameters(stdev): 19.76(0.236)
## Number of equivalent replicates : 9.11
##
## Marginal log-Likelihood:  336.14
## Posterior marginals for the linear predictor and
##  the fitted values are computed
```

Figure 4.7 shows the posterior means of the intercept and random effect (slope) of the fit line on the data using the random slope model (black line) and a line obtained by fitting a linear regression to the data of each subject (in blue).

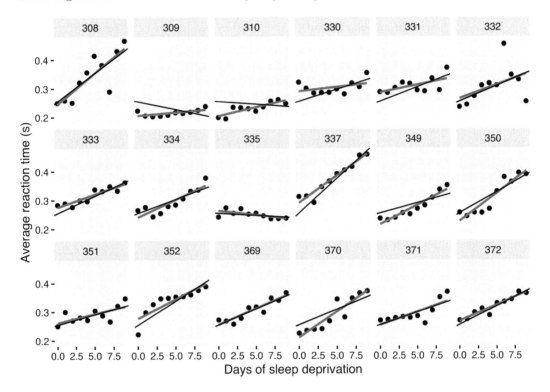

FIGURE 4.7 Posterior mean of fit line using model with a random slope. The blue line represents a fit line using linear regression and the black line represents the line with the posterior mean of the slope and group effect.

4.6 Multilevel models for binary data

The multilevel models presented in previous sections can be extended to the case of non-Gaussian responses. For the case of binary data, a logistic regression can be proposed with fixed and random effects to account for different levels of variation in the data.

As an example, we will consider data from a survey for the 1988 election in the United States of America. These data have been analyzed in Gelman and Hill (2006) and it is available from Prof. Gelman's website (see Preface for details). Note that there are no observations from two states (Alaska and Hawaii) and hence the actual number of states in the data is 49 instead of 51.

This is a subset of a dataset comprising different polls on the 1988 presidential elections in the United States of America and only the latest survey conducted by CBS News will be considered. In this election, the Republican candidate was George H. W. Bush and the Democrat candidate was Michael Dukakis. The variables in this dataset are summarized in Table 4.5.

TABLE 4.5: Summary of the variables in the dataset on the 1988 US presidential election poll.

Variable	Description
org	Organization that conducted the survey.
year	Year of survey.
survey	Survey id.
bush	Respondent will vote for Bush (1 = yes, 0 = no).
state	State id of respondent (including D.C.).
edu	Education level of respondent.
age	Age category of respondent.
female	Respondent is female.
black	Respondent is black.
weight	Survey weight.

The dataset can be loaded as follows:

```
election88 <- read.table(file = "data/polls.subset.dat")
```

Gelman and Little (1997) give more details about the categories of variables `age` and `edu` in the dataset and these are used to label the different levels:

```
election88$age <- as.factor(election88$age)
levels(election88$age) <- c("18-29", "30-44", "45-64", "65+")

election88$edu <- as.factor(election88$edu)
levels(election88$edu) <- c("not.high.school.grad", "high.school.grad",
  "some.college", "college.grad")
```

The analysis in Gelman and Hill (2006) also includes a region indicator for each state. The region indicator has been obtained from the files in Prof. Gelman's website and will be added as a new `region` column to the original dataset:

```
# Add region
election88$region <- c(3, 4, 4, 3, 4, 4, 1, 1, 5, 3, 3, 4, 4, 2, 2, 2, 2,
  3, 3, 1, 1, 1, 2, 2, 3, 2, 4, 2, 4, 1, 1, 4, 1, 3, 2, 2, 3, 4, 1, 1, 3,
  2, 3, 3, 4, 1, 3, 4, 1, 2, 4)[as.numeric(election88$state)]
```

Gelman and Hill (2006) propose a number of models to analyze this dataset. This is a multilevel dataset because respondents are nested within states, which in turn are nested within regions. In addition, we have individual covariates as well as the indicator of the state, which could be used to include random effects in the model. Here, respondents will be in level one of the model, with state being the second level of the model. Region could be considered a third level of the model.

Hence, a simple approach would be to model the probability of voting for Bush π_{ij} of respondent i in state j on gender, race and state (included as a random effect) using a logit link function, as follows:

$$\text{logit}(\pi_{ij}) = \beta_0 + \beta_1 \text{female}_{ij} + \beta_2 \text{black}_{ij} + \beta_3 \text{age}_{ij}^{30-44} + \beta_4 \text{age}_{ij}^{45-64} + \beta_5 \text{age}_{ij}^{65+} +$$

$$\beta_6 \text{edu}_{ij}^{high.school.grad} + \beta_7 \text{edu}_{ij}^{some.college} + \beta_8 \text{edu}_{ij}^{college.grad} + u_j; \ i = 1, \ldots, n_j; \ j = 1, \ldots, 51$$

$$u_j \sim N(0, \tau_u); \ j = 1, \ldots, 51$$

Note that n_j represents the number of respondents in state j. Although state j is indexed from 1 to 51 there are no data for two states that are ignored in the analysis for simplicity. Hence, the number of states considered in the model is actually 49.

This model can be easily fitted to this dataset as follows:

```
inla.elec88 <- inla(bush ~ 1 + female + black + age + edu +
    f(state, model = "iid"),
  data = election88, family = "binomial",
  control.predictor = list(link = 1))

summary(inla.elec88)
```

```
##
## Call:
##    c("inla(formula = bush ~ 1 + female + black + age + edu + f(state,
##    ", " model = \"iid\"), family = \"binomial\", data = election88,
##    control.predictor = list(link = 1))" )
## Time used:
##     Pre = 1.5, Running = 0.857, Post = 0.338, Total = 2.69
## Fixed effects:
##                      mean    sd 0.025quant 0.5quant 0.975quant   mode kld
## (Intercept)         0.312 0.192     -0.064    0.312      0.690  0.312   0
## female             -0.096 0.095     -0.284   -0.096      0.090 -0.096   0
## black              -1.740 0.210     -2.163   -1.736     -1.340 -1.728   0
## age30-44           -0.292 0.123     -0.534   -0.292     -0.052 -0.292   0
## age45-64           -0.066 0.136     -0.334   -0.065      0.202 -0.065   0
## age65+             -0.224 0.160     -0.539   -0.224      0.090 -0.225   0
## eduhigh.school.grad 0.230 0.164     -0.092    0.230      0.553  0.230   0
## edusome.college     0.514 0.178      0.165    0.513      0.863  0.513   0
## educollege.grad     0.313 0.173     -0.027    0.312      0.653  0.312   0
##
## Random effects:
##   Name       Model
##      state IID model
```

```
##
## Model hyperparameters:
##                       mean   sd 0.025quant 0.5quant 0.975quant mode
## Precision for state 7.78 4.26       3.02     6.74      18.91 5.39
##
## Expected number of effective parameters(stdev): 31.04(4.34)
## Number of equivalent replicates : 64.91
##
## Marginal log-Likelihood:  -1374.72
## Posterior marginals for the linear predictor and
##  the fitted values are computed
```

In the previous code, `control.predictor = list(link = 1)` is required to set the right link (i.e., the logit function) to have the fitted values in the appropriate scale (i.e., the expit of the linear predictor).

The results show a clear trend regarding black voters preferring Dukakis, as well as voters in the range of age 30-44. Regarding education, only the group of voters with `some.college` show a significant preference for Bush as compared to the reference group.

Figure 4.8 shows the posterior means and 95% credible intervals of the state-level random effects. Only a few states show a significant effect, with Tennessee supporting Bush and New York supporting Dukakis. The poll used in the analysis did not include any responses from Alaska or Hawaii so results are not reported for these states.

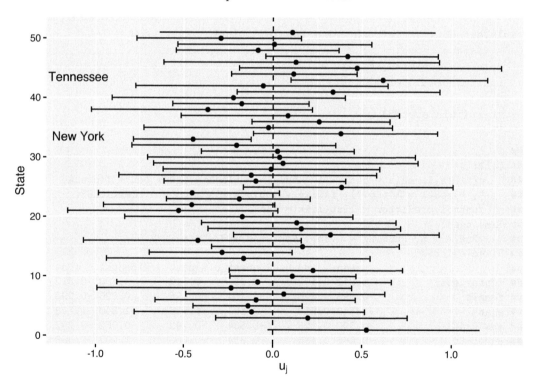

FIGURE 4.8 Posterior means and 95% credible intervals of the random effects of the US States.

Furthermore, Figure 4.9 shows a map of the point estimates of the state-level random effects, which has been created with packages `sf` (Pebesma, 2018) and `USAboundaries` (Mullen and Bratt, 2018).

State effect

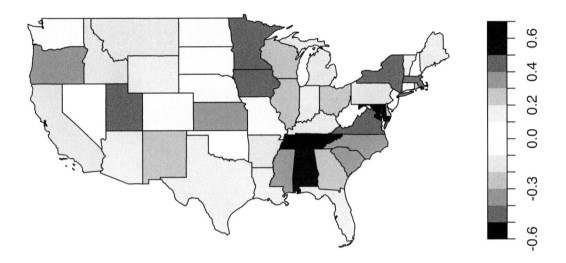

FIGURE 4.9 Point estimates of state-level random effect.

The map shows an interesting pattern. First of all, the values of the point estimates change smoothly from one state to its neighbors, which may lead us to think that there is some residual spatial variation not explained by the model. For example, several states in the south-east part have positive posterior means of the random effect, which increases the probability of voting for Bush. On the other hand, states on the west coast have a negative point estimate, which makes them have a lower probability of voting for Bush.

4.7 Multilevel models for count data

The next example will discuss the "stop-and-frisk" dataset analyzed in Gelman and Little (1997), Gelman and Hill (2006) and Gelman et al. (2007). This dataset records the number of stops between January 1998 and March 1999 and was used as part of a study to assess whether members of ethnic minorities (in particular, blacks and latinos) were more likely to be stopped by the New York City (NYC) police. Data being analyzed here have been obtained from Prof. Andrew Gelman's website (see Preface for details), who added some noise to the original data.

Table 4.6 shows the variables in the dataset. The number of stops, population and number of arrests in 1997 (as recorded by the Division of Criminal Justice Services, DCJS) is stratified by precinct, ethnicity and type of crime. The dataset contains data for 75 precincts, which excluded precinct 22 as this covers the Central Park area and it has no population.

Note that precincts are identified by an index from 1 to 75 and not by their actual NYC precinct number. Furthermore, only three ethnic groups were considered (white, black and latino) because other ethnic groups covered a small percentage of the stops (about 4%) and ambiguities in the classification (Gelman and Hill, 2006).

TABLE 4.6: Summary of variables in the NYC police stop and frisk dataset.

Variable	Description
stops	Number of stops between January 1998 and March 1999.
pop	Population.
past.arrests	Number of arrests within New York City in 1997.
precinct	Number of precinct (from 1 to 75)
eth	Ethnicity (black, hispanic or white)
crime	Crime type (violent, weapons, property or drug).

Data can be loaded as follows:

```
nyc.stops <- read.table(file = "data/frisk_with_noise.dat", skip = 6,
  header = TRUE)

# Add labels to factors
nyc.stops$eth <- as.factor(nyc.stops$eth)
levels(nyc.stops$eth) <- c("black", "hispanic", "white")
nyc.stops$eth <- relevel(nyc.stops$eth, "white")

nyc.stops$crime <- as.factor(nyc.stops$crime)
levels(nyc.stops$crime) <- c("violent", "weapons", "property", "drug")
```

Note that in the previous code labels have been assigned to factor variables eth and crime. Furthermore, white has been set as the baseline level for variable eth so that this will become the reference level when fitting models to assess any effect of the ethnicity of stops.

Given that we are not interested in crime type, the next step is to aggregate the data by precinct and ethnicity:

```
nyc.stops.agg <- aggregate(cbind(stops, past.arrests, pop) ~ precinct + eth,
  data = nyc.stops, sum)

# Population is summed 4 times
nyc.stops.agg$pop <- nyc.stops.agg$pop / 4
```

Note that now the aggregated population per precinct has been divided by 4 in the aggregated dataset because it is added up 4 times.

In this analysis, the focus is on the ethnicity effect to determine whether individuals from ethnic minorities (i.e., black and hispanic) are more likely to be stopped by the NYC police. For this reason, this effect will be included as a fixed effect in the model. Furthermore, precinct will be included as a random effect as we expect variation between precincts as well. Hence, the resulting model is:

$$\text{stops}_{ep} \sim Po(E_{ep}\theta_{ep})$$

$$\log(\theta_{ep}) = \beta_0 + \beta_1 \text{eth}_{ep}^{\text{black}} + \beta_2 \text{eth}_{ep}^{\text{hispanic}} + u_p$$

$$u_p \sim N(0, \tau_u), i = 1, \ldots, 75$$

Here, E_{ep} will be taken as a reference (e.g., expected) number of stops considering the number of stops in 1997 multiplied by 15/12 because the number of stops is recorded over a period of 15 months (January 1998 to March 1999). Furthermore, this must be introduced as an offset in the log-scale in the model.

Then, the model can be fit as:

```
nyc.inla <- inla(stops ~ eth + f(precinct, model = "iid"),
   data = nyc.stops.agg, offset = log((15 / 12) * past.arrests),
   family = "poisson")

summary(nyc.inla)
```

```
##
## Call:
##    c("inla(formula = stops ~ eth + f(precinct, model = \"iid\"),
##    family = \"poisson\", ", " data = nyc.stops.agg, offset =
##    log((15/12) * past.arrests))" )
## Time used:
##    Pre = 1.11, Running = 0.141, Post = 0.0607, Total = 1.31
## Fixed effects:
##               mean    sd 0.025quant 0.5quant 0.975quant    mode kld
## (Intercept) -1.088 0.071    -1.227   -1.087    -0.949  -1.087   0
## ethblack     0.418 0.009     0.400    0.418     0.437   0.418   0
## ethhispanic  0.429 0.010     0.410    0.429     0.448   0.429   0
##
## Random effects:
##   Name      Model
##     precinct IID model
##
## Model hyperparameters:
##                      mean    sd 0.025quant 0.5quant 0.975quant mode
## Precision for precinct 2.77 0.451      1.96     2.75       3.73 2.70
##
## Expected number of effective parameters(stdev): 77.21(0.028)
## Number of equivalent replicates : 2.91
##
## Marginal log-Likelihood:  -2864.03
```

Gelman and Hill (2006) and Gelman et al. (2007) also propose a model which includes an ethnicity-precinct noise term, which is included as a random effect and has the interpretation of adding an error term to the linear predictor. Fitting this model requires a new index for each ethnicity-precinct, with different values for each row, and the model is fitted as follows:

```
# Ethnicity precinct index
nyc.stops.agg$ID <- 1:nrow(nyc.stops.agg)
nyc.inla2 <- inla(stops ~ eth + f(precinct, model = "iid") +
    f(ID, model = "iid"),
  data = nyc.stops.agg, offset = log((15/12) * past.arrests),
  family = "poisson")

summary(nyc.inla2)
```

```
##
## Call:
##    c("inla(formula = stops ~ eth + f(precinct, model = \"iid\") +
##    f(ID, ", " model = \"iid\"), family = \"poisson\", data =
##    nyc.stops.agg, ", " offset = log((15/12) * past.arrests))")
## Time used:
##     Pre = 1.32, Running = 0.276, Post = 0.068, Total = 1.66
## Fixed effects:
##                  mean    sd 0.025quant 0.5quant 0.975quant    mode kld
## (Intercept) -1.214 0.079     -1.369   -1.214     -1.059 -1.214   0
## ethblack      0.497 0.050      0.399    0.497      0.596  0.497   0
## ethhispanic  0.516 0.050      0.417    0.516      0.615  0.516   0
##
## Random effects:
##    Name      Model
##      precinct IID model
##      ID IID model
##
## Model hyperparameters:
##                            mean      sd 0.025quant 0.5quant 0.975quant  mode
## Precision for precinct  2.82 0.498       1.94     2.79       3.89  2.73
## Precision for ID        11.87 1.539       9.06    11.80      15.10 11.70
##
## Expected number of effective parameters(stdev): 213.93(1.10)
## Number of equivalent replicates : 1.05
##
## Marginal log-Likelihood:  -1477.92
```

In both models ethnic minority groups show a clear effect to be stopped more often than white people. Regarding the precinct-level effect, posterior means and 95% credible intervals for each precinct are shown in Figure 4.10. It is clear that some precincts have a number of stops that are higher than the average in 1997 and considering ethnicity.

These results can nicely be plotted in a map using the precinct boundaries provided in the web of the City of New York (see Preface for details). Precinct 121, which was not in 1999, has been merged together with Precinct 122, but this provides slightly different results from the current boundaries of precincts 120 and 122 in Staten Islands, but this is enough for our purpose. Note that Precinct 22 in Central Park has been excluded, so that the map ends with the 75 precincts discussed in the analysis in Gelman and Hill (2006) and Gelman et al. (2007).

Furthermore, precincts in the original dataset have been matched to the NYC precinct number by using the proportion of ethnic groups in each precinct as precinct ids in the original data ranged from 1 to 75. These precinct-level data have been obtained from the original "stop-and-frisk" report (New York Attorney General, 1999). This way, we have been able to match each precinct in the original dataset to its actual NYC precinct number. It turned out that precincts in the "stop-and-frisk" dataset were already ordered by NYC precinct number (after excluding Precinct 22 and merging Precincts 121 and 122).

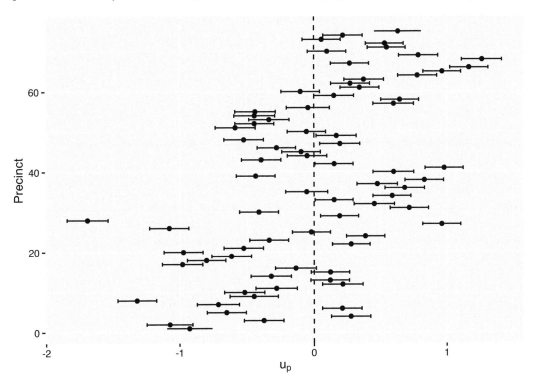

FIGURE 4.10 Posterior means and 95% credible intervals of the random effects of the 75 NYC precincts.

The next lines of code will load the precinct-level data available as Table I.A.1 in the report New York Attorney General (1999) that records NYC police stop rates by precinct from January 1998 to March 1999:

```
# Load precinct data
precinct99 <- read.csv2(file = "data/precinct_data_98-99.csv")
rownames(precinct99) <- precinct99$Precinct

# Order by precinct number
precinct99 <- precinct99[order(precinct99$Precinct), ]

# Remove Central Park
precinct99 <- subset(precinct99, Precinct != 22)
```

Next, a shapefile with the boundaries of the 75 precincts is loaded using function `readOGR()` from package rgdal (Bivand et al., 2019):

```
# Test to check boundaries of precincts
library("rgdal")
nyc.precincts <- readOGR("data/Police_Precincts", "nyc_precincts")
```

The shapefile includes the precinct number in a column. We will assign it as the polygon id in order to merge the `SpatialPolygons` object to our data:

```
# Set IDs to polygons
for(i in 1:length(nyc.precincts)) {
  slot(slot(nyc.precincts, "polygons")[[i]], "ID") <-
    as.character(nyc.precincts$precinct[i])
}
```

Finally, a `SpatialPolygonsDataFrame` is created by merging the precinct boundaries to the `precinct99` data:

```
#Merge boundaries and 1999 data
nyc.precincts99 <- SpatialPolygonsDataFrame(nyc.precincts, precinct99)
```

Then, point estimates of the precinct random effect (e.g., posterior means) can be added to the map in a simple way:

```
# Add r. eff. estimates
nyc.precincts99$u <- nyc.inla$summary.random$precinct$mean
```

Note that this is only possible because the order of the precincts is the same in the `SpatialPolygonsDataFrame` and our fit model. Figure 4.11 shows the point estimates of the random effects for the precincts.

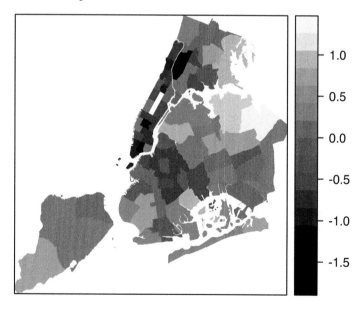

FIGURE 4.11 Point estimates of the random effects of the 75 precincts of NYC in 1999.

5

Priors in R-INLA

5.1 Introduction

Priors play an important role in Bayesian analysis and their definition should be considered very carefully. In this chapter prior definition in `INLA` is described in more detail. If no prior distribution on a given parameter is set, a default one will be used. Hence, it is important to know what the default priors are, as well as other possible alternatives.

`INLA` provides different ways to define the prior of the hyperparameters, and all of them are covered in this chapter. First of all, there is a list of implemented priors available that can be used in the models straight away. These are described in Section 5.2. New priors can easily be implemented as well, as described in Section 5.3. The new Penalized Complexity priors, or PC-priors, are introduced in Section 5.4. Given that `INLA` can fit Bayesian models very fast, sensitivity analysis on the priors can be done, as seen in Section 5.5. Finally, scaling of the latent random effects and prior definition is tackled in Section 5.6.

5.2 Selection of priors

The first thing to know about setting priors in `INLA` is that priors are set in the internal representation of the parameter, which may be different from the scale of the parameter in the model. For example, precisions are represented in the internal scale in the log-scale. This is computationally convenient because in the internal scale the parameter is not bounded. For example, the posterior mode of the hyperparameters can be obtained by maximizing the sum of the log-likelihood and the log-prior on the hyperparameters. This optimization step is used by `INLA` at the beginning of the model fitting to locate the posterior mode of the hyperparameters and find the region of high posterior density.

Note that the internal representation of the hyperparameters is described in the documentation of the `INLA` package corresponding to the relevant likelihood or latent effect. Table 5.3 below summarizes the different internal representations for different hyperparameters.

In order to use one of the prior distributions implemented in `INLA` it is necessary to set them explicitly. Priors on the hyperparameters of the likelihood must be passed by defining argument `hyper` within `control.family` in the call to INLA. Priors on the hyperparameters of the latent effects are set using the parameter `hyper`, inside the `f()` function.

Parameter `hyper` is a named list so that each element in the list defines the prior for a different hyperparameter. The names used in the list can be the names of the parameters or those used for the internal representation. These can be checked in the documentation or using function `inla.models()`, as described in Section 2.3.2. The next example focuses on the `iid` latent effect, which only has the precision hyperparameter, and shows the name in the internal representation (`"theta"`), the name of the parameter (`"log precision"`) and a short name (`"prec"`):

```
names(inla.models()$latent$iid$hyper)
```

```
## [1] "theta"
```

```
inla.models()$latent$iid$hyper$theta$name
```

```
## [1] "log precision"
## attr(,"inla.read.only")
## [1] FALSE
```

```
inla.models()$latent$iid$hyper$theta$short.name
```

```
## [1] "prec"
## attr(,"inla.read.only")
## [1] FALSE
```

Note that in order to define a prior, both the name of the internal parameter `theta` and the short name `prec` can be used in the named list passed to `hyper`. However, regardless of the name used, the prior is always set in the scale of the internal parameter, i.e., if the prior is set using `prec` it must be a prior on the log-precision.

Full details about the default prior can also be found with

```
inla.models()$latent$iid$hyper$theta
```

```
## $hyperid
## [1] 1001
## attr(,"inla.read.only")
## [1] FALSE
##
## $name
## [1] "log precision"
## attr(,"inla.read.only")
## [1] FALSE
##
## $short.name
## [1] "prec"
## attr(,"inla.read.only")
## [1] FALSE
##
## $prior
## [1] "loggamma"
## attr(,"inla.read.only")
## [1] FALSE
##
## $param
```

```
## [1] 1e+00 5e-05
## attr(,"inla.read.only")
## [1] FALSE
##
## $initial
## [1] 4
## attr(,"inla.read.only")
## [1] FALSE
##
## $fixed
## [1] FALSE
## attr(,"inla.read.only")
## [1] FALSE
##
## $to.theta
## function (x)
## log(x)
## <bytecode: 0x7ffda686e318>
## <environment: 0x7ffda6878350>
## attr(,"inla.read.only")
## [1] TRUE
##
## $from.theta
## function (x)
## exp(x)
## <bytecode: 0x7ffda686e200>
## <environment: 0x7ffda6878350>
## attr(,"inla.read.only")
## [1] TRUE
```

TABLE 5.1: Summary of arguments passed in `hyper` to set a prior in INLA.

Argument	Description
prior	Name of the prior distribution.
param	Values of the parameters of the prior.
initial	Initial value of the hyperparameter.
fixed	Whether to keep the value fixed to `initial`.

This output is better understood by looking at Table 5.1, which describes the different options to set a prior by passing a number of elements via the `hyper` argument. For example, to define a Gamma prior on the precision of a `iid` model with parameters 0.01 and 0.01, these settings can be used:

```
prec.prior <- list(prec = list(prior = "loggamma", param = c(0.01, 0.01)),
  initial = 4, fixed = FALSE)
```

Note that in the previous definition `initial` and `fixed` are set to their default values (as seen in the code above) and that, in fact, they do not need to be defined here. Value `initial` refers to the initial value of the hyperparameter and `fixed` refers to whether the hyperparameter is fixed to its initial value, in which case it is not estimated (and the prior distribution is ignored).

Then, `prec.prior` can be passed to `hyper` as follows in the definition of the latent effect to define the model formula:

```
f <- y ~ 1 + f(idx, model = "iid", hyper = prec.prior)
```

The list of different priors implemented in INLA can be obtained as:

```
names(inla.models()$prior)
```

```
##  [1] "normal"               "gaussian"
##  [3] "wishart1d"            "wishart2d"
##  [5] "wishart3d"            "wishart4d"
##  [7] "wishart5d"            "loggamma"
##  [9] "gamma"                "minuslogsqrttruncnormal"
## [11] "logtnormal"           "logtgaussian"
## [13] "flat"                 "logflat"
## [15] "logiflat"             "mvnorm"
## [17] "pc.alphaw"            "pc.ar"
## [19] "dirichlet"            "none"
## [21] "invalid"              "betacorrelation"
## [23] "logitbeta"            "pc.prec"
## [25] "pc.dof"               "pc.cor0"
## [27] "pc.cor1"              "pc.fgnh"
## [29] "pc.spde.GA"           "pc.matern"
## [31] "pc.range"             "pc.gamma"
## [33] "pc.mgamma"            "pc.gammacount"
## [35] "pc.gevtail"           "pc"
## [37] "ref.ar"               "pom"
## [39] "jeffreystdf"          "expression:"
## [41] "table:"
```

Detailed information about all these priors can be obtained with `inla.doc("prior_name")`, where `prior_name` is one of the prior names listed above.

Table 5.2 provides a summary of these prior distributions, and includes some information about the parameterzation. This is useful when defining the prior. For example, the Gaussian distribution is defined using the mean and precision (instead of the variance or the standard deviation).

TABLE 5.2: Summary of the priors implemented in INLA.

Prior	Description	Parameters
normal	Gaussian prior	mean, precision
gaussian	Gaussian prior	mean, precision
loggamma	log-Gamma	shape, rate
logtnormal	Truncated (positive) Gaussian prior	mean, precision
logtgaussian	Truncated (positive) Gaussian prior	mean, precision
flat	Flat (improper) prior on θ	

Prior	Description	Parameters
logflat	Flat (improper prior) on $\exp(\theta)$	
logiflat	Flat (improper prior) on $\exp(-\theta)$	
mvnorm	Multivarite Normal prior	
dirichlet	Dirichlet prior	α
betacorrelation	Beta prior for correlation	a, b
logitbeta	Beta prior, logit-scale	a, b
jeffreystdf	Jeffreys prior	
table	User defined prior	
expression	User defined prior	

As stated in Table 5.2, priors `expression` and `table` can be used to create user defined priors, and these priors are described in the next section.

5.3 Implementing new priors

Although the list of implemented priors in `INLA` contains a wide range of distributions used in practice other priors not in the list may be required. For this reason, `INLA` provides two options for setting user-defined priors. These are the `table` and `expression` priors. While the `table` prior is based on a tabulated density, the `expression` prior allows the user to define the actual density function for the prior.

5.3.1 Priors defined with `table`

The `table` prior essentially defines a table with the value of the hyperparameter (in the internal scale) and then associated prior density in the log-scale. For values not defined in the table, these are interpolated. For values outside of the domain defined in the table, the internal optimizer in `INLA` will give an error and stop. More information about this prior can be found by typing `inla.doc("table")` in R.

The way in which the table is defined is as a single character string that starts with `table:`, followed by the values at which the hyperparameters are evaluated and then followed by the values of the log-density. This means that the structure is

$$\text{table: } \theta_1 \ldots \theta_n \log(\pi(\theta_1)) \ldots \log(\pi(\theta_n))$$

For example, to set a Gaussian prior with zero mean and precision 0.001 on θ, the `table` prior can be defined as follows:

```
theta <- seq(-100, 100, by = 0.1)
log_dens <- dnorm(theta, 0, sqrt(1 / 0.001), log = TRUE)

gaus.prior <- paste0("table: ",
  paste(c(theta, log_dens), collapse = " ")
)
```

The first 50 characters of the prior are:

```
substr(gaus.prior, 1, 50)
```

```
## [1] "table: -100 -99.9 -99.8 -99.7 -99.6 -99.5 -99.4 -9"
```

And the last 50 characters are:

```
substr(gaus.prior, nchar(gaus.prior) - 50 + 1, nchar(gaus.prior))
```

```
## [1] "35283617269574 -9.36282117269574 -9.37281617269574"
```

Table 5.3 shows a summary of the internal representation of some parameters. Given that the prior must be set using the internal representation of the hyperparameter, the density must be $\pi(\theta)$. When the prior is set on a parameter $\tau = f(\theta)$ (i.e., $\pi_\tau(\tau)$), then the prior on the hyperparameter θ must be set as

$$\pi(\theta) = \pi_\tau(\tau)|\partial f(\theta)/\partial \theta|$$

Note that this applies in general and this should be taken into account when defining priors using the `table` and `expression` latent effects. See, for example, Ugarte et al. (2016) and Wang et al. (2018) for some examples on setting user defined priors with INLA.

For example, if the prior is defined on the standard deviation σ (note that $\sigma = \exp(-\theta/2)$), then the log-prior on θ should be

$$\log(\pi(\theta)) = \log(\pi_\sigma(\sigma)) + \log(|\partial f(\theta)/\partial \theta|) = \log(\pi_\sigma(\sigma)) + \log(\exp(-\theta/2)/2) =$$

$$= \log(\pi_\sigma(\sigma)) - \theta/2 - \log(2) = \log(\pi_\sigma(\exp(-\theta/2))) - \theta/2 - \log(2)$$

Note that constant $\log(2)$ can be omitted when defining the prior in INLA but this will affect the computation of the marginal likelihood.

TABLE 5.3: Summary of internal representation of some model hyperparameters.

Parameter	Range	Internal	$f(\theta)$	$|\partial f(\theta)/\partial \theta|$
Precision τ	$(0, \infty)$	$\theta = \log(\tau)$	$\tau = \exp(\theta)$	$\exp(\theta)$
Variance σ^2	$(0, \infty)$	$\theta = -\log(\sigma^2)$	$\sigma^2 = \exp(-\theta)$	$\exp(-\theta)$
St. dev. σ	$(0, \infty)$	$\theta = -2\log(\sigma)$	$\sigma = \exp(-\theta/2)$	$\exp(-\theta/2)/2$
Correlation ρ	$(-1, 1)$	$\theta = \log(\frac{1+\rho}{1-\rho})$	$\rho = 2\frac{\exp(\theta)}{1+\exp(\theta)} - 1$	$2\exp(\theta)/(1+\exp(\theta))^2$
Coefficient β	$(0, 1)$	$\theta = \log(\frac{\beta}{1-\beta})$	$\beta = \frac{\exp(\theta)}{1+\exp(\theta)}$	$\exp(\theta)/(1+\exp(\theta))^2$

5.3.2 Priors defined with `expression`

The `expression` prior in INLA allows the user to define directly the prior on the hyperparameter using the `muparser` library (http://beltoforion.de/article.php?a=muparser). The syntax is very similar to that of R. For example, the Gaussian prior on θ with zero mean and precision 1000 can be defined as

```
"expression:
  mean = 0;
  prec = 1000;
  logdens = 0.5 * log(prec) - 0.5 * log (2 * pi);
  logdens = logdens - 0.5 * prec * (theta - mean)^2;
  return(logdens);
"
```

When defining an expression, all variables are set by default to the value of the hyperparameter θ. Hence, any variable name that is not a reserved word can be used to get the value of θ. Here, `pi` represents number π and `log` the natural logarithm function. Note that the previous function returns the log-density of the Gaussian distribution for a value of θ.

The `muparser` has a number of common constants and functions predefined that can be used to define the prior. More information and examples can be found in the `muparser` documentation.

5.3.3   Example

For illustrative purposes, we will consider now a simple example on setting a prior on the standard deviation. Ugarte et al. (2016), Wang et al. (2018) and Gómez-Rubio et al. (2019) also develop some of the priors mentioned below.

Gelman (2006) discusses and compares different prior choices for the scale parameter of linear mixed models as better alternatives to the Gamma prior on the precision. The reason to do so is to provide a set of weakly informative priors as opposed to the typically used Gamma prior with equal and tiny parameters. Although this Gamma prior looks like a vague prior as it is centered at one and has a large prior variance, it provides more prior information as compared to other alternatives. For this reason, we have included below how to define four different priors for the standard deviation: a half-normal, a half-Cauchy, a half-t and an improper flat prior.

Note that in the following definitions, the prior is set on the internal parameter θ. Remember that the stadard deviation is $\sigma = \exp(-\theta/2)$. Hence, the prior on the internal parameter θ becomes

$$\log(\pi(\theta)) = \log(\pi_\sigma(\exp(-\theta/2))) - \theta/2 - \log(2)$$

as stated above.

Half-Normal

The half-normal distribution shown here is a normal with zero mean and precision τ_0 which is truncated at zero. Hence, its density function is:

$$\pi_{HN}(\sigma \mid \tau_0) = \frac{2\tau_0^{1/2}}{\sqrt{2\pi}} \exp(\frac{-\tau_0}{2}\sigma^2)$$

Following this and noting that $\sigma = \exp(-\theta/2)$, the following expression can be used to use this prior using the `expression` prior in INLA:

```
HN.prior = "expression:
  tau0 = 0.001;
  sigma = exp(-theta/2);
  log_dens = log(2) - 0.5 * log(2 * pi) + 0.5 * log(tau0);
  log_dens = log_dens - 0.5 * tau0 * sigma^2;
  log_dens = log_dens - log(2) - theta / 2;
  return(log_dens);
"
```

Half-Cauchy

Similarly, the half-Cauchy is a Cauchy distribution which is truncated at zero so that it can serve as a prior for the standard deviation σ. Its density, which has a scale parameter γ, is

$$\pi_{HN}(\sigma \mid \gamma) = \frac{2}{\pi\gamma(1 + (\sigma/\gamma)^2)}$$

The code to use this prior with INLA is:

```
HC.prior  = "expression:
  sigma = exp(-theta/2);
  gamma = 25;
  log_dens = log(2) - log(pi) - log(gamma);
  log_dens = log_dens - log(1 + (sigma / gamma)^2);
  log_dens = log_dens - log(2) - theta / 2;
  return(log_dens);
"
```

Here, we have set the scale parameter γ to 25 following Gelman (2006).

Half-t

The half-t is also a truncated distribution at zero. In this case, a Student's t distribution with ν degrees of freedom. The resulting density function is

$$\pi_{HN}(\sigma \mid \nu) = \frac{\Gamma((\nu + 1)/2)}{\sqrt{\nu\pi}\Gamma(\nu/2)} \left(1 + \frac{x^2}{\nu}\right)^{-\frac{\nu+1}{2}}$$

In order to implement this prior we need to precompute $\Gamma((\nu + 1)/2)$ and $\Gamma(\nu/2)$ because the Gamma function is not implemented in the muparser library. In addition, it is a good idea to compute the constant that multiplies because this will save time. For educational purposes, we have included all the terms in the constant so that all elements in the definition of the prior can be identified:

```
HT.prior = "expression:
  sigma = exp(-theta/2);
  nu = 3;
  log_dens = 0 - 0.5 * log(nu * pi) - (-0.1207822);
  log_dens = log_dens - 0.5 * (nu + 1) * log(1 + sigma * sigma);
  log_dens = log_dens - log(2) - theta / 2;
```

```
    return(log_dens);
  "
```

Note that the degrees of freedom have been set to 3 to make sure that both the mean and variance exist.

Uniform

Finally, a uniform improper prior can be set on the standard deviation:

$$\pi_{UN}(\sigma) \propto 1$$

This produces the following prior definition:

```
UN.prior = "expression:
  log_dens = 0 - log(2) - theta / 2;
  return(log_dens);
  "
```

Note that `INLA` assumes that hyperparameters in the internal scale are unbounded. For this reason, it is difficult to set a uniform prior on the standard deviation in a bounded interval.

5.4 Penalized Complexity priors

Simpson et al. (2017) describe a novel and principled approach for the construction of priors suited for additive models defined by different components (e.g., latent effects). They propose priors that penalize departure from a base model and for this reason they are called Penalized Complexity (PC) priors. In addition, the appeal of these priors is that they are defined using probability statements about the parameter.

PC priors are designed following some principles for inference. First of all, the prior favors the base model unless evidence is provided against it, following the principle of parsimony. Distance from the base model is measured using the Kullback-Leibler distance, and penalization from the base model is done at a constant rate on the distance. Finally, the PC prior is defined using probability statements on the model parameters in the appropriate scale.

For example, the PC prior for the precision τ is defined on the standard deviation $\sigma = \tau^{-1/2}$. It is defined by parameters σ_0 and α, so that

$$P(\sigma > \sigma_0) = \alpha$$

Hence, the prior can be easily used to elicit our prior belief about the parameter. The actual expression of the prior is (Simpson et al., 2017):

$$\pi(\tau) = \frac{\lambda}{2} \tau^{-3/2} \exp(-\lambda \tau^{-1/2}), \ \tau > 0$$

Here, $\lambda = -\log(\alpha)/u$.

Table 5.4 shows a summary of some of the PC priors available in `INLA`. Note that there are other PC priors implemented in `INLA` that have not been included. Detailed information about the different PC priors can be found in their respective manual pages, which can be accessed with function `inla.doc()`.

TABLE 5.4: Summary of some of the Penalized Complexity priors implemented in `INLA`.

Prior	Parameter	Hyperparameters	Base model	Definition
`pc.prec`	Precision $\tau = \sigma^{-2}$	(σ_0, α)	$\sigma = 0$	$P(\sigma > \sigma_0) = \alpha$
`pc.dof`	Degrees of freedom ν	(u, α)	$\nu = \infty$	$P(\nu < u) = \alpha$
`pc.cor0`	Correlation ρ	(ρ_0, α)	$\rho = 0$	$P(|\rho| > \rho_0) = \alpha$
`pc.cor1`	Correlation ρ	(ρ_0, α)	$\rho = 1$	$P(\rho > \rho_0) = \alpha$

In addition to implementing these priors for its use in the models, `INLA` includes a number of functions for each PC prior to compute its density, cumulative probability, quantiles and sampling random numbers. These functions follow the usual `R` naming convention for densities and probability distributions. For example, the associated functions for the `pc.prec` prior are `inla.pc.dprec()` (density), `inla.pc.pprec()` (cumulative probability), `inla.pc.qprec` (quantile) and `inla.pc.rprec` (sampling). Functions associated with other PC priors follow a similar naming convention.

Figure 5.1 shows different PC priors for the precision using $P(\sigma > 1) = \alpha$, for several values of α. Note how large values of α lead to a greater prior belief on large values of σ, which in turn leads to a larger prior belief on small values of τ.

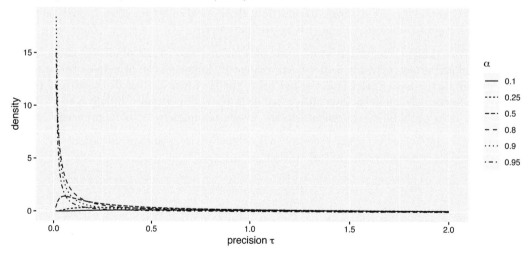

FIGURE 5.1 PC priors for the precision τ.

5.5 Sensitivity analysis with R-INLA

Given the speed at which models are fitted with `INLA` it is possible to conduct a sensitivity analysis on the priors in the model. This is important because the choice of the priors can have an important impact on the posterior distributions of the model parameters.

We will go back to the dataset described in Section 4.4 on the performance of children at school. The dataset can be loaded as follows:

```
csize_data <- read.csv (file = "data/class_size_data.txt", header = FALSE,
  sep = "", dec = ".")

#Set names
names(csize_data) <- c("clsnr", "pupil", "nlitpre", "nmatpre", "nlitpost",
  "nmatpost", "csize")

#Set NA's
csize_data [csize_data < -1e+29 ] <- NA

#Set class size levels
csize_data$csize <- as.factor(csize_data$csize)
levels(csize_data$csize) <- c("<=19", "20-24", "25-29", ">=30")
```

In the sensitivity analysis we will compare the default prior with INLA and the priors defined in the previous section. All these priors will be put together in a list so that different models are fit by looping over this list.

```
prior.list = list(
  default = list(prec = list(prior = "loggamma", param = c(1, 0.00005))),
  half.normal = list(prec = list(prior = HN.prior)),
  half.cauchy = list(prec = list(prior = HC.prior)),
  h.t = list(prec = list(prior = HT.prior)),
  uniform = list(prec = list(prior = UN.prior)),
  pc.prec = list(prec = list(prior = "pc.prec", param = c(5, 0.01)))
)
```

Before proceeding to fit the models with `INLA`, the rows with missing values in the first 4 columns of the dataset are removed. `INLA` will remove them anyway, but we prefer to make this step explicit and create a new dataset `csize_data2` for model fitting:

```
#Remove rows with NA's
csize_data2 <- na.omit(csize_data[, -5])
```

Model fitting is done with the `lapply()` function so that each prior in list `prior.list` is used in turn:

```
csize.models <- lapply(prior.list, function(tau.prior) {
  inla(nmatpost ~ 1 + nmatpre + nlitpre + csize +
```

```
      f(clsnr, model = "iid", hyper = tau.prior), data = csize_data2,
    control.family = list(hyper = tau.prior))
})
```

The posterior marginals of the error precision τ_e and the iid random effect τ_u for the different priors used have been plotted in Figure 5.2. In this particular case no differences can be appreciated.

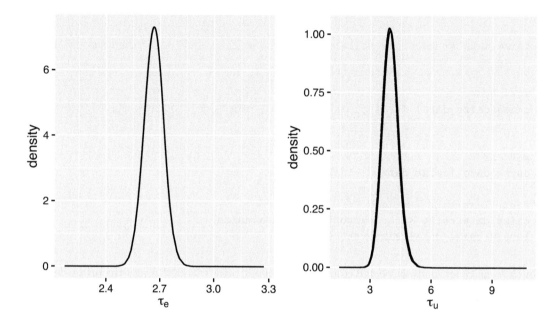

FIGURE 5.2 Sensitivity analysis on the priors of the precisions of the model.

5.6 Scaling effects and priors

As mentioned in Chapter 3, latent effects in INLA can be scaled in different ways and this may require a different prior setting. Scaling is particularly important for intrinsic models, such as the random walk latent effects or some of the spatial models described in Section 7.2.2. Sørbye (2013) and Sørbye and Rue (2014) provide more details on how the scaling is done in INLA.

Briefly, scaling a model means that the generalized variance of the latent effect is one (see Sørbye, 2013, for details). This scaling will take the values of the scale hyperparameter to a different range, which implies that different priors should be used for scaled and unscaled models. In addition, this also means that precision estimates are comparable between different models and that estimates are less affected by re-scaling covariates in the linear predictor. Furthermore, re-scaling makes the precision invariant to changes in the shape and size of the latent effect.

Scaling is done through arguments `scale` and `scale.model` in the definition of the latent effects via the `f()` function. See Table 5.5.

TABLE 5.5: Arguments that can be passed to the `f()` function for model scaling.

Argument	Default	Description
`scale`	NULL	A scaling vector.
`scale.model`	NULL	Scale model (if TRUE).

Scaling latent effects means that the generalized variance is taken to be equal to one. As a result, precision parameters in the latent effects are comparable and they can take the same prior distribution.

In order to show how scaling affects model fitting we will use the `lidar` dataset described in detail in Chapter 9. We will consider the same non-parametric models using `rw1` and `rw2` latent effect with and without re-scaling the models:

```
library("SemiPar")
data(lidar)

#Data for prediction
xx <- seq(390, 720, by = 5)
# Add data for prediction
new.data <- cbind(range = xx, logratio = NA)
new.data <- rbind(lidar, new.data)

# Set prior on precision
prec.prior <- list(prec = list(param = c(0.001, 0.001)))

#RW1 latent effect
m.rw1 <- inla(logratio ~ 1 + f(range, model = "rw1", constr = FALSE,
    hyper = prec.prior),
  data = new.data, control.predictor = list(compute = TRUE))
#RW1 scaled latent effect
m.rw1.sc <- inla(logratio ~ 1 + f(range, model = "rw1", constr = FALSE,
    scale.model = TRUE, hyper = prec.prior),
  data = new.data, control.predictor = list(compute = TRUE))

#RW2 latent effect
m.rw2 <- inla(logratio ~ 1 + f(range, model = "rw2", constr = FALSE,
    hyper = prec.prior),
  data = new.data, control.predictor = list(compute = TRUE))
#RW2 scaled latent effect
m.rw2.sc <- inla(logratio ~ 1 + f(range, model = "rw2", constr = FALSE,
    scale.model = TRUE,  hyper = prec.prior),
  data = new.data, control.predictor = list(compute = TRUE))
```

Note that in the previous code, the priors for the precision parameters of the scaled models is a Gamma with parameters 0.001 and 0.001, instead of the default values of 1 and 0.00005 to provide a vague prior (as discussed in Chapter 3). This is required because the precision parameters in the scaled models are in a completely different scale and the default prior does not make much sense now as it provides an extremely large prior variance of the precision parameter. Also, by setting the same prior for all models we can appreciate the effects of scaling a model better.

Table 5.6 shows the different estimates of the precisions of the `rw1` and `rw2` latent effects. As can be seen, the precision parameters of the scaled models are comparable, while the corresponding parameters for the un-scaled models are in completely different ranges (Sørbye, 2013). This scaling effect is similar to the one observed in the examples on scaling random effects in Chapter 3.

TABLE 5.6: Summary of the posterior distribution of the precision hyperparameters for different scaled and un-scaled intrinsic latent effects.

Model	Scaled	Mean	St. dev.	0.025 quant.	0.975 quant.
rw1	No	1427.80	57.81	1317.86	1547.80
rw1	Yes	39.12	0.56	38.02	40.25
rw2	No	16450.29	1005.96	14981.05	18812.76
rw2	Yes	133.52	0.88	131.70	135.22

Regarding the fitted model, Figure 5.3 shows the different models fit to the data. Both scaled and unscaled models produce very similar estimates. However, scaled models seem to produce smoother curves, which may also be an effect of the priors used.

5.7   Final remarks

Prior definition in `INLA` is flexible enough to consider many different types of approaches which in turn allow us to fit wider types of models. In particular, PC priors are particularly well suited for the INLA methodology and the modular model definition of additive models. `INLA` also has the capability of re-scaling intrinsic latent effects so that the estimates of the precision do not depend on the shape and size of the latent effect and re-scaled covariates in the model.

Other priors may be implemented in `INLA` in a number of ways. For example, when new latent effects are implemented (as explained in Section 11) priors need to be set explicitly using appropriate `R` functions. This means that priors not implemented in `INLA` but available in `R` can be used. This includes, for example, multivariate priors or priors that do not fit within the INLA framework (Gómez-Rubio and Rue, 2018).

Multivariate priors could, in principle, be used with `INLA` and a few latent effects have them implemented. However, most of the priors available in `INLA` are univariate. Multivariate priors could be included in the latent effects by implementing them using the methods described in Chapter 11. This is so because the prior of the hyperparameters needs to be explicitly computed using `R` code and, hence, this will allow us to include multivariate priors. Palmí-Perales et al. (2019) use the `rgeneric` feature described in Chapter 11 to implement new latent effects for multivariate data and some of the models require multivariate priors.

Those examples can be used as a template to implement latent effects that use multivariate priors.

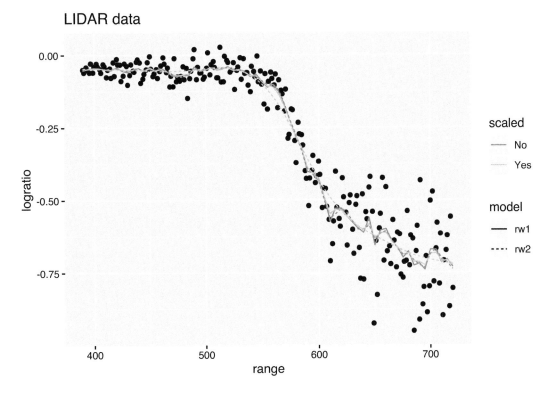

FIGURE 5.3 Fitted values of the `lidar` dataset using scaled and unscaled latent effects.

6

Advanced Features

6.1 Introduction

As seen in previous chapters, INLA is a methodology to fit Bayesian hierarchical models by computing approximations of the posterior marginal distributions of the model parameters. In order to build more complex models and compute the posterior marginal distribution of some quantities of interest, the INLA package has a number of *advanced* features that are worth knowing. Some of these features are also described in detail in Krainski et al. (2018).

In this chapter we will describe some of these features. In particular, Section 6.2 shows how to define a *predictor* matrix that multiplies all terms in the linear predictor, so that the actual linear predictor of the model is a linear combination of the effects in the model formula. Next, Section 6.3 presents how to define linear combinations of the latent effects to compute their posterior distribution. Section 6.4 introduces the use of models with several likelihoods. Models with several likelihoods that share some terms are in Section 6.5, where the `copy` and `replicate` features are described in detail. These features are very useful when working with, for example, joint models (see Chapter 10).

6.2 Predictor Matrix

The formula passed to the `inla()` function defines the model to be fit by INLA, i.e., the formula defines the terms in the linear predictor. However, sometimes we need to modify the model so that linear combinations of these terms are used instead of simply the ones set in the formula. INLA allows this by defining a matrix A, which is called *predictor matrix* so that the actual linear predictor η^* used is

$$\eta^* = A\eta$$

Here, η is the linear predictor defined in the formula. By default, this matrix is the identity matrix.

Matrix A that defines the linear combinations to be used is passed using element A in the list passed to argument `control.predictor` (see Section 2.5 for details). Matrix A can be a dense matrix or a sparse one of the types implemented in the Matrix package (Bates and Maechler, 2019). The dimension of the A matrix must be $n \times n$, with n the number of observations in the model.

In order to provide a simple example we will consider the `cement` dataset described in Section 2.3. A very simple use of the A matrix is to re-scale the linear predictor used in the model (see Krainski et al., 2018, for a similar example), for example, to have it multiplied by a constant. In this case, we will take the A matrix as a diagonal matrix with values equal to 5. This means that the linear predictors, as defined by the formula, will be multiplied by 5, and that the estimates of the terms in the linear predictor will shrink in a similar way so that the actual linear predictor $A\eta$ remains the same as in the example in Section 2.3. Note that the fitted values will also remain the same.

```r
library("MASS")
library("Matrix")

data(cement)
A <- Diagonal(n = nrow(cement), x = 5)
summary(A)
```

```
## 13 x 13 diagonal Matrix of class "ddiMatrix"
##    Min. 1st Qu.  Median    Mean 3rd Qu.    Max.
##       5       5       5       5       5       5
```

Note how in the code above matrix A is a sparse matrix. Hence, the model using this *predictor* matrix can be fit:

```r
m1.A <- inla(y ~ x1 + x2 + x3 + x4, data = cement,
   control.predictor = list(A = A))
summary(m1.A)
```

```
##
## Call:
##     "inla(formula = y ~ x1 + x2 + x3 + x4, data = cement,
##     control.predictor = list(A = A))"
## Time used:
##     Pre = 1.16, Running = 0.0934, Post = 0.0688, Total = 1.32
## Fixed effects:
##               mean     sd 0.025quant 0.5quant 0.975quant   mode kld
## (Intercept) 12.482 14.083    -15.705   12.481     40.627 12.482   0
## x1           0.310  0.150      0.011    0.310      0.609  0.310   0
## x2           0.102  0.145     -0.189    0.102      0.393  0.102   0
## x3           0.020  0.152     -0.283    0.020      0.324  0.020   0
## x4          -0.029  0.143     -0.314   -0.029      0.256 -0.029   0
##
## Model hyperparameters:
##                                           mean    sd 0.025quant 0.5quant
## Precision for the Gaussian observations 0.209 0.093      0.068    0.195
##                                          0.975quant  mode
## Precision for the Gaussian observations      0.429 0.167
##
## Expected number of effective parameters(stdev): 5.00(0.00)
## Number of equivalent replicates : 2.60
##
## Marginal log-Likelihood:  -67.54
```

Note how the estimates of the fixed effects are divided by 5 as compared to the estimates obtained with the model fit in Section 2.3. This is because of the effect of the A matrix.

In general, the predictor matrix can be useful for non-trivial examples. For example, the predictor matrix plays an important role in the development of spatial models based on stochastic partial differential equations (Krainski et al., 2018). See Chapter 7 for details.

6.3   Linear combinations

The use of the predictor matrix introduced in the previous section allows us to define models where the actual linear predictors are linear combinations of the effects in the model formula. However, in some situations we are only interested in computing linear combinations on some effects without altering model fitting.

With `INLA`, linear combinations on the different latent effects can be defined and their posterior marginals estimated. Note that these linear combinations do not alter the fit model (as the use of a predictor matrix did). Linear combinations are passed using argument `lincomb` to the `inla()` function. Furthermore, argument `control.lincomb` can be used to set the parameters that control how posterior marginals of linear combinations are computed. Table 6.1 shows the options available to control how the linear combinations are fit.

TABLE 6.1: Summary of options in `control.lincomb`.

Argument	Default	Description
precision	1e09	Tiny noise added to compute approximation
verbose	TRUE	Use verbose if verbose is enabled globally.

Linear combinations are defined by setting the effects and the associated coefficients that they have to make the linear combination. Two functions are available to define linear combinations: `inla.make.lincomb()`, to define a single linear combination, and `inla.make.lincombs()`, to define several linear combinations at once.

Function `inla.make.lincomb()` takes named arguments with the values of the coefficients of the linear combination. The names are the names of the effects to be used in the linear combination. For fixed effects, values must be a single number, while for random effects it is a vector of coefficients of the same length as the index of the random effect. For those values of the random effect not in the linear combination, `NA` must be used.

For example, in the analysis of the `cement` data above we might be interested in computing the difference between coefficients of covariates `x1` and `x2`. This could be defined as follows:

```
inla.make.lincomb(x1 = 1, x2 = -1)
```

If the linear combination involves a random effect index from 1 to p, the linear combination can be defined by including a term with the name of the latent random effect. The value now is not a single number, but a vector of length p with the coefficients of the different elements of the random effects. Those elements that do not appear in the linear combination must have a value of `NA`.

For example, if a random effect named `u` of length 4 is included in a model and we want to compute the difference between its two terms, this can be set up as:

```
inla.make.lincomb(u = c(1, -1, NA, NA))
```

Function `inla.make.lincombs()` can be used to set more than one linear combination at a time. Instead of using a single value for the linear combinations on the fixed effects, a vector of coefficients can be passed.

For example, say that we are interested in comparing the coefficient of variable `x1` to the other three coefficients. In the design of experiments literature these types of comparisons are often referred to as contrasts. This can be set as several differences using linear combinations as follows:

```
inla.make.lincomb(
  x1 = c( 1,   1,   1),
  x2 = c(-1,   0,   0),
  x3 = c( 0,  -1,   0),
  x4 = c( 0,   0,  -1)
)
```

Once the model has been fit, summaries of the linear combinations are available in `summary.lincomb.derived` in the `inla` object returned. Similarly, posterior marginals densities are available in `marginals.lincomb`.

Finally, two arguments can be passed through `control.inla` to control how linear combinations are computed: `lincomb.derived.only` and `lincomb.derived.correlation.matrix`. The first option indicates whether the linear combinations are to be computed, and the second controls the computation of the correlation matrix of the linear combinations. See Table 6.2 for a summary.

TABLE 6.2: Options in `control.inla` to control how the linear combinations are computed.

Argument	Default	Description
`lincomb.derived.only`	TRUE	Compute full graph of derived linear combinations.
`lincomb.derived.correlation.matrix`	FALSE	Compute correlations for derived linear combinations.

Linear combinations can be used for a number of issues, such as computing the posterior marginal of the linear predictor for a given set of covariate values. Another interesting application is to compare whether two effects are equal.

In order to provide a simple example, we will consider the **abrasion** dataset (Davies, 1954) from package `faraway` (Faraway, 2016). This dataset records data from an industrial experiment about wear of four different types of materials after being fed into a wear testing machine. In each run, four samples are processed, and the position of the samples may be important. The different variables in this dataset are described in Table 6.3.

TABLE 6.3: Variables in the `abrasion` dataset.

Variable	Description
run	Run number (from 1 to 4).
position	Position number (from 1 to 4).
material	Type of material (A, B, C or D).
wear	Weight loss (in 0.1mm) over testing period.

Given that the main interest is in the wear depending on the type of material, `material` will be introduced into the model as a fixed effect, while `run` and `position` are introduced as `iid` random affects. In addition, we have noticed that default INLA priors produce too much shrinkage of the coefficients and random effects towards zero, and the results do not reproduce those in Faraway (2006). In particular, we have considered a larger precision on the coefficients of the fixed effects. For the prior on the precisions we have followed Faraway (2019b) and taken a Gamma prior with parameters 0.5 and 95. This is an informative prior that has a mean value half the variance of the residuals of a linear regression on `wear` using `material` as predictor. The posterior means of precisions of the random effects should be lower than this value. Furthermore, function `inla.hyperpar()` has been used to obtain better estimates of the hyperparameters once the model has been fit with INLA.

```
library("faraway")
data(abrasion)

# Prior prec. of random effects
prec.prior <- list(prec = list(param = c(0.5, 95)))
# Model formula
f.wear <- wear ~ -1 + material +
    f(position, model = "iid", hyper = prec.prior) +
    f(run, model = "iid", hyper = prec.prior)

# Model fitting
m0 <- inla(f.wear, data = abrasion,
  control.fixed = list(prec = 0.001^2)
)
# Improve estimates of hyperparameters
m0 <- inla.hyperpar(m0)
summary(m0)
```

```
##
## Call:
##    "inla(formula = f.wear, data = abrasion, control.fixed = list(prec
##    = 0.001^2))"
## Time used:
##     Pre = 1.16, Running = 0.252, Post = 0.0708, Total = 1.49
## Fixed effects:
##              mean    sd 0.025quant 0.5quant 0.975quant  mode kld
## materialA 265.7 9.773      246.1    265.7      285.2 265.7   0
## materialB 219.9 9.773      200.3    219.9      239.5 219.9   0
## materialC 241.7 9.773      222.1    241.7      261.2 241.7   0
```

```
## materialD 230.4 9.773      210.8    230.4      250.0 230.4    0
##
## Random effects:
##   Name      Model
##     position IID model
##     run IID model
##
## Model hyperparameters:
##                                          mean    sd 0.025quant 0.5quant
## Precision for the Gaussian observations 0.022 0.011      0.006    0.020
## Precision for position                  0.008 0.006      0.001    0.006
## Precision for run                       0.009 0.007      0.001    0.007
##                                          0.975quant  mode
## Precision for the Gaussian observations      0.048 0.016
## Precision for position                       0.025 0.004
## Precision for run                            0.027 0.005
##
## Expected number of effective parameters(stdev): 9.34(0.428)
## Number of equivalent replicates : 1.71
##
## Marginal log-Likelihood:  -96.48
```

Then, we may be interested in comparing whether there is any difference between material A and any of the others. For example, the following linear constraint will compute the difference of the effects between material A and B:

```
lc <- inla.make.lincomb(materialA = 1, materialB = -1)
```

This model can now be fit to compare materials A and B:

```
m0.lc <- inla.hyperpar(inla(f.wear, data = abrasion, lincomb = lc,
   control.fixed = list(prec = 0.001^2)))
summary(m0.lc)
```

```
##
## Call:
##    "inla(formula = f.wear, data = abrasion, lincomb = lc,
##    control.fixed = list(prec = 0.001^2))"
## Time used:
##    Pre = 1.12, Running = 0.28, Post = 0.072, Total = 1.47
## Fixed effects:
##          mean    sd 0.025quant 0.5quant 0.975quant  mode kld
## materialA 265.7 9.773     246.1    265.7     285.2 265.7   0
## materialB 219.9 9.773     200.3    219.9     239.5 219.9   0
## materialC 241.7 9.773     222.1    241.7     261.2 241.7   0
## materialD 230.4 9.773     210.8    230.4     250.0 230.4   0
##
## Linear combinations (derived):
##    ID  mean    sd 0.025quant 0.5quant 0.975quant  mode kld
## lc  1 45.75 5.297      35.07    45.75      56.44 45.75   0
##
```

```
## Random effects:
##   Name      Model
##     position IID model
##     run IID model
##
## Model hyperparameters:
##                                          mean    sd 0.025quant 0.5quant
## Precision for the Gaussian observations 0.022 0.011      0.006    0.020
## Precision for position                  0.008 0.006      0.001    0.006
## Precision for run                       0.009 0.007      0.001    0.007
##                                         0.975quant  mode
## Precision for the Gaussian observations      0.048 0.016
## Precision for position                       0.025 0.004
## Precision for run                            0.027 0.005
##
## Expected number of effective parameters(stdev): 9.34(0.428)
## Number of equivalent replicates : 1.71
##
## Marginal log-Likelihood:  -96.48
```

Note that summary statistics of the posterior marginal of the linear combination can be accessed with

```
m0.lc$summary.lincomb.derived
```

```
##    ID  mean    sd 0.025quant 0.5quant 0.975quant  mode kld
## lc  1 45.75 5.297      35.07    45.75      56.44 45.75   0
```

This shows a positive posterior means and 95% credible interval that is above 0, which means that wear in material A is higher than in material B.

This can be extended to compare material A to all the other materials. This can be represented by a 3×4 matrix to represent the 3 linear combinations required. Now `inla.make.lincombs` must be used in order to define 3 different linear combinations.

```
lcs <- inla.make.lincombs(
  materialA = c( 1,  1,  1),
  materialB = c(-1,  0,  0),
  materialC = c( 0, -1,  0),
  materialD = c( 0,  0, -1)
)
```

The model is fit similarly to the previous example:

```
m0.lcs <- inla.hyperpar(inla(f.wear, data = abrasion, lincomb = lcs,
  control.fixed = list(prec = 0.001^2)))
summary(m0.lcs)
```

```
##
## Call:
##    "inla(formula = f.wear, data = abrasion, lincomb = lcs,
```

```
##       control.fixed = list(prec = 0.001^2))"
## Time used:
##       Pre = 1.15, Running = 0.318, Post = 0.0713, Total = 1.54
## Fixed effects:
##               mean      sd 0.025quant 0.5quant 0.975quant  mode kld
## materialA 265.7 9.773        246.1    265.7       285.2 265.7   0
## materialB 219.9 9.773        200.3    219.9       239.5 219.9   0
## materialC 241.7 9.773        222.1    241.7       261.2 241.7   0
## materialD 230.4 9.773        210.8    230.4       250.0 230.4   0
##
## Linear combinations (derived):
##     ID  mean     sd 0.025quant 0.5quant 0.975quant   mode kld
## lc1  1 45.75 5.297      35.07    45.75      56.44 45.75   0
## lc2  2 24.00 5.297      13.32    24.00      34.69 24.00   0
## lc3  3 35.25 5.297      24.57    35.25      45.94 35.25   0
##
## Random effects:
##   Name      Model
##     position IID model
##     run IID model
##
## Model hyperparameters:
##                                             mean      sd 0.025quant 0.5quant
## Precision for the Gaussian observations 0.022 0.011      0.006    0.020
## Precision for position                  0.008 0.006      0.001    0.006
## Precision for run                       0.009 0.007      0.001    0.007
##                                        0.975quant  mode
## Precision for the Gaussian observations     0.048 0.016
## Precision for position                      0.025 0.004
## Precision for run                           0.027 0.005
##
## Expected number of effective parameters(stdev): 9.34(0.428)
## Number of equivalent replicates : 1.71
##
## Marginal log-Likelihood:  -96.48
```

Linear combinations can also be used to compare the levels of the random effects. For example, let's consider a comparison between positions 1 and 2. Variable `position` is an `iid` random effect with four different levels, and the weights must be set in a vector of the same length. For those levels that must be ignored in the linear combination, `NA` can be used.

Hence, to define a linear combination to compare levels 1 and 2 of variable `position` we can define the linear combination as follows:

```
lc.pos <- inla.make.lincomb(position = c(1, -1, NA, NA))

m0.pos <- inla.hyperpar(inla(f.wear, data = abrasion, lincomb = lc.pos,
  control.fixed = list(prec = 0.001^2)))
summary(m0.pos)
```

```
##
```

```
## Call:
##    "inla(formula = f.wear, data = abrasion, lincomb = lc.pos,
##    control.fixed = list(prec = 0.001^2))"
## Time used:
##       Pre = 1.12, Running = 0.275, Post = 0.0712, Total = 1.47
## Fixed effects:
##               mean    sd 0.025quant 0.5quant 0.975quant  mode kld
## materialA 265.7 9.773       246.1    265.7      285.2 265.7   0
## materialB 219.9 9.773       200.3    219.9      239.5 219.9   0
## materialC 241.7 9.773       222.1    241.7      261.2 241.7   0
## materialD 230.4 9.773       210.8    230.4      250.0 230.4   0
##
## Linear combinations (derived):
##    ID  mean     sd 0.025quant 0.5quant 0.975quant   mode kld
## lc  1 -23.6 5.356     -33.64   -23.85     -12.05 -24.27   0
##
## Random effects:
##   Name     Model
##     position IID model
##     run IID model
##
## Model hyperparameters:
##                                             mean    sd 0.025quant 0.5quant
## Precision for the Gaussian observations 0.022 0.011      0.006    0.020
## Precision for position                  0.008 0.006      0.001    0.006
## Precision for run                       0.009 0.007      0.001    0.007
##                                             0.975quant  mode
## Precision for the Gaussian observations      0.048 0.016
## Precision for position                       0.025 0.004
## Precision for run                            0.027 0.005
##
## Expected number of effective parameters(stdev): 9.34(0.428)
## Number of equivalent replicates : 1.71
##
## Marginal log-Likelihood:  -96.48
```

Fixed and random effects can be combined together to create more complex linear combinations. For example, the following linear combination considers the sum of the effect of material A, position 1 and run 2:

```
lc.eff <- inla.make.lincomb(materialA = 1, position = c(1, NA, NA, NA),
  run = c(NA, 1, NA, NA))
m0.eff <- inla.hyperpar(inla(f.wear, data = abrasion, lincomb = lc.eff,
  control.fixed = list(prec = 0.001^2)))
summary(m0.eff)
```

```
##
## Call:
##    "inla(formula = f.wear, data = abrasion, lincomb = lc.eff,
##    control.fixed = list(prec = 0.001^2))"
## Time used:
```

```
##      Pre = 1.13, Running = 0.275, Post = 0.0706, Total = 1.47
## Fixed effects:
##              mean    sd 0.025quant 0.5quant 0.975quant  mode kld
## materialA 265.7 9.773      246.1    265.7      285.2 265.7   0
## materialB 219.9 9.773      200.3    219.9      239.5 219.9   0
## materialC 241.7 9.773      222.1    241.7      261.2 241.7   0
## materialD 230.4 9.773      210.8    230.4      250.0 230.4   0
##
## Linear combinations (derived):
##    ID  mean    sd 0.025quant 0.5quant 0.975quant  mode kld
## lc  1 253.9 5.746      242.8    253.7      265.9 253.5   0
##
## Random effects:
##   Name      Model
##     position IID model
##     run IID model
##
## Model hyperparameters:
##                                            mean    sd 0.025quant 0.5quant
## Precision for the Gaussian observations 0.022 0.011      0.006    0.020
## Precision for position                  0.008 0.006      0.001    0.006
## Precision for run                       0.009 0.007      0.001    0.007
##                                         0.975quant  mode
## Precision for the Gaussian observations   0.048 0.016
## Precision for position                    0.025 0.004
## Precision for run                         0.027 0.005
##
## Expected number of effective parameters(stdev): 9.34(0.428)
## Number of equivalent replicates : 1.71
##
## Marginal log-Likelihood:  -96.48
```

6.4   Several likelihoods

So far, we have considered models with a single likelihood but INLA can handle models with more than one likelihood. This is useful to define joint models (see Chapter 10) in which one likelihood models survival time and the second one models longitudinal data. The first likelihood will be that of a survival model, while the second one will be of the types used to model longitudinal data.

When using several likelihoods data must be stored in a very particular way. First of all, the response variable must be a matrix with as many columns as likelihoods. Hence, the first column will be the response used by the first likelihood and so on. Data must be stored so that there is one variable per column and a single value of any of the variables per row. All the empty elements in the matrix are set to NA.

For example, let us consider a joint model with response variables $\mathbf{y} = (y_1 \ldots, y_n)$ and $\mathbf{z} = (z_1, \ldots, z_m)$. Then, data must be stored in a matrix like the following:

$$\begin{bmatrix} y_1 & \text{NA} \\ \vdots & \text{NA} \\ y_n & \text{NA} \\ \text{NA} & z_1 \\ \text{NA} & \vdots \\ \text{NA} & z_m \end{bmatrix}$$

Note that the dimension of this matrix is $(n + m) \times 2$, i.e., the number of rows is the total number of observations and the number of columns is equal to the number of variables. This can be easily generalized to any number of response variables.

When multiple likelihoods are used in a model, these are passed in a vector to argument `family`. For example, the following code could be used to fit a model with a Gaussian and a Poisson likelihood:

```
family = c("gaussian", "poisson")
```

As stated above, the response variables need to be formatted in a particular way. A matrix with as many likelihoods as columns is required. The number of rows is the total number of observations for all likelihoods. If in the example above there are 30 observations from a Gaussian likelihood and 20 from a Poisson one, then the response must be a matrix with 2 columns and 50 rows.

Then, observations are stacked in a matrix so that the observations from the Gaussian likelihood are in the first column and rows 1 to 30. Then, observations for the Poisson likelihood are in the second column and rows 31 to 50. All the other elements in the matrix are filled with `NA`. This ensures that every row has only a single observed value. Note that then there is an implicit index from 1 to 50 to identify each one of the observations, regardless of the likelihood they belong to.

In order to define the model, all terms for both likelihoods need to be included in the linear predictor. Hence, when defining indices for the latent random effects, this can go (for example) from 1 to the total number of rows in the response matrix. When a covariate only affects observations in a single likelihood, the values for the observations in the other likelihoods must be set to `NA`. Similarly, the indices of the latent random effects must be set to `NA` for those observations that do not depend on the latent random effect.

6.4.1 Simulated example

To illustrate the use of several likelihoods we will develop an example here using two (independent) variables from a Gaussian and Poisson likelihood, respectively. First of all, 30 observations from a standard Gaussian distribution and 20 observations from a Poisson with mean 10 will be drawn:

```
set.seed(314)
# Gaussian data
d1 <- rnorm(30)

# Poisson data
d2 <- rpois(20, 10)
```

Next, the two response variables will be put in a 2-column matrix as required by INLA:

```
# Data
d <- matrix(NA, ncol = 2, nrow = 30 + 20)
d[1:30, 1] <- d1
d[30 + 1:20, 2] <- d2
```

In order to have two different intercepts in the model it is necessary to add them as two separate covariates. In this case, both intercepts have all values equal to one, but the same principle would apply when two separate coefficients are required for the same covariate or when random effects only apply to data in one the likelihoods. Values NA mean that the covariate does not appear in the linear predictor of the response.

```
# Define a different intercept for each likelihood
Intercept1 <- c(rep(1, 30), rep(NA, 20))
Intercept2 <- c(rep(NA, 30), rep(1, 20))
```

If the coefficient is to be the same, shared between both likelihoods, then the covariate is replicated as many times as likelihoods in the model, so that it is a vector. For example, the next variable x will be shared by both terms because it is a vector of simulated data of length 50 (the total number of observations):

```
x <- rnorm(30 + 20)
```

Finally, the model is defined and fit below. Note how the data is now passed using a list as a data.frame would not be suitable in this case because the response is a matrix.

```
mult.lik <- inla(Y ~ -1 + I1 + I2 + x,
  data = list(Y = d, I1 = Intercept1, I2 = Intercept2, x = x),
  family = c("gaussian", "poisson"))

summary(mult.lik)
```

```
##
## Call:
##    c("inla(formula = Y ~ -1 + I1 + I2 + x, family = c(\"gaussian\",
##    \"poisson\"), ", " data = list(Y = d, I1 = Intercept1, I2 =
##    Intercept2, x = x))" )
## Time used:
##     Pre = 1.01, Running = 0.0998, Post = 0.0589, Total = 1.17
## Fixed effects:
##       mean    sd 0.025quant 0.5quant 0.975quant    mode kld
## I1 -0.316 0.161     -0.635   -0.316      0.003 -0.316   0
## I2  2.222 0.077      2.067    2.223      2.369  2.225   0
## x   0.021 0.071     -0.118    0.021      0.159  0.021   0
##
## Model hyperparameters:
##                                           mean    sd 0.025quant 0.5quant
## Precision for the Gaussian observations   1.36 0.346      0.769     1.33
```

```
##                                       0.975quant mode
## Precision for the Gaussian observations    2.12 1.27
##
## Expected number of effective parameters(stdev): 3.00(0.00)
## Number of equivalent replicates : 16.66
##
## Marginal log-Likelihood:  -117.94
```

Note that the second intercept (for the Poisson likelihood) is close to the logarithm of the actual mean and not the actual mean of the Poisson likelihood. Also, there is a single coefficient for x because it is shared by both parts of the model. The point estimate is very close to zero because the covariate had no effect on the response when the data were simulated.

6.5 Shared terms

When a model with several likelihoods is defined, it may be necessary to share some terms among the different parts of the model. This can be implemented using the `copy` and `replicate` features. In both cases the linear predictors of the different likelihoods will share the same type of latent effect. The main differences between the `copy` and `replicate` features is that with the `copy` effect the values of the random effects are the same but copied effects can be scaled by a parameter. This also means that all copies of the random effects will share the same hyperparameters. The `replicate` effect will have different hyperparameters for each replicate of the effect. These two features are described in more detail below.

6.5.1 Copy feature

The `copy` feature allows for the inclusion of a shared term among several linear predictors. In practice, this is implemented by defining the effect as part of a linear predictor and then making a copy of it in another linear predictor. The copy is the copied effect plus some tiny noise. Optionally, the copied effect can be multiplied by a scale parameter that can be set to a fixed value or estimated from the data.

More formally, let's assume that we have a latent effect $\mathbf{u} = (u_1, \ldots, u_p)$, where p is the length of the latent effect. Then, the copied effect $\mathbf{u}^*$ is defined to be

$$u_j^* = \beta u_{j(i)} + \varepsilon_j, \; j = 1, \ldots, n$$

Here, n is the number of data observations, and $j(i)$ is the index (between 1 and p) of the copied latent effect. Note that the copied effect does not necessarily have the same indexing as the original effect and that, in fact, only parts of it can be copied. ε_j is a tiny error that is added with a large precision for computational reasons. This precision is set in option `precision` in the call to the `f()` function when the copied effect is defined, with a default value of $\exp(14)$ (see Chapter 3).

Note that several copies of the same effect can be made and that all these effects (e.g., original and copies) will share the same hyperparameters. This means that the effect will be estimated from all the data observations that share this effect.

The `copy` effect is defined as:

```
f(idx2, copy = "idx")
```

Here, `"idx"` is the name of the index variable used in the original effect (as a character variable) and `idx2` is another index that must take values in the same set as `idx`. However, the values in `idx2` do not necessarily have the same ordering and that only the elements of **u** indexed in `idx2` will be copied.

Coefficient β of the copied effects can be estimated or set to a fixed number by using argument `hyper` to define its prior distribution (see Chapter 5 for details). By setting `fixed` to `TRUE` in the definition of the prior, β will be set to the value specified in `initial`. Table 6.4 shows the default values of the prior on β, which is setting the hyperparameter to a fixed value of 1. Thus, the part of the definition that sets a Gaussian prior distribution with parameters 1 and 10 is ignored (unless `fixed` is set to `FALSE`).

TABLE 6.4: Default values of the prior setting for parameter β of the `copy` latent effect.

Argument	Default value
initial	1
fixed	TRUE
prior	"normal"
params	c(1, 10)

As a simple example on the use of the `copy` feature we will use a simulated dataset that shares a common coefficient. The data set is made of Gaussian and Poisson observations that depend on a common covariate. In particular, this is the model:

$$y_i \sim N(\mu_i, \tau = 1) \quad i = 1, \dots, 150$$
$$\mu_i = 2 \cdot x_i \quad i = 1, \dots, 150$$
$$y_i \sim Po(\lambda_i) \quad i = 151, \dots, 200$$
$$\log(\lambda) = 2 \cdot x_i \quad i = 151, \dots, 200$$

Note that in this case, the copied effect is the coefficient of covariate x_i in the linear predictors. This coefficient is the same in the two parts of the model and parameter β of the `copy` effect should be close to 1.

First of all, data are simulated from the model above:

```
set.seed(271)
#Covariate
xx <- runif(200, 1, 2)
#Gaussian data
y.gaus <- rnorm(150, mean = 2 * xx[1:150])
#Poisson data
y.pois <- rpois(50, lambda = exp(2 * xx[151:200]))
```

Note that in the previous code the mean of the Poisson takes into account that the effect of the covariate included in the linear predictor is linked to the mean using a non-linear function.

Next, the response variable must be stored in a two-column matrix as this is a model with two likelihoods (see Section 6.4).

```
y <- matrix(NA, ncol = 2, nrow = 200)
y[1:150, 1] <- y.gaus
y[151:200, 2] <- y.pois
```

Note that in order to be able to use the `copy` feature, the latent effect must be defined through the `f()` function. Hence, the latent effect will be an `iid` with an index vector with all values equal to 1, which will be the coefficient of the covariate. For this reason, the values of the covariates are introduced as weights in the latent effect inside the `f()` function. This requires the creation of two indices for the Gaussian and Poisson observations:

```
idx.gaus <- c(rep(1, 150), rep(NA, 50))
idx.pois <- c(rep(NA, 150), rep(1, 50))
```

Note that index `idx.gaus` is 1 for all Gaussian observations and `NA` for the Poisson ones. This makes that the latent effect defined with this one only affect the Gaussian observations. Index `idx.pois` works in a similar way but only affects the Poisson observations.

Given that both indices only have a single value, the latent effect will only be u_1, that appears in the linear predictor multiplying covariate x_i, i.e., the linear predictor in the Gaussian likelihood will be $u_1 \cdot x_i$. The copied part of the model will then be $\beta \cdot (u_1 \cdot x_i)$, in the linear predictor of the Poisson likelihood. Note that in the example we also want to estimate β; we need to set `fixed` to `FALSE` in its prior definition so that it is actually estimated.

Finally, the model is fit with `INLA`. The call to `inla()` and summary of the resulting model are:

```
m.copy <- inla(y ~ -1 + f(idx.gaus, xx, model = "iid") +
  f(idx.pois, xx, copy = "idx.gaus",
    hyper = list(beta = list(fixed = FALSE))),
  data = list(y = y, xx = xx),
  family = c("gaussian", "poisson")
)
summary(m.copy)
```

```
##
## Call:
##    c("inla(formula = y ~ -1 + f(idx.gaus, xx, model = \"iid\") +
##    f(idx.pois, ", " xx, copy = \"idx.gaus\", hyper = list(beta =
##    list(fixed = FALSE))), ", " family = c(\"gaussian\", \"poisson\"),
##    data = list(y = y, xx = xx))" )
## Time used:
##     Pre = 1.38, Running = 0.25, Post = 0.0642, Total = 1.7
## Random effects:
##   Name      Model
##     idx.gaus IID model
##     idx.pois Copy
##
```

```
## Model hyperparameters:
##                                                   mean    sd 0.025quant 0.5quant
## Precision for the Gaussian observations 0.984 0.113      0.778    0.979
## Precision for idx.gaus                  0.744 0.599      0.089    0.590
## Beta for idx.pois                       1.025 0.029      0.969    1.024
##                                               0.975quant  mode
## Precision for the Gaussian observations            1.22 0.969
## Precision for idx.gaus                             2.31 0.261
## Beta for idx.pois                                  1.08 1.022
##
## Expected number of effective parameters(stdev): 1.01(0.00)
## Number of equivalent replicates : 198.22
##
## Marginal log-Likelihood:  -390.85
```

The estimates of the coefficients of the model are not shown in the model summary because they are included now as a random effect. Note that parameter β of the `copy` feature has a posterior mean very close to 1.

The estimates of the coefficient (original and copy) are shown as:

```
m.copy$summary.random
```

```
## $idx.gaus
##   ID  mean      sd 0.025quant 0.5quant 0.975quant  mode       kld
## 1  1 1.987 0.05353      1.886    1.989      2.088 1.989 1.047e-06
##
## $idx.pois
##   ID  mean      sd 0.025quant 0.5quant 0.975quant  mode       kld
## 1  1 2.032 0.01604          2    2.032      2.063 2.032 6.163e-07
```

Two important things should be noted now. First of all, the estimates are almost identical, with the only difference that the effect `idx.pois` is a copy of `idx.gaus` which includes some tiny added noise. Secondly, both point estimates are very close to the actual value of the coefficient, which is 2. Hence, the model works as expected.

6.5.2   Replicate feature

The `replicate` effect is similar to the `copy` effect but now the replicated effects only share the hyperparameters. This means that the values of the random effects in the different replicates can be different. Replicates of the same latent effect are defined with argument `replicate` in the definition of the latent effect, which takes a vector of integer values with the different groups that define the replicas. Hence, the hyperparameters will be informed by all the observations but the actual estimates of the latent effects can vary between groups.

Given a set of K replicated random effects $\mathbf{u}_1, \ldots, \mathbf{u}_K$ and hyperparameters θ_r, the distribution of the random effects can be written down as

$$\mathbf{u}_k \sim f(\theta_r), \; k = 1, \ldots, K$$

Note that each of the $\mathbf{u}_k$ is a vector of values and that the hyperparameters θ_r may be a vector as well. Also, $f(\theta_r)$ represents the distribution of the random effects given the hyperparameters θ_r, that are shared by all replicated effects. Note that the length of the different $\mathbf{u}_k$ is the same as the length of the longest replicated random effect. For example, if two random effects are replicated and $\mathbf{u}_1$ is indexed from 1 to 30 and $\mathbf{u}_2$ only from 1 to 20, then $\mathbf{u}_2$ will have 10 extra elements that will not be estimated from the data (and treated as modeling missing observations).

The replicate index must take consecutive integer values starting from 1 to K, the number of replicas, and the number of replicated effects created is the maximum value in the index of the replicate effect.

The `NelPlo` dataset (Koop and Steel, 1994) in the `dlm` package (Petris et al., 2009; Petris, 2010) contains a subset of the dataset with the same name in the `tseries` package that will be used to show the use of the `replicate` feature. The two variables included in the time series measure industrial production (`ip`), using a transformation of the original time series, and stock prices (`stock.prices`), as measured by the S&P500 index. The variables in the dataset are summarized in Table 6.5.

TABLE 6.5: Variables in the `NelPlo` dataset from package `dlm`.

Variable	Description
ip	Industrial production from 1946 to 1988. Transformed from the original series by taking `100 * diff(log())`.
stock.prices	Stock prices (S&P500 index) from 1946 and 1988.

The dataset can be loaded and summarized with the following code:

```
library("dlm")
data(NelPlo, package = "dlm")
summary(NelPlo)
```

```
##       ip              stock.prices
##  Min.   :-4.390    Min.   :-5.71
##  1st Qu.: 0.261    1st Qu.:-0.58
##  Median : 1.065    Median : 1.56
##  Mean   : 0.791    Mean   : 1.67
##  3rd Qu.: 1.854    3rd Qu.: 3.71
##  Max.   : 3.914    Max.   : 8.76
```

Figure 6.1 shows the two times series in the dataset, which seem to have a similar behavior. For this reason, a model with different intercepts but replicated `ar1` latent effect will be fit. Hence, this model assumes that the temporal correlation of the data is similar.

The model will be fit using a single Gaussian likelihood so the data needs to be put as a single vector as well.

```
nelplo <- as.vector(NelPlo)
```

Next, the indices for the `ar1` latent effect and the replicate effects are defined. This is done by taking the number of year first, `n`, and then creating the required indices. The index for the `ar1` latent effect will go from 1 to n (and will be repeated once to cover both time

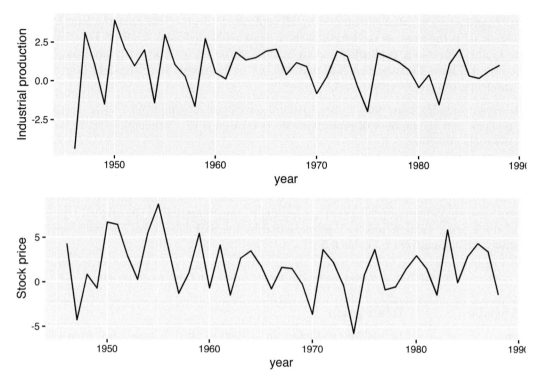

FIGURE 6.1 Time series of industrial production and stock prices in the `NelPlo` dataset.

series). The index for the `replicate` effect will go from 1 to 2, with the first n values having an index of 1 and the last n values of the data having an index of 2.

```
#Number of years
n <- nrow(NelPlo)

#Index for the ar1 latent effect
idx.ts <- rep(1:n, 2)

# Index for the replicate effect
idx.rep <- rep(1:2, each = n)
```

Two new variables are created to include two different intercepts for each part of the data:

```
# Intercepts
i1 <- c(rep(1, n), rep(NA, n))
i2 <- c(rep(NA, n), rep(1, n))
```

Finally, the model is fit as seen below. The fitted values are also computed (using the options in `control.compute`) and a vague prior on the precision of the random effects has been used (as described in Chapter 3).

```
m.rep <- inla(nelplo ~ -1 + i1 + i2 +
  f(idx.ts, model = "ar1", replicate = idx.rep,
    hyper = list(prec = list(param = c(0.001, 0.001)))),
  data = list(nelplo = nelplo, i1 = i1, i2 = i2, idx.ts = idx.ts,
    idx.rep = idx.rep),
  control.predictor = list(compute = TRUE)
)
```

```
summary(m.rep)
```

```
##
## Call:
##    c("inla(formula = nelplo ~ -1 + i1 + i2 + f(idx.ts, model =
##    \"ar1\", ", " replicate = idx.rep, hyper = list(prec = list(param
##    = c(0.001, ", " 0.001)))), data = list(nelplo = nelplo, i1 = i1,
##    i2 = i2, ", " idx.ts = idx.ts, idx.rep = idx.rep),
##    control.predictor = list(compute = TRUE))" )
## Time used:
##     Pre = 1.08, Running = 0.357, Post = 0.0681, Total = 1.51
## Fixed effects:
##      mean    sd 0.025quant 0.5quant 0.975quant  mode kld
## i1 0.789 0.381      0.030    0.790      1.538 0.793   0
## i2 1.673 0.381      0.919    1.673      2.425 1.673   0
##
## Random effects:
##   Name      Model
##     idx.ts AR1 model
##
## Model hyperparameters:
##                                                mean        sd 0.025quant
## Precision for the Gaussian observations 1.86e+04 1.83e+04    1260.409
## Precision for idx.ts                    1.71e-01 2.60e-02       0.124
## Rho for idx.ts                          1.10e-02 1.10e-01      -0.203
##                                         0.5quant 0.975quant      mode
## Precision for the Gaussian observations 1.32e+04   6.71e+04 3442.528
## Precision for idx.ts                    1.70e-01   2.28e-01     0.167
## Rho for idx.ts                          1.10e-02   2.28e-01     0.008
##
## Expected number of effective parameters(stdev): 86.00(0.002)
## Number of equivalent replicates : 1.00
##
## Marginal log-Likelihood:  -216.10
## Posterior marginals for the linear predictor and
##   the fitted values are computed
```

The model fit shows different estimates of the intercepts, which we had anticipated. However, the hyperparameters of the ar1 are shared between both time series.

Figure 6.2 shows the fitted values together with the observed values. It seems that the fitted values overfit the observed data, but see Chapter 8 and Chapter 9 for a discussion of these models and how to avoid overfitting. In general, overfitting can be avoided by setting specific priors on the model hyperparameters.

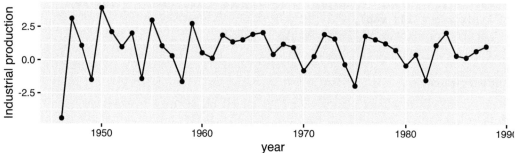

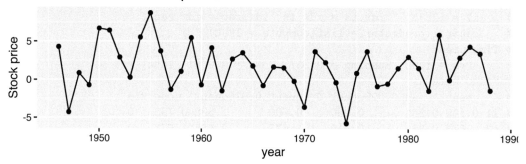

FIGURE 6.2 Fitted values (i.e., posterior means) to the variables in the `NelPlo` dataset using the `replicate` feature in INLA.

6.6   Linear constraints

As introduced in Chapter 3, additional linear constraints on the latent effects can be imposed. Given a latent effect $\mathbf{u}$, the linear constraint is defined as

$$\mathbf{A}\mathbf{u}^\top = \mathbf{e}^\top$$

where $\mathbf{A}$ is a matrix with the same number of columns as the length of the latent effect $\mathbf{u}$. Hence, the number of rows represents the number of linear constraints on the latent effect and $\mathbf{e}$ is a vector of values that is defined accordingly.

Both $\mathbf{A}$ and $\mathbf{e}$ are passed through argument `extraconstr` using a named list with values $\mathbf{A}$ and $\mathbf{e}$ in the the definition of the latent effect using function `f()`. Note that there is another argument `constr` which can be used to add a sum-to-zero constraint on the latent effect by setting it to `TRUE`. This argument is set to `TRUE` for some latent effects (such as, for example, the `rw1` and `besag` latent effects and other intrinsic effects). In case of doubt, the default option can be seen in the documentation available via the `inla.doc()` function.

TABLE 6.6: Arguments to be passed to the `f()` function to add constraints on the random effect.

Argument	Default	Description
constr	Depends on latent effect.	Add sum-to-zero constraint.
extraconstr	list(A = NULL, e = NULL)	Add extra constraints on the random effect.

Adding linear constraints is important in some cases as this makes the different effects in a model identifiable. Rue and Held (2005) describe this topic in detail. Furthermore, see Knorr-Held (2000) and Ugarte et al. (2014) on the role of imposing linear constraints to spatio-temporal latent effects, but these principles could also be applied to other types of latent effects. Also, Goicoa et al. (2018) note that adding additional constraints on the latent effects may produce different estimates than expected and caution should be taken when setting additional linear constraints.

As a simple example, we will add a sum to zero constraint to the `ar1` model fit to the `NelPLo` dataset. In this case only the industrial production will be considered. We will also remove the intercept to show the effect of constraining the random effect.

First, the matrix `A` and vector `e` need to be defined:

```
# Define values of A and e to set linear constraints
A <- matrix(1, ncol = n, nrow = 1)
e <- matrix(0, ncol = 1)
```

Next, the model is fit using argument `extraconstr` in the call to the `f()` function that defines the latent effect. Remember that the intercept has the sole purpose of making the effect of the sum-to-zero constraint more evident.

```
m.unconstr <- inla(ip ~ -1 + f(idx, model = "ar1"),
  data = list(ip = NelPlo[, 1], idx = 1:n),
  control.family = list(hyper = list(prec = list(initial = 10,
    fixed = TRUE))),
  control.predictor = list(compute = TRUE)
)
```

```
m.constr <- inla(ip ~ -1 + f(idx, model = "ar1",
    extraconstr = list(A = A, e = e)),
  data = list(ip = NelPlo[, 1], idx = 1:n),
  control.family = list(hyper = list(prec = list(initial = 10,
    fixed = TRUE))),
  control.predictor = list(compute = TRUE)
)
```

Figure 6.3 shows the estimates of the random effects from both models. Note how now imposing the sum-to-zero constraint seems to provide slightly different estimates from the unconstrained estimates. It is possible that the estimates of other parameters in the model also change as a result of imposing a constraint on the random effects, as described in Goicoa et al. (2018).

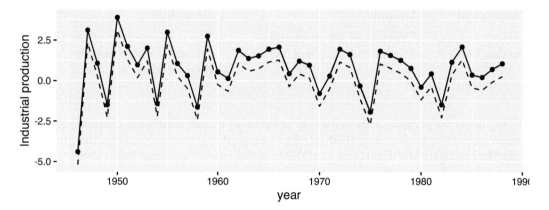

FIGURE 6.3 Comparison between two random effects estimates using a sum-to-zero constraint (solid line) and no constraint (dashed lines).

6.7   Final remarks

The features presented in this chapter can help to build more complex models using `INLA`. These are extensively used in some of the models used in other parts of the book. When the latent effect has a very complex structure that does not fit any of the latent effects described so far with the help of these additional features, there are a number of ways to implement custom latent effects for `INLA`. These methods are described in Chapter 11.

7

Spatial Models

7.1 Introduction

Many models assume that observations are obtained independently of each other. However, this is seldom the case. In Chapter 4 we have already seen how to account for correlated observations within groups. Distance between observations can also be a source of correlation. For example, in a city housing value usually changes smoothly between too contiguous neighborhoods. Pollution also shows a spatial smooth pattern and measurements close in space will likely be very similar. Also, the location of trees in a forest may follow a spatial pattern, depending on ground conditions, soil nutrients, etc.

All these examples have in common the spatial nature of the data. Observations that are close in space are likely to show similar values and a high degree of *spatial* autocorrelation. Spatial models will take into account this spatial autocorrelation in order to separate the general trend (usually depending on some covariates) from the purely spatial random variation.

Spatial statistics is traditionally divided into three main areas depending on the type of problem and data: lattice data, geostatistics and point patterns (Cressie, 2015). Sometimes, spatial data is also measured over time and spatio-temporal models can be proposed (Cressie and Wikle, 2011). In the next sections models for the different types of spatial data will be considered. In Section 8.6 models for spatio-temporal data will be described. Blangiardo and Cameletti (2015) and Krainski et al. (2018) provide a thorough description of most of the models described in this section. Bivand et al. (2013) and Lovelace et al. (2019) provide general description on handling spatial data in R and are recommended reads.

Spatial models for spatial data are introduced in Section 7.2. Geostatistical models for continuous spatial processes are presented in Section 7.3. Next, the analysis of point patterns is described in 7.4.

7.2 Areal data

Areal data, also known as lattice data, usually refers to data that are observed within given boundaries. For example, administrative boundaries are often used and the variables of study aggregated over these regions. Administrative boundaries will produce a lattice which will often have an irregular structure. Lattices with regular structures are difficult to find, but they may appear when spatial data come from an experiment (as described below).

In either case, spatial adjacency is often represented by a (sparse) adjacency matrix, with non-zero entries at the intersection of rows and columns of neighbouring areas. This matrix will play an important role when building spatial models as spatial correlation structures will be built upon it. In particular, spatially correlated random effects will be modeled using a multivariate Gaussian distribution with a precision matrix that depends on an adjacency matrix.

7.2.1 Regular lattice

A regular lattice occurs when areas are structured as a matrix in rows and columns. It is often the case that spatial data is in a regular lattice as a result of an experimental design or data collection structure. For example, a regular lattice is a convenient way of modeling a count process, so that the study region is divided into small squares and the number of events in each cell is recorded. Because of the spatially inhomogeneous distribution of the events, cells which are neighbors will tend to have a similar number of events and this is how spatial autocorrelation appears in these data.

The `bei` dataset in the `spatstat` package (Baddeley et al., 2015) records the locations of 3605 trees in a tropical rain forest (Condit, 1998; Condit et al., 1996; Hubbell and Foster, 1983; Møller and Waagepetersen, 2007). This is stored as a `ppp` object, that essentially contains the boundary of the study region, a 1000×500 meters region in this case, and the coordinates of the points. Furthermore, the `bei.extra` dataset includes the elevation and slope in the study region. These are available as `im` objects, which are raster images that cover the study area. Each raster is made of 201×101 pixels that represent the study area.

A regular lattice can be created from the original data by considering a matrix of 5×10 squares in which the number of trees inside is computed. The following code makes extensive use of function in the `sp` and `spatstat` packages.

First of all, dataset `bei` is loaded and converted into a `SpatialPoints` object to represent the point pattern using classes in the `sp` package:

```
library("spatstat")
library("sp")
library("maptools")

data(bei)

# Create SpatialPoints object
bei.pts <- as(bei, "SpatialPoints")
```

Next, a grid over the rectangular study region is created to count the number of trees inside each of the cells in the grid:

```
#Create grid
bei.poly <- as(as.im(bei$window, dimyx=c(5, 10)), "SpatialGridDataFrame")
bei.poly <- as(bei.poly, "SpatialPolygons")
```

Function `over()` is used now to overlay the point pattern and the cells in the grid, so that the number of points in each cell of the grid is obtained.

```
#Number of observations per cell
idx <- over(bei.pts, bei.poly)
tab.idx <- table(idx)
```

```
#Add number of trees
d <- data.frame(Ntrees = rep(0, length(bei.poly)))
row.names(d) <- paste0("g", 1:length(bei.poly))
d$Ntrees[as.integer(names(tab.idx))] <- tab.idx
```

Finally, a `SpatialPolygonsDataFrame` is created by putting together the polygon representation of the cells in the grid and the number of trees in each cell:

```
#SpatialPolygonsDataFrame
bei.trees <- SpatialPolygonsDataFrame(bei.poly, d)
```

At this point, it is important to highlight how spatial data is internally stored in a `SpatialGridDataFrame` and the latent effects described in Table 7.1. For some models, INLA considers data sorted by column, i.e., a vector with the first column of the grid from top to bottom, followed by the second column and so on. In order to have this mapping we need to reorder the data as follows:

```
#Mapping
idx.mapping <- as.vector(t(matrix(1:50, nrow = 10, ncol = 5)))
bei.trees2 <- bei.trees[idx.mapping, ]
```

Figure 7.1 shows the order in which observations are internally stored in a `SpatialGridDataFrame` and how they are considered by the models in Table 7.1.

1	2	3	4	5	6	7	8	9	10
11	12	13	14	15	16	17	18	19	20
21	22	23	24	25	26	27	28	29	30
31	32	33	34	35	36	37	38	39	40
41	42	43	44	45	46	47	48	49	50

1	6	11	16	21	26	31	36	41	46
2	7	12	17	22	27	32	37	42	47
3	8	13	18	23	28	33	38	43	48
4	9	14	19	24	29	34	39	44	49
5	10	15	20	25	30	35	40	45	50

FIGURE 7.1 Mapping of cells in a SGDF (left) and mapping required by INLA (right).

Figure 7.2 represents the cells into which we have divided the study region, that have been colored according to the number of trees inside. Furthermore, the actual location of the points has been plotted as an extra spatial layer to assess that the counts are correct.

In addition to the counts, we will obtain summary statistics of the covariates to be used in our model fitting.

```
#Summary statistics of covariates
covs <- lapply(names(bei.extra), function(X) {
  layer <- bei.extra[[X]]
    res <- lapply(1:length(bei.trees2), function(Y) {
      summary(layer[as.owin(bei.trees2[Y, ])])})
    res <- as.data.frame(do.call(rbind, res))
```

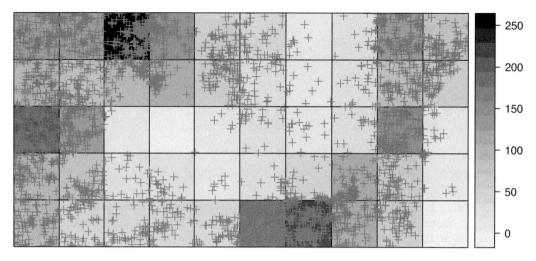

FIGURE 7.2 Spatial distribution of trees in a rain forest.

```
    names(res) <- paste0(X, ".", c("min", "1Q", "2Q", "mean", "3Q", "max"))
    return(res)
    })

covs <- do.call(cbind, covs)

#Add to SPDF
bei.trees2@data <- cbind(bei.trees2@data, covs)
```

Figure 7.3 shows the average values of the elevation and gradient in the cells. When areal data are considered, aggregating individual data over areas is useful to build regression models. However, this aggregation process may blur the underlying point process.

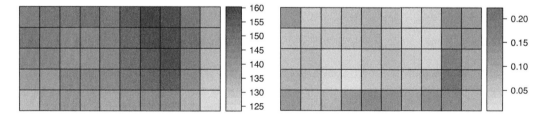

FIGURE 7.3 Average values of elevation (left) and gradient (right).

Spatial models for lattice data are often defined as random effects with a variance-covariance structure that depends on the neighborhood structure of the areas. In general, two areas will be neighbors if they share some boundaries. This could be just a single point (i.e., *queen* adjacency) or at least a segment (*rook* adjacency). For the current dataset, this is illustrated in Figure 7.4. The neighborhood structure has been obtained with function `poly2nb` from package `spdep` (Bivand and Wong, 2018), which will return an `nb` object.

```
library("spdep")
bei.adj.q <- poly2nb(bei.trees2)
bei.adj.r <- poly2nb(bei.trees2, queen = FALSE)
```

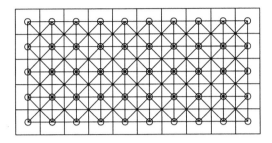 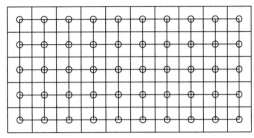

FIGURE 7.4 Queen (left) versus rook (right) adjacency.

For n regions, adjacency can be represented as a $n \times n$ matrix with non-zero entries if the regions in that row and column are neighbors. This is often represented as a binary indicator, but other types of weights can be used. Function nb2listw can be used to transform an nb object into a matrix of spatial weights using different specifications. A matrix of spatial weights will be denoted by W.

The following code will create two adjacency matrices with binary weights (style = "B") and row-standardized (style = "W"), so that the values in each row sum up to one:

```
W.bin <- nb2listw(bei.adj.q, style = "B")
W.rs <- nb2listw(bei.adj.q, style = "W")
W.bin
```

```
## Characteristics of weights list object:
## Neighbour list object:
## Number of regions: 50
## Number of nonzero links: 314
## Percentage nonzero weights: 12.56
## Average number of links: 6.28
##
## Weights style: B
## Weights constants summary:
##    n   nn  S0  S1   S2
## B 50 2500 314 628 8488
```

```
W.rs
```

```
## Characteristics of weights list object:
## Neighbour list object:
## Number of regions: 50
## Number of nonzero links: 314
## Percentage nonzero weights: 12.56
## Average number of links: 6.28
```

```
##
## Weights style: W
## Weights constants summary:
##    n   nn S0    S1    S2
## W 50 2500 50 16.82 203.4
```

Spatial latent effects are multivariate Gaussian distribution with zero mean and precision matrix $\tau\Sigma$, where τ is an hyperparameter (i.e., the precision) and Σ a matrix that depends on the spatial adjacency matrix W. Depending on the complexity of the spatial effect, matrix Σ may also depend on further hyperparameters (Banerjee et al., 2014).

A summary of the main spatial latent effects available in INLA for regular lattice data is available in Table 7.1.

TABLE 7.1: Latent models in INLA for regular lattice data.

Model	Precision
rw2d	Random walk of order 2.
matern2d	Gaussian field with Matérn correlation.

First of all, non-spatial models using the covariates and i.i.d. Gaussian random effects will be fit. This will serve as a baseline in order to assess whether spatial dependence is really needed in the model.

```
library("INLA")

#Log-Poisson regression
m0 <- inla(Ntrees ~ elev.mean + grad.mean, family = "poisson",
  data = as.data.frame(bei.trees2) )

#Log-Poisson regression with random effects
bei.trees2$ID <- 1:length(bei.trees2)
m0.re <- inla(Ntrees ~ elev.mean + grad.mean + f(ID), family = "poisson",
  data = as.data.frame(bei.trees2) )
```

As noted above, INLA assumes that the lattice is stored by columns, i.e., a vector with the first column, then followed by the second column and so on. Hence, a proper mapping between the spatial object with the data and the data.frame used in the call to inla is required.

In this case, data have already been reordered to the right mapping and the model can be fitted:

```
#RW2d
m0.rw2d <- inla(Ntrees ~ elev.mean + grad.mean +
    f(ID, model = "rw2d", nrow = 5, ncol = 10),
  family = "poisson", data = as.data.frame(bei.trees2),
  control.predictor = list(compute = TRUE),
  control.compute = list(dic = TRUE) )
```

```
summary(m0.rw2d)
```

```
##
## Call:
##    c("inla(formula = Ntrees ~ elev.mean + grad.mean + f(ID, model =
##    \"rw2d\", ", " nrow = 5, ncol = 10), family = \"poisson\", data =
##    as.data.frame(bei.trees2), ", " control.compute = list(dic =
##    TRUE), control.predictor = list(compute = TRUE))" )
## Time used:
##       Pre = 1.13, Running = 0.137, Post = 0.0663, Total = 1.34
## Fixed effects:
##                 mean    sd 0.025quant 0.5quant 0.975quant    mode kld
## (Intercept) -10.862 7.781    -26.360  -10.821      4.392 -10.736   0
## elev.mean     0.094 0.053     -0.010    0.094      0.200   0.094   0
## grad.mean    12.652 3.566      5.618   12.647     19.703  12.637   0
##
## Random effects:
##   Name      Model
##     ID Random walk 2D
##
## Model hyperparameters:
##                   mean    sd 0.025quant 0.5quant 0.975quant mode
## Precision for ID 0.242 0.066      0.135    0.235      0.393 0.22
##
## Expected number of effective parameters(stdev): 45.08(0.862)
## Number of equivalent replicates : 1.11
##
## Deviance Information Criterion (DIC) ...............: 385.18
## Deviance Information Criterion (DIC, saturated) ....: 109.39
## Effective number of parameters ....................: 45.27
##
## Marginal log-Likelihood:  -319.68
## Posterior marginals for the linear predictor and
##   the fitted values are computed
```

```
#Matern2D
m0.m2d <- inla(Ntrees ~ elev.mean + grad.mean +
    f(ID, model = "matern2d", nrow = 5, ncol = 10),
  family = "poisson", data = as.data.frame(bei.trees2),
  control.predictor = list(compute = TRUE) )
```

```
summary(m0.m2d)
```

```
##
## Call:
##    c("inla(formula = Ntrees ~ elev.mean + grad.mean + f(ID, model =
##    \"matern2d\", ", " nrow = 5, ncol = 10), family = \"poisson\",
##    data = as.data.frame(bei.trees2), ", " control.predictor =
##    list(compute = TRUE))")
```

```
## Time used:
##     Pre = 1.11, Running = 0.253, Post = 0.0657, Total = 1.43
## Fixed effects:
##                 mean    sd 0.025quant 0.5quant 0.975quant    mode kld
## (Intercept) -8.470 3.976   -16.444   -8.424    -0.756 -8.336   0
## elev.mean    0.079 0.028     0.026    0.079     0.134  0.078   0
## grad.mean   14.128 3.353     7.594   14.099    20.819 14.044   0
##
## Random effects:
##   Name     Model
##     ID Matern2D model
##
## Model hyperparameters:
##                     mean    sd 0.025quant 0.5quant 0.975quant  mode
## Precision for ID 0.417 0.254     0.064    0.373     0.997 0.202
## Range for ID     6.985 4.088     3.035    5.782    17.924 4.114
##
## Expected number of effective parameters(stdev): 45.94(0.718)
## Number of equivalent replicates : 1.09
##
## Marginal log-Likelihood:  -274.24
## Posterior marginals for the linear predictor and
##   the fitted values are computed
```

Once the models have been fit, the posterior means of the fitted values are added to the SpatialPolygonsDataFame for plotting:

```
bei.trees2$RW2D <- m0.rw2d$summary.fitted.values[, "mean"]

bei.trees2$MATERN2D <- m0.m2d$summary.fitted.values[, "mean"]
```

As a summary of the fit models, Figure 7.5 shows the posterior means of the spatial random effects for the rw2d and matern2d models. The results support the hypothesis of a non-uniform distribution of the trees in the region.

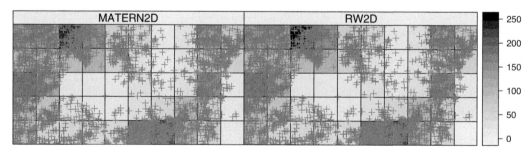

FIGURE 7.5 Posterior means of fitted values for regular lattices for the bei dataset.

7.2.2 Irregular lattice

Lattice data are seldom in a regular grid. For example, administrative boundaries usually lead to an irregular lattice. The `boston` dataset, available in the `spData` package, records housing values in Boston census tracts (Harrison and Rubinfeld, 1978) corrected for a few errors (Gilley and Pace, 1996) and including longitude and latitude of the observations (Bivand, 2017). Table 7.2 describes the variables in the dataset.

TABLE 7.2: Summary of some variables in the `boston` dataset, obtained from the its manual page.

Variable	Description
TOWN	Town name
CMEDV	Corrected median of owner-occupied housing (in USD 1,000)
CRIM	Crime per capita
ZN	Proportions of residential land zoned for lots over 25,000 sq. ft per town
INDUS	Proportions of non-retail business acres per town
CHAS	Whether the tract borders Charles river (1 = yes, 0 = no)
NOX	Nitric oxides concentration (in parts per 10 million)
RM	Average number of rooms per dwelling
AGE	Proportions of owner-occupied units built prior to 1940
DIS	Weighted distances to five Boston employment centres
RAD	Index of accesibility to radial highways per town
TAX	Full-value property-tax rate per USD 10,000 per town
PTRATIO	Pupil-teacher ratios per town
B	$1000 * (Bk - 0.63)^2$, where Bk is the proportion of blacks
LSTAT	Percentage values of lower status population

This dataset is available as a shapefile in the `spData` package, that can be loaded as follows:

```
library("rgdal")
boston.tr <- readOGR(system.file("shapes/boston_tracts.shp",
  package="spData")[1])
```

In order to compute the adjacency matrix, function `poly2nb` can be used:

```
boston.adj <- poly2nb(boston.tr)
```

By default, it will create a binary adjacency matrix, so that two regions are neighbors only if they share at least one point in common boundary (i.e., it is a *queen* adjacency). Figure 7.6 shows Boston census tracts in the data and the adjacency matrix.

Because of the irregular nature of the adjacency structure of the census tracts, the models introduced in the previous section cannot be used. Furthermore, binary and row-standardized adjacency matrices will be computed as they will be needed by the spatial models presented below:

```
W.boston <- nb2mat(boston.adj, style = "B")
W.boston.rs <- nb2mat(boston.adj, style = "W")
```

This dataset contains a few censored observations in the response, which correspond to tracts with a higher median housing value then $50,000. For this reason, we will set all values equal to 50.0 to NA. This means that these areas will not be used for model fitting, but the predictive distribution will be computed by INLA so that inference on the housing value in these areas is still possible. See Section 12.3 for more details about how the predictive distribution is computed.

```
boston.tr$CMEDV2 <- boston.tr$CMEDV
boston.tr$CMEDV2 [boston.tr$CMEDV2 == 50.0] <- NA
```

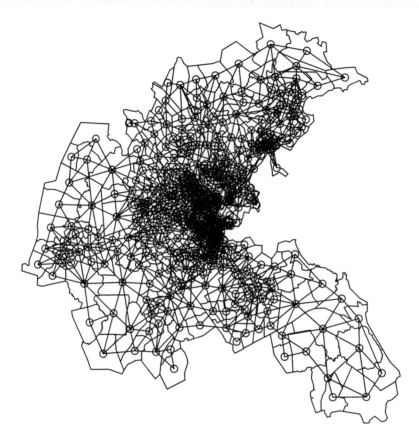

FIGURE 7.6 Boston tracts and adjacency matrix.

The model that we will be fitting will consider the response in the log-scale as this will make the response less skewed. The formula with the 13 covariates included in the model can be seen below. This is similar to the analysis performed in Harrison and Rubinfeld (1978) but other random effects will be considered as well to illustrate the use of the different models. In addition, a new column with the a region ID will be added to be used when defining random effects.

```
boston.form  <- log(CMEDV2) ~ CRIM + ZN + INDUS + CHAS + I(NOX^2) + I(RM^2) +
    AGE + log(DIS) + log(RAD) + TAX + PTRATIO + B + log(LSTAT)
boston.tr$ID <- 1:length(boston.tr)
```

First of all, a model with i.i.d. random effects will be fit to the data. This will provide a baseline to assess whether spatial random effects are really required when modeling these

data. The estimates of the random effects (i.e., posterior means) will be added to the
SpatialPolygonsDataFrame to be plotted later.

```
boston.iid <- inla(update(boston.form, . ~. + f(ID, model = "iid")),
  data = as.data.frame(boston.tr),
  control.compute = list(dic = TRUE, waic = TRUE, cpo = TRUE),
  control.predictor = list(compute = TRUE)
)
summary(boston.iid)
```

```
##
## Call:
##    c("inla(formula = update(boston.form, . ~ . + f(ID, model =
##    \"iid\")), ", " data = as.data.frame(boston.tr), control.compute =
##    list(dic = TRUE, ", " waic = TRUE, cpo = TRUE), control.predictor
##    = list(compute = TRUE))" )
## Time used:
##     Pre = 1.74, Running = 2.52, Post = 0.116, Total = 4.37
## Fixed effects:
##               mean    sd 0.025quant 0.5quant 0.975quant   mode kld
## (Intercept)  4.376 0.151      4.079    4.376      4.673  4.376   0
## CRIM        -0.011 0.001     -0.013   -0.011     -0.009 -0.011   0
## ZN           0.000 0.000     -0.001    0.000      0.001  0.000   0
## INDUS        0.001 0.002     -0.003    0.001      0.006  0.001   0
## CHAS1        0.056 0.034     -0.011    0.056      0.123  0.056   0
## I(NOX^2)    -0.540 0.108     -0.751   -0.540     -0.329 -0.540   0
## I(RM^2)      0.007 0.001      0.005    0.007      0.010  0.007   0
## AGE          0.000 0.001     -0.001    0.000      0.001  0.000   0
## log(DIS)    -0.143 0.032     -0.207   -0.143     -0.080 -0.143   0
## log(RAD)     0.082 0.018      0.047    0.082      0.118  0.082   0
## TAX          0.000 0.000     -0.001    0.000      0.000  0.000   0
## PTRATIO     -0.031 0.005     -0.040   -0.031     -0.021 -0.031   0
## B            0.000 0.000      0.000    0.000      0.001  0.000   0
## log(LSTAT)  -0.329 0.027     -0.382   -0.329     -0.277 -0.329   0
##
## Random effects:
##   Name      Model
##      ID IID model
##
## Model hyperparameters:
##                                           mean   sd 0.025quant 0.5quant
## Precision for the Gaussian observations  73.89 8.51      57.33    73.98
## Precision for ID                         64.25 6.85      52.59    63.58
##                                          0.975quant  mode
## Precision for the Gaussian observations       90.50 74.79
## Precision for ID                              79.40 61.93
##
## Expected number of effective parameters(stdev): 281.92(87.93)
## Number of equivalent replicates : 1.74
##
## Deviance Information Criterion (DIC) ...............: -565.61
```

```
## Deviance Information Criterion (DIC, saturated) ....: 657.62
## Effective number of parameters ....................: 227.57
##
## Watanabe-Akaike information criterion (WAIC) ...: -486.03
## Effective number of parameters .................: 238.63
##
## Marginal log-Likelihood:   36.79
## CPO and PIT are computed
##
## Posterior marginals for the linear predictor and
##   the fitted values are computed
```

Note that the model is fit on the logarithm of CMEDV2. Hence, in order to make inference about CMEDV2 directly, the posterior marginals of the fitted values need to be transform with function inla.tmarginal() and then the posterior mean computed with inla.emarginal() (see Section 2.6 for details on manipulating marginals distributions). A new function tmarg() will be created to be used by other models as well.

```
# Use 4 cores to process marginals in parallel
library("parallel")
options(mc.cores = 4)
# Transform marginals and compute posterior mean
#marginals: List of `marginals.fitted.values` from inla model
tmarg <- function(marginals) {
  post.means <- mclapply(marginals, function (marg) {
  # Transform post. marginals
  aux <- inla.tmarginal(exp, marg)
  # Compute posterior mean
  inla.emarginal(function(x) x, aux)
  })

  return(as.vector(unlist(post.means)))
}


# Add posterior means to the SpatialPolygonsDataFrame

boston.tr$IID <- tmarg(boston.iid$marginals.fitted.values)
```

Regarding spatial models for data in an irregular lattice, Table 7.3 summarizes some of the models available in INLA.

TABLE 7.3: Latent models in INLA for irregular lattice data.

Model	Precision
besagproper	Proper version of Besag's spatial model
besag	Besag's spatial model (improper prior)
bym	Convolution model, i.e., besag plus iid models

Three models will be considered: Besag's proper spatial model, Besag's improper spatial model and the one by Besag, York and Mollié, that is a convolution of an intrinsic CAR model and i.i.d. Gaussian model:

```
#Besag's improper
boston.besag <- inla(update(boston.form, . ~. +
    f(ID, model = "besag", graph = W.boston)),
  data = as.data.frame(boston.tr),
  control.compute = list(dic = TRUE, waic = TRUE, cpo = TRUE),
  control.predictor = list(compute = TRUE)
)
boston.tr$BESAG <- tmarg(boston.besag$marginals.fitted.values)


#Besag proper
boston.besagprop <- inla(update(boston.form, . ~. +
    f(ID, model = "besagproper", graph = W.boston)),
  data = as.data.frame(boston.tr),
  control.compute = list(dic = TRUE, waic = TRUE, cpo = TRUE),
  control.predictor = list(compute = TRUE)
)
boston.tr$BESAGPROP <- tmarg(boston.besagprop$marginals.fitted.values)


#BYM
boston.bym <- inla(update(boston.form, . ~. +
    f(ID, model = "bym", graph = W.boston)),
  data = as.data.frame(boston.tr),
  control.compute = list(dic = TRUE, waic = TRUE, cpo = TRUE),
  control.predictor = list(compute = TRUE)
)
boston.tr$BYM <- tmarg(boston.bym$marginals.fitted.values)
```

A convenient model when the aim is to assess spatial dependence in the data is the one proposed in Leroux et al. (1999). In this model, the structure of the precision matrix is a convex combination of an identity matrix I (to represent i.i.d. spatial effect) and the precision of an intrinsic CAR Q (to represent a spatial pattern):

$$(1 - \lambda)I + \lambda Q$$

Parameter λ lies between 0 and 1 and it controls the amount of spatial structure in the data. Small values indicate a non-spatial pattern, while large values indicate a strong spatial pattern.

Although this model is not directly implemented in INLA it can be noted that it is possible to fit this model using the generic1 (see Section 3.3) by taking matrix C equal to $I - Q$, where Q is the precision matrix of an intrinsic CAR specification (Ugarte et al., 2014; Bivand et al., 2015).

```
Q <- Diagonal(x = sapply(boston.adj, length))
for(i in 2:nrow(boston.tr)) {
  Q[i - 1, i] <- -1
  Q[i, i - 1] <- -1
}

C <- Diagonal(x = 1, n = nrow(boston.tr)) - Q

boston.ler <- inla(update(boston.form, . ~. +
    f(ID, model = "generic1", Cmatrix = C)),
  data = as.data.frame(boston.tr),
  control.compute = list(dic = TRUE, waic = TRUE, cpo = TRUE),
  control.predictor = list(compute = TRUE)
)
boston.tr$LER <- tmarg(boston.ler$marginals.fitted.values)
```

Figure 7.7 displays the observed values of `CMEDV2` and the point estimates obtained with the different models. In the plot for `CMEDV2` a few holes can be seen, which are filled with the prediction from the different models in the other plots. In the models with spatially correlated random effects this prediction is based on the covariates plus the spatially correlated random effects.

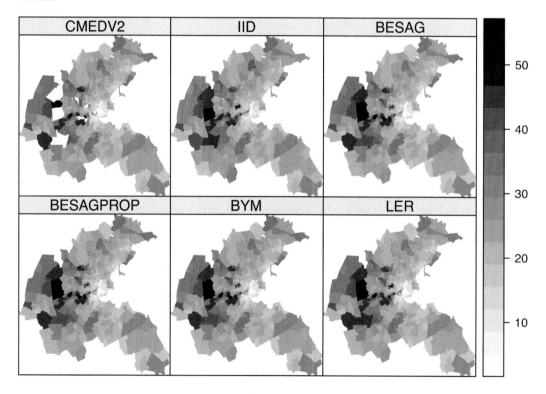

FIGURE 7.7 Summary of observed data and posterior means obtained with different models for the Boston housing dataset.

In general, all models provide similar posterior point estimates of the median housing value. For the areas with censored data, the predictive distributions also provide very similar estimates.

In terms of model selection criteria (see Section 2.4), Table 7.4 shows the different values for each model. All criteria point to the model by Leroux et al. (1999) as the best one.

TABLE 7.4: Summary of model selection criteria of the models fit to the Boston housing dataset .

Model	DIC	WAIC	CPO
iid	-565.6	-486	-158.5
besag	-2180.2	-2180	-695.3
besagproper	-2814.1	-2814	-886.4
bym	-2823.6	-2824	-928.8
leroux	-2876.5	-2877	-1006.6

7.3 Geostatistics

Geostatistics deals with the analysis of continuous processes in space. A typical example is the spatial distribution of temperature or pollutants in the air. In this case, the variable of interest is only observed at a finite number of points and statistical methods are required for estimation all over the study region.

A geostatistical process is often represented as a continuous stochastic process $y(x)$ with $x \in \mathcal{D}$, where $\mathcal{D}$ is the study region. This stochastic process is often assumed to follow a Gaussian distribution and $y(x)$ is then called a Gaussian Process (GP, Cressie, 2015).

In principle, dependence between two observations of the GP can be modeled by using an appropriate covariance function. However, quite often the GP is assumed to fulfill two important properties. First of all, the GP is assumed to be *stationary*, which means that the covariance between two points is the same even if they are shifted in space. Furthermore, the GP is assumed to be *isotropic*, which means that the correlation between two observations only depends on the distance between them. Making these two assumptions simplifies modeling of the geostatistics process as the covariance between two points will only depend on the relative distance between them regardless of their relative positions.

A commonly used covariance function is the Matérn covariance function (Cressie, 2015). The covariance of two points which are a distance d apart is:

$$C_\nu(d) = \sigma^2 \frac{2^{1-\nu}}{\Gamma(\nu)} \left(\sqrt{2\nu}\frac{d}{\rho}\right)^\nu K_\nu \left(\sqrt{2\nu}\frac{d}{\rho}\right)$$

Here, $\Gamma(\cdot)$ is the gamma function and $K_\nu(\cdot)$ is the modified Bessel function of the second kind. Parameters σ^2, ρ and ν are non-negative values of the covariance function.

Parameter σ^2 is a general scale parameter. The range of the spatial process is controlled by parameter ρ. Large values will imply a fast decay in the correlation with distance, which imply a small range spatial process. Small values will indicate a spatial process with a large range. Finally, parameter ν controls smoothness of the spatial process.

7.3.1   The `meuse` dataset

The `meuse` dataset in package `gstat` (Pebesma, 2004) contains measurements of heavy metals concentrations in the fields next to the Meuse river, near the village of Stein (The Netherlands). In addition, the `meuse.grid` dataset records several of the covariates in the `meuse` dataset in a regular grid over the study region. These can be used in order to estimate the concentration of heavy metals at any point of the study region.

TABLE 7.5: Variables in the `meuse` dataset, obtained from its manual page.

Variable	Description
x	Easting (in meters).
y	Northing (in meters).
cadmium	Topsoil cadmium concentration (in ppm).
copper	Topsoil copper concentration (in ppm).
lead	Topsoil lead concentration (in ppm).
zinc	Topsoil zinc concentration (in ppm).
elev	Relative elevation above local river bed (in meters).
dist	Distance to the Meuse river (normalized to $[0, 1]$).
om	Organic matter (in percentage).
ffreq	Flooding frequency (1 = once in two years; 2 = once in ten years; 3 = once in 50 years).
soil	Soil type (1 = Rd10A; 2 = Rd90C/VII; 3 = Bkd26/VII).
lime	Lime class (0 = absent; 1 = present).
landuse	Land use class.
dist.m	Distance to the river (in meters).

These two datasets can be loaded by following the commands listed in their respective manual pages:

```
library("gstat")
data(meuse)

summary(meuse)
```

```
##       x                y              cadmium          copper
##  Min.   :178605   Min.   :329714   Min.   : 0.20   Min.   : 14.0
##  1st Qu.:179371   1st Qu.:330762   1st Qu.: 0.80   1st Qu.: 23.0
##  Median :179991   Median :331633   Median : 2.10   Median : 31.0
##  Mean   :180005   Mean   :331635   Mean   : 3.25   Mean   : 40.3
##  3rd Qu.:180630   3rd Qu.:332463   3rd Qu.: 3.85   3rd Qu.: 49.5
##  Max.   :181390   Max.   :333611   Max.   :18.10   Max.   :128.0
##
##       lead            zinc            elev            dist
##  Min.   : 37.0   Min.   : 113   Min.   : 5.18   Min.   :0.0000
##  1st Qu.: 72.5   1st Qu.: 198   1st Qu.: 7.55   1st Qu.:0.0757
##  Median :123.0   Median : 326   Median : 8.18   Median :0.2118
##  Mean   :153.4   Mean   : 470   Mean   : 8.16   Mean   :0.2400
##  3rd Qu.:207.0   3rd Qu.: 674   3rd Qu.: 8.96   3rd Qu.:0.3641
```

```
## Max.    :654.0  Max.   :1839  Max.    :10.52  Max.    :0.8804
##
##          om      ffreq soil  lime     landuse       dist.m
## Min.    : 1.00  1:84  1:97  0:111  W       :50  Min.    :   10
## 1st Qu.: 5.30  2:48  2:46  1: 44  Ah      :39  1st Qu.:   80
## Median : 6.90  3:23  3:12         Am      :22  Median :  270
## Mean    : 7.48                    Fw      :10  Mean    :  290
## 3rd Qu.: 9.00                     Ab      : 8  3rd Qu.:  450
## Max.    :17.00                    (Other):25  Max.    :1000
## NA's    :2                        NA's    : 1
```

Next, we will create a `SpatialPointsDataFrame` and assign the data its coordinate reference system (obtained from the manual page):

```
coordinates(meuse) <- ~x+y
proj4string(meuse) <- CRS("+init=epsg:28992")
```

A similar operation will be performed on the grid. Note that now the resulting object is a `SpatialPixelsDataFrame`, which is one of the objects in the `sp` package to represent spatial grids:

```
#Code from gstat
data(meuse.grid)
coordinates(meuse.grid) = ~x+y
proj4string(meuse.grid) <- CRS("+init=epsg:28992")
gridded(meuse.grid) = TRUE
```

Note that function `proj4string` is used to set the correct coordinate reference system (CRS) for the data, which essentially sets the units of the coordinates of the points as these do not necessarily need to be longitude and latitude. In this case, the CRS is Netherlands topographical map coordinates and they are measured in meters.

7.3.2 Kriging

As a preliminary analysis of this dataset, kriging will be used to obtain an estimation of the concentration of zinc in the study region. In particular, universal kriging (Cressie, 2015; Bivand et al., 2013) will be used in order to include covariates in the prediction.

First of all, the empirical variogram will be computed using function `variogram()` and a spherical variogram fitted using function `fit.variogram`.

```
# Variogram and fit variogram
vgm <- variogram(log(zinc) ~ dist, meuse)
fit.vgm <- fit.variogram(vgm, vgm("Sph"))
```

Next, universal kriging will provide an estimate of the concentration of zinc at all points of the grid defined in `meuse.grid`. In addition to the point estimates, the square root of the prediction variance (which can be used as a measure of the error in the prediction) will be added as well.

```
# Kriging
krg <- krige(log(zinc) ~ dist, meuse, meuse.grid, model = fit.vgm)
```

```
## [using universal kriging]
```

```
#Add estimates to meuse.grid
meuse.grid$zinc.krg <- krg$var1.pred
meuse.grid$zinc.krg.sd <- sqrt(krg$var1.var)
```

Figure 7.8 shows the concentration of zinc, in the log-scale, estimated using universal kriging. The plot shows a clear spatial pattern, with higher concentrations in points closer to the Meuse river. These estimates will be compared later to other estimates obtained with spatial models fit with INLA. Note that the standard errors of the estimates have been computed and will be compared later to their analogous Bayesian estimates.

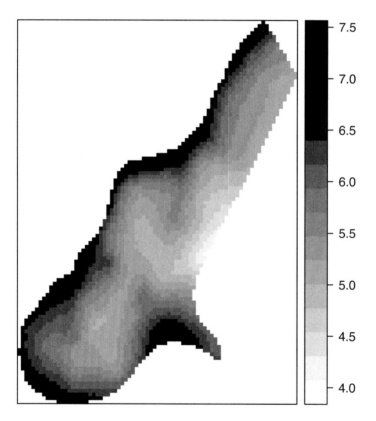

FIGURE 7.8 Concentration of zinc (log-scale) estimated with universal kriging for the meuse dataset.

7.3.3 Spatial Models using Stochastic Partial Differential Equations

Continuous spatial processes using a Matérn covariance function can be easily fitted with INLA. Lindgren et al. (2011) note that a spatial process with a Matérn covariance can be obtained as the weak solution to a stochastic partial differential equation (SPDE). Hence, they provide a solution to the equation and they are able to work with a sparse representation of the solution that fits within the INLA framework.

The solution $u(s)$ can be represented as:

$$u(s) = \sum_{k=1}^{K} \psi_k(s) w_k, \ s \in \mathcal{D}$$

In the previous equation, $\{\psi_k(s)\}_{k=1}^{K}$ is a basis of functions needed to approximate the solution and w_k are associate coefficients, which are assumed to have a Gaussian distribution.

This spatial model is implemented as the `spde` latent effect in `INLA`. However, defining this model to be used with `INLA` requires more work than previous spatial models. In particular, a mesh needs to be defined over the study region and it will be used to compute the approximation to the solution (i.e., the spatial process). Krainski et al. (2018) describe SPDE models in detail, but here we will summarize the different steps require to fit these models.

As a previous step, the boundary of the study region needs to be defined. For this, the boundaries of the pixels in the `meuse.grid` will be joined into a single region. This will provide a reasonable approximation to the boundary of the study region.

```
#Boundary
meuse.bdy <- unionSpatialPolygons(
  as(meuse.grid, "SpatialPolygons"), rep (1, length(meuse.grid))
)
```

Next, a two-dimensional mesh will be defined to define the set of basis functions using function `inla.mesh.2d()`. This will take the boundary of the study region, as well as the dimensions of the maximum edge of the triangles in the mesh and the length of the inner and outer offset.

```
#Define mesh
pts <- meuse.bdy@polygons[[1]]@Polygons[[1]]@coords
mesh <- inla.mesh.2d(loc.domain = pts, max.edge = c(150, 500),
  offset = c(100, 250) )
```

Figure 7.9 displays the boundary of the study region and the mesh created to approximate the solution of the SPDE to obtain the spatial model. A thick line separates the outer offset from the inner offset and the boundary of the study region. The figure has been obtained with the following code:

This triangulation defines the basis of functions that will be used to approximate the spatial process with Matérn covariance. In particular, the basis of functions is defined such as each function is one at a given vertex and zero outside the triangles that meet at that vertex. Hence, the functions have a compact support and they decay linearly from the vertex (where the value is 1) to the the boundary of the support (where it takes a value of zero). This means that for any given triangle in the mesh, only three functions in the basis will have non-zero values, which simplifies the computation of the estimates of the random effect at any given point because its estimate will be a linear combination of only three functions in the basis. See Chapter 2 in Krainski et al. (2018) for full details on how the basis functions are defined].

```
par(mar = c(0, 0, 0, 0))
plot(mesh, asp = 1, main = "")
lines(pts, col = 3, with = 2)
```

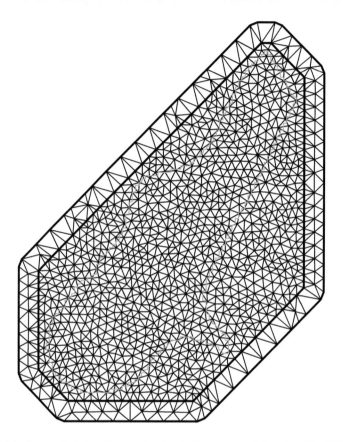

FIGURE 7.9 Mesh created for the analysis of the `meuse` dataset with INLA and SPDEs.

Function `inla.spde2.matern()` is used next to create an object for a Matérn model. Furthermore, `inla.spde.make.A` is also used to create the projector matrix A to map the projection of the SPDE to the observed points and `inla.spde.make.index` a necessary list of named index vectors for the SPDE model.

```
#Create SPDE
meuse.spde <- inla.spde2.matern(mesh = mesh, alpha = 2)
A.meuse <- inla.spde.make.A(mesh = mesh, loc = coordinates(meuse))
s.index <- inla.spde.make.index(name = "spatial.field",
  n.spde = meuse.spde$n.spde)
```

The previous steps will define how the solution to the SPDE that defined the spatial process with a Matérn covariance is computed. This will be used later when defining the spatial random effect using the `f()` function in the `formula` that defines the INLA model.

Data passed to `inla()` when a SPDE is used needs to be in a particular format. For this, the `inla.stack` function is provided. It will take data in different ways, including the SPDE indices, and arrange them conveniently for model fitting. In short, `inla.stack` will be a list with the following named elements:

- `data`: a list with data vectors.

- `A`: a list of projector matrices.

- `effects`: a list of effects (e.g., the SPDE index) or predictors (i.e., covariates).

- `tag`: a character with a label for this group of data.

For example, in order to define the data to be used for model fitting, we could do the following:

```
#Create data structure
meuse.stack <- inla.stack(data  = list(zinc = meuse$zinc),
  A = list(A.meuse, 1),
  effects = list(c(s.index, list(Intercept = 1)),
    list(dist = meuse$dist)),
  tag = "meuse.data")
```

Here, `data` is simply a list with a vector of the values of zinc. `A` is a list with projector matrix `A.meuse` (used in the spatial model) and the value 1. These two elements are associated with the two elements in `effects`, which is a list of some information about the definition of the SPDE and some effects with covariate `dist`. Finally, `tag` is a label to indicate that this is the data in the `meuse` dataset.

This is all that is required to fit the model with an intercept, a covariate (distance to the river) plus the spatial random effect defined with a SPDE. However, given that we are studying a continuous spatial process, obtaining an estimate of the variable of interest (and the underlying spatial effect) in the study region is of interest.

For this reason, another stack of data can be defined for prediction. In this case, the values of the response variable will be set to `NA` and the predictive distributions computed. In addition, a different projector matrix will be required in order to map the estimates of the spatial process to the prediction points. This can be done using function `inla.spde.make.A` as before using the points in the grid.

```
#Create data structure for prediction
A.pred <- inla.spde.make.A(mesh = mesh, loc = coordinates(meuse.grid))
meuse.stack.pred <- inla.stack(data = list(zinc = NA),
  A = list(A.pred, 1),
  effects = list(c(s.index, list (Intercept = 1)),
    list(dist = meuse.grid$dist)),
  tag = "meuse.pred")
```

Note that now a different tag (`"meuse.pred"`) has been used in order to be able to identify this part of the data in the stack to retrieve the fitted values and other quantities of interest at the grid points.

Finally, both stacks of data can be put together into a single object with `inla.stack` again. The resulting object will be the one passed to function `inla` when fitting the model.

```
#Join stack
join.stack <- inla.stack(meuse.stack, meuse.stack.pred)
```

To define the model that will be fitted, the spatial effects need to be added using the
f() function. The index passed to this function will be the one created before with
inla.spde.make.index and whose name is spatial.field. In addition, the model will be
of type spde.

```
#Fit model
form <- log(zinc) ~ -1 + Intercept + dist + f(spatial.field, model = spde)
```

Data passed to the inla function needs to be joined with the definition of the SPDE
to fit the spatial model. This is done with function inla.stack.data. Furthermore,
control.predictor will need to take the projector matrix for the whole dataset (model
fitting and prediction) using function inla.stack.A in join.stack.

```
m1 <- inla(form, data = inla.stack.data(join.stack, spde = meuse.spde),
   family = "gaussian",
   control.predictor = list(A = inla.stack.A(join.stack), compute = TRUE),
   control.compute = list(cpo = TRUE, dic = TRUE))
```

```
#Summary of results
summary(m1)
```

```
##
## Call:
##    c("inla(formula = form, family = \"gaussian\", data =
##    inla.stack.data(join.stack, ", " spde = meuse.spde),
##    control.compute = list(cpo = TRUE, dic = TRUE), ", "
##    control.predictor = list(A = inla.stack.A(join.stack), compute =
##    TRUE))" )
## Time used:
##     Pre = 1.59, Running = 7.03, Post = 0.72, Total = 9.34
## Fixed effects:
##              mean    sd 0.025quant 0.5quant 0.975quant    mode kld
## Intercept   6.598 0.168      6.267    6.595      6.945   6.589   0
## dist       -2.777 0.413     -3.585   -2.781     -1.944  -2.787   0
##
## Random effects:
##    Name      Model
##      spatial.field SPDE2 model
##
## Model hyperparameters:
##                                          mean    sd 0.025quant 0.5quant
## Precision for the Gaussian observations 13.03 3.034       8.02    12.71
## Theta1 for spatial.field                 4.77 0.260       4.26     4.76
## Theta2 for spatial.field                -5.28 0.307      -5.90    -5.28
##                                          0.975quant  mode
## Precision for the Gaussian observations       19.90 12.11
```

```
## Theta1 for spatial.field                      5.29  4.75
## Theta2 for spatial.field                     -4.69 -5.26
##
## Expected number of effective parameters(stdev): 69.26(13.39)
## Number of equivalent replicates : 2.24
##
## Deviance Information Criterion (DIC) ...............: 118.22
## Deviance Information Criterion (DIC, saturated) ....: 228.58
## Effective number of parameters ....................: 69.95
##
## Marginal log-Likelihood:   -110.05
## CPO and PIT are computed
##
## Posterior marginals for the linear predictor and
##  the fitted values are computed
```

According to the model fitted there is a clear reduction in the concentration of zinc as distance to the river increases. This is consistent with previous findings and the results from the universal kriging.

Obtaining the fitted values at the prediction points requires first getting the index for the points in the `meuse.pred` part of the stack. This can be easily done with function `inla.stack.index` (see code below). Similarly, fitted values for the `meuse.data` can be obtained. Next, the index is used to obtain the posterior means and other summary statistics computed on the predictive distributions and these added to the `meuse.grid` object for plotting.

```
#Get predicted data on grid
index.pred <- inla.stack.index(join.stack, "meuse.pred")$data

meuse.grid$zinc.spde <- m1$summary.fitted.values[index.pred, "mean"]
meuse.grid$zinc.spde.sd <- m1$summary.fitted.values[index.pred, "sd"]
```

Figure 7.10 shows the posterior means of the concentrations of zinc in the log-scale and Figure 7.11 the prediction standard deviations, which are a measure of the uncertainty about the predictions. Point estimates of the concentration seem to be very similar between universal kriging and the model fitted with INLA. However, prediction uncertainty seems to be smaller with the SPDE model. Note that here we are comparing results from two different inference methods. Furthermore, these differences in the uncertainty may be due to the different ways in which the covariance of the spatial effect is computed and a shrinkage effect due to the priors in the Bayesian model.

Besides the estimation of the concentration of zinc, studying the underlying spatial process may be of interest. For this reason, it is important to study the estimates of the parameters of the spatial effect. INLA reports summary estimates of the parameters in the internal scale, but the marginals of the variance and range parameters can be obtained using function `inla.spde2.result`. Then, summary statistics on the parameters using their respective posterior marginals can be computed with function `inla.zmarginal`.

```
#Compute statistics in terms or range and variance
spde.est <- inla.spde2.result(inla = m1, name = "spatial.field",
```

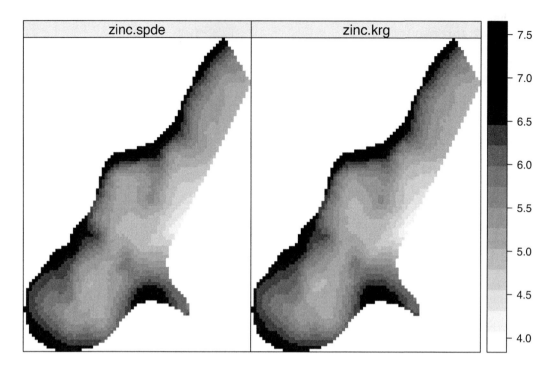

FIGURE 7.10 Posterior means of log-concentration of zinc.

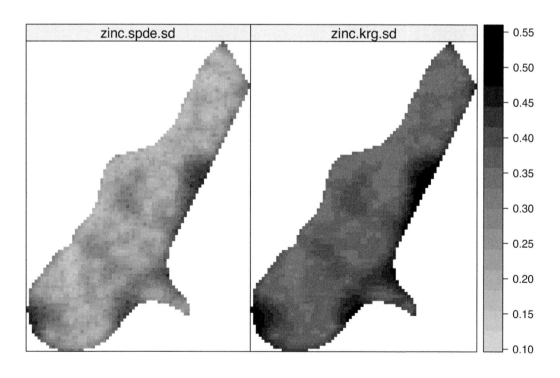

FIGURE 7.11 Posterior prediction standard deviations of log-concentration of zinc.

```
    spde = meuse.spde, do.transf = TRUE)

#Kappa
#inla.zmarginal(spde.est$marginals.kappa[[1]])
#Variance
inla.zmarginal(spde.est$marginals.variance.nominal[[1]])
```

```
## Mean               0.234397
## Stdev              0.0732946
## Quantile  0.025 0.123512
## Quantile  0.25  0.18169
## Quantile  0.5   0.223108
## Quantile  0.75  0.274691
## Quantile  0.975 0.408933
```

```
#Range
inla.zmarginal(spde.est$marginals.range.nominal[[1]])
```

```
## Mean               583.193
## Stdev              183.875
## Quantile  0.025 309.442
## Quantile  0.25  451.237
## Quantile  0.5   553.144
## Quantile  0.75  682.498
## Quantile  0.975 1025.16
```

A similar summary for the variogram used in the universal kriging can be obtained as follows:

```
#Summary stats; nugget is a 'random' effect with a variance
fit.vgm
```

```
##    model   psill range
## 1    Nug 0.07643   0.0
## 2    Sph 0.20529 728.7
```

The sill and range of the variogram are very similar to the estimates obtained for the Matérn covariance computed using SPDE. The nugget effect in the variogram can be regarded as a measurement error or the variance in the Gaussian likelihood. A rough comparison can be done between the sill of the nugget effect in the variogram and the inverse of the mode of the precision of the Gaussian likelihood:

```
#Precision of nugget term (similar to precision of error term)
1 / fit.vgm$psill[1]
```

```
## [1] 13.08
```

The resulting value is very similar to the posterior mean of the precision of the Gaussian likelihood. Hence, both universal kriging and the SPDE model provide similar estimates of the underlying spatial process.

As a final remark, it is worth mentioning that the `inlabru` package (Bachl et al., 2019) can simplify the way in which the model is defined and fit. Furthermore, the `meshbuilder()` function in the `INLA` package can help to define and assess the adequacy of a mesh in an interactive way (Krainski et al., 2018).

7.4   Point patterns

In Section 7.2 we considered the analysis of a point pattern using a discrete representation of the process. However, point patterns can also be studied as a continuous process. In particular, we will consider inhomogeneous Poisson point processes defined by a given intensity $\lambda(x)$ which varies spatially and may also be modulated by some covariates.

Hence, the intensity can be represented as

$$\lambda(x) = \lambda_0(x) \exp(\beta \mathbf{x})$$

Here, $\lambda_0(x)$ is an underlying spatial distribution modulated by a vector of covariates $\mathbf{x}$ with associated coefficients β.

The intensity can be estimated semi-parametrically by using a non-parametric estimate of $\lambda_0(x)$ (Diggle, 2013). For example, Diggle et al. (2007) use kernel smoothing to estimate $\lambda_0(x)$ and a logistic regression (conditional of the locations of the observed events) to obtain estimates of the vector of coefficients β. Below we will show how to model $\log(\lambda(x))$ using a Gaussian process to define a log-Gaussian Cox process (Krainski et al., 2018).

7.4.1   Log-Gaussian Cox processes

Simpson et al. (2016) describe the use of SPDE to estimate $\lambda(x)$ using log-Gaussian Cox models. In particular, $\lambda_0(x)$ is estimated using a SPDE, i.e.,

$$\log(\lambda_0(x)) = S(x)$$

Here, $S(x)$ is a stationary and isotropic Gaussian spatial process with a Matérn covariance. This spatial process can be estimated using the SPDE approach described in Section 7.3.

Simpson et al. (2016) show how fitting the previous model is similar to fitting a Poisson process on an extended data set using the locations of the events and the integration points of the SPDE mesh. This extended dataset needs to be created as follows:

- The value of the response is 0 at the integration points and 1 at the observed points.
- Each data point will have an associated weight, which will be 0 for the observed data and the area of its associated polygon in a Voronoi tessellation using the integration points.
- Weights required to estimate the model (see below).

The `inlabru` package (Bachl et al., 2019) provides a simple interface for the analysis of point patterns with INLA and SPDE models. However, we provide here full details on the whole process to fit the model according to Simpson et al. (2016). The construction of the expanded dataset as well as the steps required for model fitting are described in the next example. The `meshbuilder()` function in the `INLA` package can also be used to test the adequacy of the mesh created for a SPDE latent effect (see also Krainski et al., 2018).

7.4.2 Castilla-La Mancha forest fires

The `clmfires` dataset in the `spatstat` package records the occurrence of forest fires in the region of Castilla-La Mancha (Spain) from 1998 to 2007. This dataset has been put together by Prof. Jorge Mateu. and Table 7.6 provides a summary of the variables in the dataset.

TABLE 7.6: Summary of variables in the `clmfires` dataset.

Variable	Description
cause	Cause of the fire (lightning, accident, intentional or other)
burnt.area	Total area burned (in hectares)
date	Date of fire
julian.date	Date of fire, as days elapsed since 1 January 1998

Furthermore, the `clmfires.extra` dataset contains two objects with covariate information for the study region. These two objects are named `clmcov100` and `clmcov200` because they provide the information in several `im` objects (that represents raster data in the `spatstat` package) in a raster of size 100x100 and 200x200 pixels, respectively. Each one is a named list of four `im` objects with the variables in Table 7.7. Covariate `landuse` is a factor with levels: 'urban', 'farm' (which includes farms and orchards), 'meadow', 'denseforest', 'conifer' (which includes conifer forests and plantations), 'mixedforest', 'grassland', 'bush', 'scrub' and 'artifgreen' (such as golf courts).

TABLE 7.7: Summary of variables in the `clmfires.extra` dataset.

Variable	Description
elevation	Elevation of the terrain (in meters).
orientation	Orientation of the terrain (in degrees).
slope	Slope.
landuse	Land use (a factor, see text for details).

First of all, the data will be loaded and the observed points in the period 2004 to 2007 selected. This is done because of the concern about how the location of the fires was done prior to 2004.

```
library("spatstat")
data(clmfires)

#Subsect to 2004 to 2007
clmfires0407 <- clmfires[clmfires$marks$date >= "2004-01-01"]
```

Next, given that the pixels classified as `artifgreen` are just a few, we have merged this category with urban (because both are human-built):

```
# Set `urban` instead of `artifgreen`
idx <- which(clmfires.extra$clmcov100$landuse$v %in% c("artifgreen",
  "farm"))
```

```
clmfires.extra$clmcov100$landuse$v[idx] <- "urban"

# Convert to factor
clmfires.extra$clmcov100$landuse$v <-
factor(as.character(clmfires.extra$clmcov100$landuse$v))
# Set right dimension of raster object

dim(clmfires.extra$clmcov100$landuse$v) <- c(100, 100)
```

Note that the reference category now is bush so the effects of all the other levels will be relative to this category (unless the intercept is removed from the model):

```
clmfires.extra$clmcov100$landuse
```

```
## factor-valued pixel image
## factor levels:
## [1] "bush"        "conifer"     "denseforest" "grassland"   "meadow"
## [6] "mixedforest" "scrub"       "urban"
## 100 x 100 pixel array (ny, nx)
## enclosing rectangle: [-2.1, 397.9] x [-2.1, 397.9] kilometres
```

Covariates elevation and orientation are rescaled so that they are expressed in kilometers and radians. This is done in order to avoid problems when fitting the spatial model with INLA. This is particularly important for elevation because it is originally in meters.

```
#In addition, we will rescale `elevation` (to express it in kilometers) and
#`orientation` (to be in radians) so that fixed effects are better estimated:
clmfires.extra$clmcov100$elevation <-
  clmfires.extra$clmcov100$elevation / 1000
clmfires.extra$clmcov100$orientation <-
  clmfires.extra$clmcov100$orientation / (2 * pi)
```

Juan et al. (2010) provide an analysis of the forest fires in 1998 alone and they suggest analyzing this type of data using log-Gaussian Cox processes. In addition, they show that forest fires due to lightning have a different pattern. Hence, we will focus our analysis of these type of fires and subset these points from the original dataset:

```
clmfires0407 <- clmfires0407[clmfires0407$marks$cause == "lightning", ]
```

Figure 7.12 shows the boundary of Castilla-La Mancha and the location of the forest fires due to lightning. Note how most of them appear in the east part of the region.

Next, the boundary of the study region will be extracted from the ppp object and it will be used to create a mesh over the study region. This mesh will be used to estimate the latent stationary and isotropic Gaussian process with Matérn covariance using the SPDE approach in INLA.

```
clm.bdy <- do.call(cbind, clmfires0407$window$bdry[[1]])
#Define mesh
```

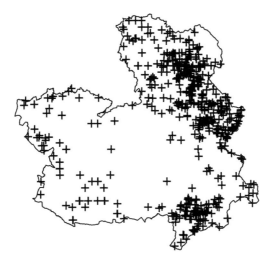

FIGURE 7.12 Location of forest fires due to a lightning in Castilla-La Mancha in the period.

```
clm.mesh <- inla.mesh.2d(loc.domain = clm.bdy, max.edge = c(15, 50),
   offset = c(10, 10))
```

As discussed before, model fitting requires an expanded dataset with the locations of the forest fires and the integration points in the mesh.

```
#Points
clm.pts <- as.matrix(coords(clmfires0407))
clm.mesh.pts <- as.matrix(clm.mesh$loc[, 1:2])
allpts <- rbind(clm.pts, clm.mesh.pts)

# Number of vertices in the mesh
nv <- clm.mesh$n
# Number of points in the data
n <- nrow(clm.pts)
```

Next, the SPDE latent effect needs to be defined. In this case, penalized complexity priors (see Section 5.4) are used for the range and standard deviation of the Matérn covariance. In particular, the prior of the range r is set by defining (r_0, p_r) such that

$$P(r < r_0) = p_r.$$

Similarly, the penalized complexity prior for the standard deviation σ is defined by pair (σ_0, p_s), such that

$$P(\sigma > \sigma_0) = p_s.$$

As a prior assumption the probability of the range being higher than 50 is small (i.e., $r_0 = 50$ and $p_r = 0.9$) and that the probability of σ being higher than 5 is also small (i.e.,

$\sigma_0 = 1$ and $p_s = 0.01$). A SPDE latent effect with this type of prior is created with function `inla.spde2.pcmatern()` as follows:

```
#Create SPDE
clm.spde <- inla.spde2.pcmatern(mesh = clm.mesh, alpha = 2,
  prior.range = c(50, 0.9), # P(range < 50) = 0.9
  prior.sigma = c(1, 0.01) # P(sigma > 10) = 0.01
)
```

See also Sørbye et al. (2019) for some comments on setting priors when fitting log-Gaussian Cox processes to point patterns using SPDEs.

The weights associated with the mesh points are equal to the area of the surrounding polygon in a Voronoi tessellation that falls inside the study region. This is computed below using packages `deldir` (Turner, 2019), `rgeos` (Bivand and Rundel, 2019) and `SDraw` (McDonald and McDonald, 2019). Note that spatial data must be in one of the objects in the `sp` package and, for this reason, the boundary is converted into a `SpatialPolygons` object and function `voronoi.polygons()` is used as it returns the Voronoi tessellation as a `SpatialPolygons` object as well.

```
library("deldir")
library("SDraw")

# Voronoi polygons (as SpatialPolygons)
mytiles <- voronoi.polygons(SpatialPoints(clm.mesh$loc[, 1:2]))

# C-LM bounday as SpatialPolygons
clmbdy.sp <- SpatialPolygons(list(Polygons(list(Polygon (clm.bdy)),
  ID = "1")))

#Compute weights
require(rgeos)

w <- sapply(1:length(mytiles), function(p) {
  aux <- mytiles[p, ]

  if(gIntersects(aux, clmbdy.sp) ) {
    return(gArea(gIntersection(aux, clmbdy.sp)))
  } else {
    return(0)
  }
})
```

Note how the sum of the weights is equal to the area of the study region:

```
# Sum of weights
sum(w)
```

```
## [1] 79355
```

```
# Area of study region
gArea(clmbdy.sp)
```

[1] 79355

Figure 7.13 shows the mesh points (black dots) as well as the resulting Voronoi tessellation and the boundary of Castilla-La Mancha. The weight associated with each point is the area of the associated Voronoi polygon inside the region of Castilla-La Mancha.

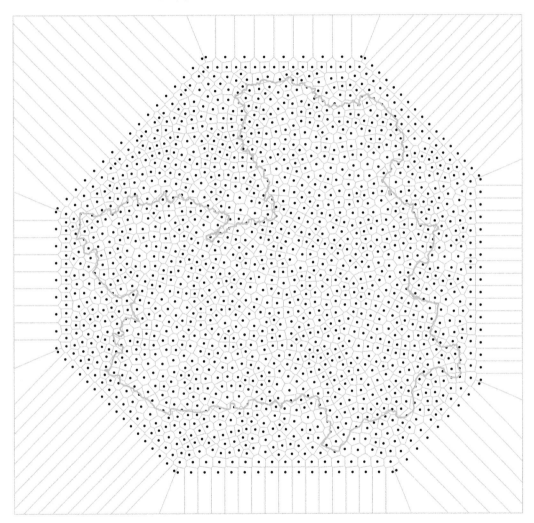

FIGURE 7.13 Voronoi tesselletation used in the analysis of forest fires in Castilla-La Mancha.

Once the weights associated with the mesh points have been computed, the expanded dataset can be put together. Values of the covariates at the integration points are required to fit the model. These are obtained from the raster data available in the `clmfires.extra` dataset.

```
#Prepare data
y.pp = rep(0:1, c(nv, n))
e.pp = c(w, rep(0, n))

lmat <- inla.spde.make.A(clm.mesh, clm.pts)
imat <- Diagonal(nv, rep(1, nv))

A.pp <-rbind(imat, lmat)

clm.spde.index <- inla.spde.make.index(name = "spatial.field",
  n.spde = clm.spde$n.spde)
```

Covariates required in the analysis are obtained by using different functions in the `spatstat` package. In particular, function `nearest.pixel()` is used below to assign to each point (in the expanded dataset) the values of the covariates of the nearest pixel in the raster object.

```
#Covariates
allpts.ppp <- ppp(allpts[, 1], allpts[, 2], owin(xrange = c(-15.87, 411.38),
  yrange = c(-1.44, 405.19)))

# Assign values of covariates to points using value of nearest pixel
covs100 <- lapply(clmfires.extra$clmcov100, function(X){
  pixels <- nearest.pixel(allpts.ppp$x, allpts.ppp$y, X)
  sapply(1:npoints(allpts.ppp), function(i) {
    X[pixels$row[i], pixels$col[i]]
  })
})
covs100$b0 <- rep(1, nv + n)
```

Once all the required data have been obtained, the data stack for model fitting is created:

```
#Create data structure
clm.stack <- inla.stack(data = list(y = y.pp, e = e.pp),
  A = list(A.pp, 1),
  effects = list(clm.spde.index, covs100),
  tag = "pp")
```

Similarly, another stack of data will be put together for prediction. This will require the locations of the points in a regular grid as well as the values of the covariates at the grid points (now using the subsetting operator in the `spatstat` package). The grid used will be the same as the one used in the raster data with the covariates.

```
#Data structure for prediction
library("maptools")
sgdf <- as(clmfires.extra$clmcov100$elevation, "SpatialGridDataFrame")
sp.bdy <- as(clmfires$window, "SpatialPolygons")
idx <- over(sgdf, sp.bdy)
spdf <- as(sgdf[!is.na(idx), ], "SpatialPixelsDataFrame")
```

```
pts.pred <- coordinates(spdf)
n.pred <- nrow(pts.pred)

#Get covariates (using subsetting operator in spatstat)
ppp.pred <- ppp(pts.pred[, 1], pts.pred[, 2], window = clmfires0407$window)
covs100.pred <- lapply(clmfires.extra$clmcov100, function(X) {
  X[ppp.pred]
})
covs100.pred$b0 <- rep(1, n.pred)

#Prediction points
A.pred <- inla.spde.make.A (mesh = clm.mesh, loc = pts.pred)
clm.stack.pred <- inla.stack(data = list(y = NA),
   A = list(A.pred, 1),
   effects = list(clm.spde.index, covs100.pred),
   tag = "pred")
```

Finally, all data stacks will be put together into a single object:

```
#Join data
join.stack <- inla.stack(clm.stack, clm.stack.pred)
```

Model fitting will be carried out similarly as in the geostatistics case. However, now the likelihood to be used in a Poisson and the weights associated to the points in the expanded dataset need to be passed using parameter E. The integration strategy is set to "eb" in order to reduce computation time (Krainski et al., 2018).

The first model estimates the intensity of the point process using an intercept and the SPDE latent effect. This estimate should be similar to a kernel density smoothing (Gómez-Rubio et al., 2015).

```
pp.res0 <- inla(y ~ 1 +
    f(spatial.field, model = clm.spde),
  family = "poisson", data = inla.stack.data(join.stack),
  control.predictor = list(A = inla.stack.A(join.stack), compute = TRUE,
    link = 1),
  control.inla = list(int.strategy = "eb"),
  E = inla.stack.data(join.stack)$e)
```

Next, the model is defined to include covariates and the SPDE latent effect.

```
pp.res <- inla(y ~ 1 + landuse + elevation + orientation + slope +
    f(spatial.field, model = clm.spde),
  family = "poisson", data = inla.stack.data(join.stack),
  control.predictor = list(A = inla.stack.A(join.stack), compute = TRUE,
    link = 1), verbose = TRUE,
  control.inla = list(int.strategy = "eb"),
  E = inla.stack.data(join.stack)$e)
```

```
summary(pp.res)
```

```
##
## Call:
##    c("inla(formula = y ~ 1 + landuse + elevation + orientation +
##       slope + ", " f(spatial.field, model = clm.spde), family =
##       \"poisson\", data = inla.stack.data(join.stack), ", " E =
##       inla.stack.data(join.stack)$e, verbose = TRUE, control.predictor =
##       list(A = inla.stack.A(join.stack), ", " compute = TRUE, link = 1),
##       control.inla = list(int.strategy = \"eb\"))" )
## Time used:
##       Pre = 1.77, Running = 57.4, Post = 0.836, Total = 60
## Fixed effects:
##                       mean    sd 0.025quant 0.5quant 0.975quant    mode  kld
## (Intercept)         -2.113 0.268     -2.640   -2.113     -1.587  -2.112    0
## landuseconifer      -0.067 0.220     -0.504   -0.066      0.362  -0.063    0
## landusedenseforest   0.323 0.272     -0.223    0.327      0.845   0.335    0
## landusegrassland    -0.170 0.263     -0.696   -0.166      0.337  -0.159    0
## landusemeadow       -0.573 0.272     -1.116   -0.570     -0.049  -0.563    0
## landusemixedforest  -0.700 0.400     -1.535   -0.682      0.037  -0.647    0
## landusescrub         0.303 0.204     -0.098    0.303      0.704   0.303    0
## landuseurban        -0.124 0.175     -0.462   -0.125      0.223  -0.128    0
## elevation           -1.496 0.197     -1.885   -1.495     -1.110  -1.494    0
## orientation          0.001 0.003     -0.006    0.001      0.007   0.001    0
## slope                0.006 0.011     -0.015    0.006      0.027   0.006    0
##
## Random effects:
##   Name      Model
##     spatial.field SPDE2 model
##
## Model hyperparameters:
##                         mean      sd 0.025quant 0.5quant 0.975quant
## Range for spatial.field 114.44 21.405     80.303   111.64     163.72
## Stdev for spatial.field   1.27  0.172      0.974     1.25       1.65
##                          mode
## Range for spatial.field 105.68
## Stdev for spatial.field   1.22
##
## Expected number of effective parameters(stdev): 106.43(0.00)
## Number of equivalent replicates : 20.48
##
## Marginal log-Likelihood:  -3043.35
## Posterior marginals for the linear predictor and
##   the fitted values are computed
```

The summary of the model with covariates provides some insight on the factors associated to the location of forest fires in this region. High elevation is associated with a lower incidence of forest fires. Orientation and slope do not seem to have an effect. Regarding land use, bush is the baseline and it does not seem that there are differences between the different types of land use. Meadows seems to have a reduced number of forest fires due to lightning as compared to the baseline level. The fitted values of the intensity with both models can be retrieved from the model fits and added to the `SpatialPixelsDataFrame` with the data to be plotted:

```
#Prediction
idx <- inla.stack.index(join.stack, 'pred')$data
# MOdel with no covariates
spdf$SPDE0 <- pp.res0$summary.fitted.values[idx, "mean"]
#Model with covariates
spdf$SPDE <- pp.res$summary.fitted.values[idx, "mean"]
```

Figure 7.14 displays the posterior means of the estimated intensity at the grid points for both models and it can be used to assess fire risk. For example, a region of high risk can be found in the southeast part of Castilla-La Mancha (municipalities of Yeste, Letur and Nerpio).

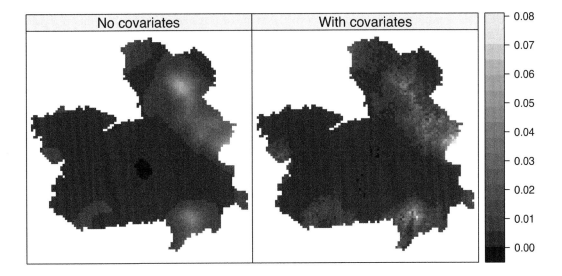

FIGURE 7.14 Intensity of forest fires in Castilla-La Mancha (Spain). The region is about 400 x 400 km.

In order to understand the latent spatial pattern, the marginals of its parameters can be estimated similarly as in the geostatistics example:

```
#Compute statistics in terms or range and variance
spde.clm.est <- inla.spde2.result(inla = pp.res, name = "spatial.field",
  spde = clm.spde, do.transf = TRUE)

#Variance
inla.zmarginal(spde.clm.est$marginals.variance.nominal[[1]])
```

```
## Mean            1.63333
## Stdev           0.448467
## Quantile  0.025 0.952454
## Quantile  0.25  1.31148
```

```
## Quantile  0.5    1.56322
## Quantile  0.75   1.88061
## Quantile  0.975  2.70111
```

```
#Range
inla.zmarginal(spde.clm.est$marginals.range.nominal[[1]])
```

```
## Mean              114.412
## Stdev             21.2312
## Quantile  0.025  80.4262
## Quantile  0.25   99.1748
## Quantile  0.5    111.598
## Quantile  0.75   126.79
## Quantile  0.975  163.388
```

Note that the output from the model already provided summary statistics for the range and variance of the spatial process. According to the value of the spatial range, it seems that the spatial random effect accounts for medium-scale spatial variation (remember that the region covers an area of about 400 x 400 km). The estimate of the spatial variance seems to be small, which makes the spatial variation not have too extreme peaks.

8

Temporal Models

8.1 Introduction

The analysis of time series refers to the analysis of data collected sequentially over time. Time can be indexed over a discrete domain (e.g., years) or a continuous one. In this section we will consider models to analyze both types of temporal data. The discrete case will be tackled with some of the autoregressive models covered in Chapter 3. The analysis of temporal data over a continuous domain will be done with smoothing methods described in Chapter 9. The analysis of space-time data will also be considered in the last part of this chapter. INLA provides a number of options to model data collected in space and time. Krainski et al. (2018) provides examples on space-time models for geostatistical data and point patterns, that we have omitted here.

This chapter starts with an introduction to the analysis of time series using autoregressive models in Section 8.2. Non-Gaussian time series are discussed in Section 8.3. Forecasting of time series is described in Section 8.4. Space-state models are in Section 8.5. Finally, Section 8.6 covers different types of space-time models.

8.2 Autoregressive models

When time is indexed over a discrete domain autoregressive models are a convenient way to model the data. Autoregressive models are described in Section 3.3 and in this chapter we will focus on providing some applications to temporal data.

As a first example of time series we will consider the climate reconstruction dataset analyzed in Fahrmeir and Kneib (2011). The original data is described in Moberg et al. (2005) and values represent the temperature anomalies (in Celsius degrees) from the Northern Hemisphere annual mean temperature 1961-90 average. Climate reconstruction is often based on indirect measurements from tree rings and other sources.

The variables in the dataset are available in Table 8.1. The original file has been obtained from the associated website of Fahrmeir and Kneib (2011). See Preface for details.

TABLE 8.1: Variables in the climate reconstruction dataset (Moberg et al., 2005; Fahrmeir and Kneib, 2011).

Variable	Description
year	Year of measurement (from AD 1 to 1979).
temp	Temperature anomaly.

```
climate <- read.table(file = "data/moberg2005.raw.txt", header = TRUE)
summary(climate)
```

```
##       year            temp
##  Min.   :   1   Min.   :-1.263
##  1st Qu.: 496   1st Qu.:-0.489
##  Median : 990   Median :-0.353
##  Mean   : 990   Mean   :-0.354
##  3rd Qu.:1484   3rd Qu.:-0.208
##  Max.   :1979   Max.   : 0.372
```

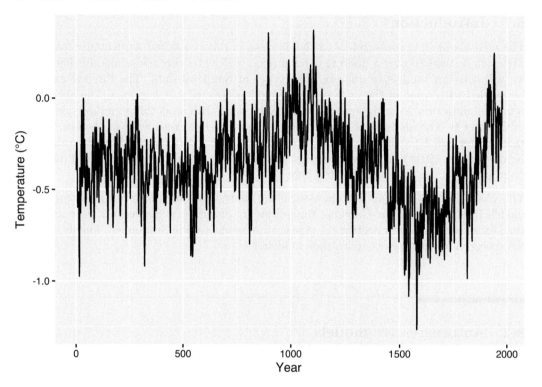

FIGURE 8.1 Plot of the climate reconstrution dataset (Moberg et al., 2005, Fahrmeir and Kneib (2011)).

The analysis will focus on estimating the main trend in the climate reconstruction time series. The model to be fit is an AR(1) on the year:

$$y_t = \alpha + u_t + \varepsilon_t, \ t = 1, \dots, 1979$$

$$u_1 \sim N(0, \tau_u(1 - \rho^2)^{-1})$$

$$u_i = \rho u_{t-1} + \epsilon_t, \ t = 2, \dots, 1979$$

$$\varepsilon_t \sim N(0, \tau_\varepsilon, t = 1, \dots 1979$$

Here, α is an intercept, ρ a temporal correlation term (with $|\rho| < 1$) and ϵ_t is a Gaussian error term with zero mean and precision τ_u. Note that variable y_t can be regarded as a Gaussian response with mean $\alpha + u_t$ and a fixed large precision so that the error term is close to zero.

First of all, an AR(1) model will be fit:

```
climate.ar1 <- inla(temp ~ 1 + f(year, model = "ar1"), data = climate,
  control.predictor = list(compute = TRUE)
)
summary(climate.ar1)
```

```
##
## Call:
##    c("inla(formula = temp ~ 1 + f(year, model = \"ar1\"), data =
##    climate, ", " control.predictor = list(compute = TRUE))")
## Time used:
##      Pre = 1.18, Running = 1.45, Post = 0.343, Total = 2.97
## Fixed effects:
##               mean    sd 0.025quant 0.5quant 0.975quant    mode kld
## (Intercept) -0.352 0.023     -0.397   -0.352     -0.308 -0.353   0
##
## Random effects:
##    Name       Model
##      year AR1 model
##
## Model hyperparameters:
##                                              mean        sd 0.025quant
## Precision for the Gaussian observations 5.96e+04 2.82e+04   21706.53
## Precision for year                      2.06e+01 2.09e+00      16.58
## Rho for year                            9.09e-01 9.00e-03       0.89
##                                         0.5quant 0.975quant      mode
## Precision for the Gaussian observations 5.40e+04   1.30e+05  4.41e+04
## Precision for year                      2.05e+01   2.48e+01  2.06e+01
## Rho for year                            9.09e-01   9.27e-01  9.09e-01
##
## Expected number of effective parameters(stdev): 1970.41(3.99)
## Number of equivalent replicates : 1.00
##
## Marginal log-Likelihood:  1895.38
## Posterior marginals for the linear predictor and
##   the fitted values are computed
```

This model does not provide a good fit because it fits the observed data exactly, i.e., it overfits the data. For this reason, it is necessary to provide some prior information about what we expect the variation of the process to be. In the next example a prior Gamma with parameters 10 and 100 is used, so that the precision is centered at 0.1 and has a small variance of 0.001. Note that this prior is closer to the scale of the actual data than the default prior as the variance of temp is 0.0484. The prior is set by using the hyper argument inside the f() function where the ar1 latent effect is defined and in the control.family argument (for the precision of the likelihood).

```
climate.ar1 <- inla(temp ~ 1 + f(year, model = "ar1",
    hyper = list(prec = list(param = c(10, 100)))), data = climate,
  control.predictor = list(compute = TRUE),
  control.compute = list(dic = TRUE, waic = TRUE, cpo = TRUE),
  control.family = list(hyper = list(prec = list(param = c(10, 100))))
)
summary(climate.ar1)
```

```
##
## Call:
##    c("inla(formula = temp ~ 1 + f(year, model = \"ar1\", hyper =
##    list(prec = list(param = c(10, ", " 100)))), data = climate,
##    control.compute = list(dic = TRUE, ", " waic = TRUE, cpo = TRUE),
##    control.predictor = list(compute = TRUE), ", " control.family =
##    list(hyper = list(prec = list(param = c(10, ", " 100)))))")
## Time used:
##     Pre = 1.03, Running = 4.37, Post = 0.396, Total = 5.8
## Fixed effects:
##               mean    sd 0.025quant 0.5quant 0.975quant   mode kld
## (Intercept) -0.288 2.969     -6.171   -0.288      5.585 -0.288   0
##
## Random effects:
##   Name     Model
##     year AR1 model
##
## Model hyperparameters:
##                                            mean    sd 0.025quant 0.5quant
## Precision for the Gaussian observations  8.036 0.259      7.537    8.033
## Precision for year                       0.122 0.035      0.065    0.118
## Rho for year                             1.000 0.000      1.000    1.000
##                                          0.975quant mode
## Precision for the Gaussian observations      8.557 8.03
## Precision for year                           0.202 0.11
## Rho for year                                 1.000 1.00
##
## Expected number of effective parameters(stdev): 42.35(6.64)
## Number of equivalent replicates : 46.73
##
## Deviance Information Criterion (DIC) ...............: -50.77
## Deviance Information Criterion (DIC, saturated) ....: 435.96
## Effective number of parameters ....................: 43.37
##
## Watanabe-Akaike information criterion (WAIC) ...: -85.55
## Effective number of parameters ................: 8.43
##
## Marginal log-Likelihood:  -757.86
## CPO and PIT are computed
##
## Posterior marginals for the linear predictor and
##   the fitted values are computed
```

The next model to fit is a random walk of order 1:

$$y_t = \alpha + u_t + \varepsilon_t, \ t = 1, \ldots 1979$$

$$u_t - u_{t-1} \sim N(0, \tau_u), \ t = 2, \ldots, 1979$$

$$\varepsilon_t \sim N(0, \tau_\varepsilon), t = 1, \ldots 1979$$

The model is fit similar to the **ar1** models and we fix the precision of the Gaussian likelihood:

```
climate.rw1 <- inla(temp ~ 1 + f(year, model = "rw1", constr = FALSE,
    hyper = list(prec = list(param = c(10, 100)))), data = climate,
  control.predictor = list(compute = TRUE),
  control.compute = list(dic = TRUE, waic = TRUE, cpo = TRUE),
  control.family = list(hyper = list(prec = list(param = c(10, 100))))
)
summary(climate.rw1)
```

```
##
## Call:
##    c("inla(formula = temp ~ 1 + f(year, model = \"rw1\", constr =
##    FALSE, ", " hyper = list(prec = list(param = c(10, 100)))), data =
##    climate, ", " control.compute = list(dic = TRUE, waic = TRUE, cpo
##    = TRUE), ", " control.predictor = list(compute = TRUE),
##    control.family = list(hyper = list(prec = list(param = c(10, ", "
##    100)))))")
## Time used:
##     Pre = 1.02, Running = 2.72, Post = 0.227, Total = 3.97
## Fixed effects:
##               mean  sd 0.025quant 0.5quant 0.975quant mode kld
## (Intercept) 0.001 647      -1439   -0.054       1438    0   0
##
## Random effects:
##   Name      Model
##     year RW1 model
##
## Model hyperparameters:
##                                         mean    sd 0.025quant 0.5quant
## Precision for the Gaussian observations 5.12 0.241       4.59     5.15
## Precision for year                      4.40 0.103       4.17     4.41
##                                         0.975quant mode
## Precision for the Gaussian observations       5.51 5.27
## Precision for year                            4.58 4.45
##
## Expected number of effective parameters(stdev): 944.67(11.54)
## Number of equivalent replicates : 2.10
##
## Deviance Information Criterion (DIC) ...............: 2250.84
## Deviance Information Criterion (DIC, saturated) ....: 1910.09
## Effective number of parameters ....................: 946.68
```

```
##
## Watanabe-Akaike information criterion (WAIC) ...: 1593.92
## Effective number of parameters ................: 233.94
##
## Marginal log-Likelihood:   -2097.64
## CPO and PIT are computed
##
## Posterior marginals for the linear predictor and
##   the fitted values are computed
```

The model summary shows a strong temporal correlation, with a posterior mean of the parameter of 1.

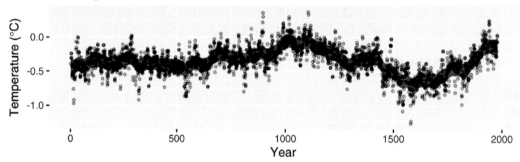

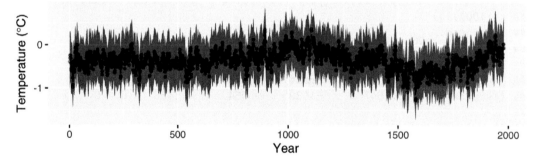

FIGURE 8.2 Models fit to the climate reconstruction dataset.

Figure 8.2 shows the posterior means and 95% credible intervals of the autoregressive and random walks models fit to the temperature data. The ar1 model produces smoother estimates than the rw1 model, which seems to overfit the data. Although both models use the same priors on the model precisions it is difficult to compare them directly unless the latent effects are scaled (see Section 5.6).

For both models the AIC and WAIC have been computed, and these clearly favor the ar1 model (probably because the rw1 overfits the data). Similarly, the CPO has been computed and they can be compared (see Section 2.4):

```
# ar1
- sum(log(climate.ar1$cpo$cpo))
```

[1] -42.77

```
# rw1
- sum(log(climate.rw1$cpo$cpo))
```

[1] 829.9

Again, this criterion shows a preference for the `ar1` model.

8.3   Non-Gaussian data

Similar models can be fit to non-Gaussian data. The next example uses the number of yearly major earthquakes from 1900 to 2006 (Zucchini et al., 2016). A major earthquake is one with a magnitude of 7 or greater. These are available in the `earthquake` dataset provided by the `MixtureInf` (Li et al., 2016) package.

TABLE 8.2: Variables in the `earthquake` dataset.

Variable	Description
number	Number of major earthquakes (magnitude 7 or greater).

The `earthquake` data can be loaded and summarized as follows (norte that a new column with the year has been added as well):

```
library("MixtureInf")
data(earthquake)

#Add year
earthquake$year <- 1900:2006

#Summary of the data
summary(earthquake)
```

```
##      number          year
##  Min.   : 6.0   Min.   :1900
##  1st Qu.:15.0   1st Qu.:1926
##  Median :18.0   Median :1953
##  Mean   :19.4   Mean   :1953
##  3rd Qu.:23.0   3rd Qu.:1980
##  Max.   :41.0   Max.   :2006
```

Figure 8.3 shows the time series of the number of major earthquakes from 1900 to 2006.

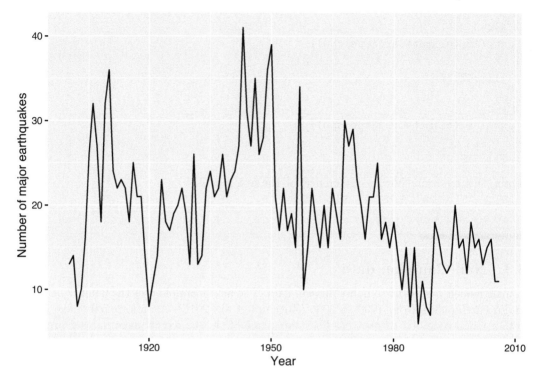

FIGURE 8.3 Number of major earthquakes from 1900 to 2006 in the `earthquake` dataset.

The first model to be fit to the `earthquake` data is an `ar1`:

$$y_t \sim Po(\mu_t), \; t = 1900, \ldots, 2006$$

$$\log(\mu_t) = \alpha + u_t, \; t = 1900, \ldots, 2006$$

$$u_1 \sim N(0, \tau_u(1 - \rho^2)^{-1})$$

$$u_i = \rho u_{t-1} + \epsilon_t, \; t = 2, \ldots, 1979$$

$$\epsilon_t \sim N(0, \tau_\varepsilon), \; t = 2, \ldots, 1979$$

Note that now the distribution of the observed number of earthquakes is modeled using a Poisson distribution and that the linear predictor is linked to the mean using the natural logarithm.

```
quake.ar1 <- inla(number ~ 1 + f(year, model = "ar1"), data = earthquake,
   family = "poisson", control.predictor = list(compute = TRUE))
summary(quake.ar1)
```

```
##
## Call:
##    c("inla(formula = number ~ 1 + f(year, model = \"ar1\"), family =
##    \"poisson\", ", " data = earthquake, control.predictor =
##    list(compute = TRUE))" )
## Time used:
##     Pre = 1.01, Running = 0.323, Post = 0.0664, Total = 1.4
## Fixed effects:
##              mean    sd 0.025quant 0.5quant 0.975quant   mode   kld
## (Intercept) 2.863 0.189      2.439    2.878       3.19 2.891 0.001
##
## Random effects:
##   Name      Model
##     year AR1 model
##
## Model hyperparameters:
##                     mean    sd 0.025quant 0.5quant 0.975quant   mode
## Precision for year 12.041 4.615      4.990   11.425     22.851 10.112
## Rho for year        0.889 0.051      0.771    0.896      0.966  0.915
##
## Expected number of effective parameters(stdev): 31.30(5.97)
## Number of equivalent replicates : 3.42
##
## Marginal log-Likelihood:  -343.44
## Posterior marginals for the linear predictor and
##  the fitted values are computed
```

Similar to the climate example, a random walk of order one can be fit to the data:

$$y_t \sim Po(\mu_t), \ t = 1900, \ldots, 2006$$

$$\log(\mu_t) = \alpha + u_t$$

$$u_t - u_{t-1} \sim N(0, \tau_u), \ t = 2, \ldots, 1979$$

This model is fit using the code below:

```
quake.rw1 <- inla(number ~ 1 + f(year, model = "rw1"), data = earthquake,
  family = "poisson", control.predictor = list(compute = TRUE))
summary(quake.rw1)
```

```
##
## Call:
##    c("inla(formula = number ~ 1 + f(year, model = \"rw1\"), family =
##    \"poisson\", ", " data = earthquake, control.predictor =
##    list(compute = TRUE))" )
## Time used:
##     Pre = 1.01, Running = 0.15, Post = 0.0661, Total = 1.22
## Fixed effects:
##              mean    sd 0.025quant 0.5quant 0.975quant  mode kld
```

```
## (Intercept) 2.923 0.023        2.877      2.923         2.968 2.923    0
##
## Random effects:
##    Name      Model
##      year RW1 model
##
## Model hyperparameters:
##                         mean     sd 0.025quant  0.5quant  0.975quant  mode
## Precision for year 82.47 34.24      36.22     75.84       167.32 64.66
##
## Expected number of effective parameters(stdev): 26.71(4.91)
## Number of equivalent replicates : 4.01
##
## Marginal log-Likelihood:   -342.67
## Posterior marginals for the linear predictor and
##   the fitted values are computed
```

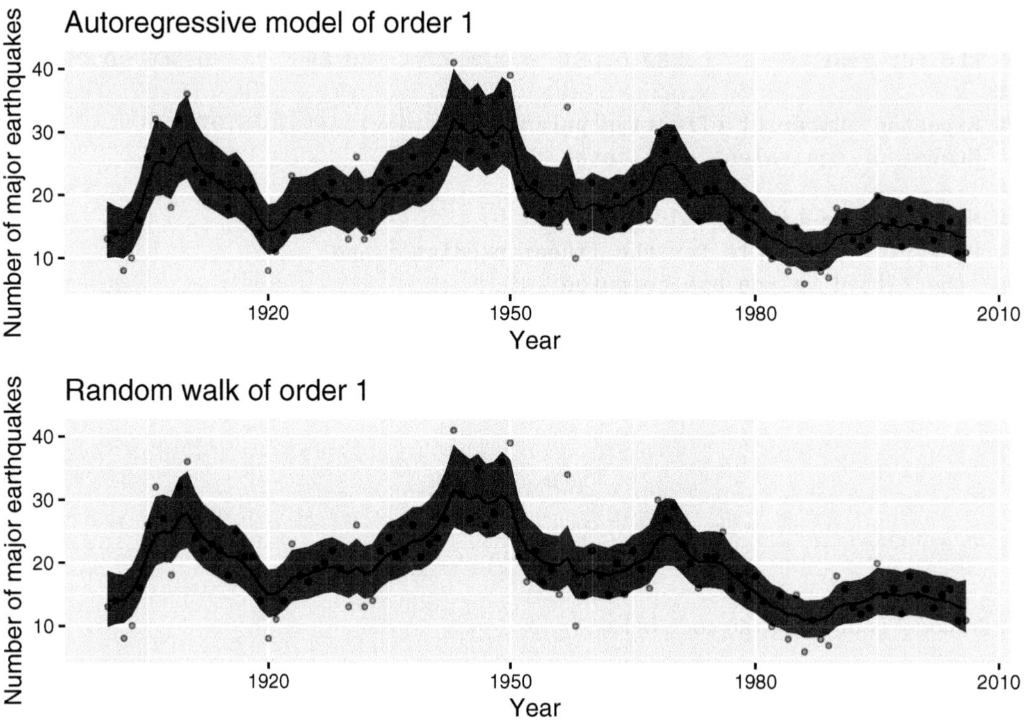

FIGURE 8.4 Models fit to the `earthquake` dataset.

Figure 8.4 shows the models fit to the `earthquake` dataset. This includes the posterior means and 95% credible intervals. Apparently, both models provide a similar fit to the data.

8.4   Forecasting

Time series forecasting in Bayesian inference can be regarded as fitting a model with some missing observations in the response, which requires computing the predictive distribution (see Section 12.3) at future times. If the model being fit includes covariates these must also be available as well for the years to be predicted. We will illustrate forecasting in time series with the `earthquake` dataset to try to estimate the future number of major earthquakes and the uncertainty about these estimates. First of all, we use a few new lines (from year 2007 to 2020) to forecast the number of major earthquakes. These lines include the new time points (i.e., years) at which the prediction will be made and the number of earthquakes is set to `NA` for these new time points:

```
quake.pred <- rbind(earthquake,
  data.frame(number = rep(NA, 14), year = 2007:2020))
```

Next, we fit the `ar1` model to the new dataset so that the predictive distributions are computed:

```
quake.ar1.pred <- inla(number ~ 1 + f(year, model = "ar1"), data = quake.pred,
  family = "poisson", control.predictor = list(compute = TRUE, link = 1))
summary(quake.ar1.pred)
```

```
##
## Call:
##    c("inla(formula = number ~ 1 + f(year, model = \"ar1\"), family =
##    \"poisson\", ", " data = quake.pred, control.predictor =
##    list(compute = TRUE, ", " link = 1))")
## Time used:
##     Pre = 1.07, Running = 0.35, Post = 0.0671, Total = 1.49
## Fixed effects:
##             mean    sd 0.025quant 0.5quant 0.975quant  mode   kld
## (Intercept) 2.864 0.181      2.456    2.878      3.182 2.891 0.001
##
## Random effects:
##   Name     Model
##     year AR1 model
##
## Model hyperparameters:
##                      mean    sd 0.025quant 0.5quant 0.975quant   mode
## Precision for year 11.99 4.615      4.952   11.374     22.816 10.054
## Rho for year        0.89 0.051      0.771    0.897      0.966  0.915
##
## Expected number of effective parameters(stdev): 31.33(5.98)
## Number of equivalent replicates : 3.42
##
## Marginal log-Likelihood:  -343.43
## Posterior marginals for the linear predictor and
##  the fitted values are computed
```

In the previous code, the use of `link = 1` is required so that predicted values are in the scale of the response, i.e., they are transformed taking the inverse of the link function. See 4.6 for details about the use of `link` in non-Gaussian models.

The mode fit is the same as the one obtained without the missing observations. Figure 8.5 shows the fitted and predicted values together with 95% credible intervals. Note how these get wider in the period from 2007 to 2020 as time progresses from the last year with observed data (i.e., 2006).

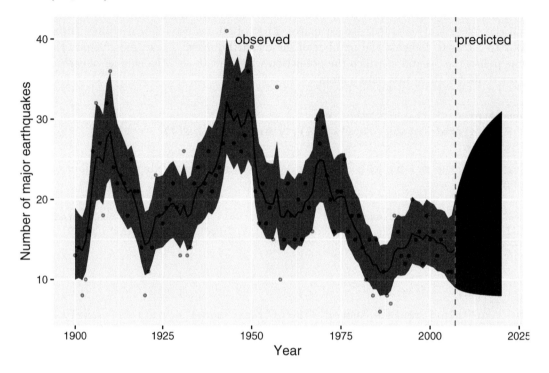

FIGURE 8.5 Prediction from the earthquake dataset from 2007 to 2020.

8.5 Space-state models

A class of temporal models where coefficients and other latent effects are allowed to change in time is that of dynamic models (Ruiz-Cárdenas et al., 2012). These models can be summarized as follows:

$$y_t = \beta_t x_t + \epsilon_t, \; \epsilon_t \sim N(0, \tau_t), \; t = 1, \dots, n$$

$$x_t = \gamma_t x_{t-1} + \omega_t, \; \omega_t \sim N(0, \nu_t), \; t = 2, \dots, n$$

Here, y_t is a temporal observation, x_t is a state latent parameter, β_t and γ_t are temporally varying coefficients, and ϵ_t and ω_t are temporal errors or perturbations which follow a Gaussian distribution with 0 mean and precisions τ_t and ν_t, respectively.

Latent effects $\mathbf{x} = (x_1, \ldots, x_n))$ represent different states which need to be estimated. Note that they are not assigned a stochastic distribution because they are constants to be estimated. This will be simulated by modeling them using an `iid` distribution with a very large variance to conform to the unconstrained nature of these values.

Ruiz-Cárdenas et al. (2012) describe how to use `INLA` to fit some classes of dynamic models when the data are fully observed. We will illustrate model fitting using a simple model.

$$y_t = x_t + \nu_t, \ \nu_t \sim N(0, V), \ t = 1, \ldots, n$$

$$x_t = x_{t-1} + \omega_t, \ \omega_t \sim N(0, w), \ t = 2, \ldots, n$$

Note that in this case the temporal coefficients are constant and equal to one. Also, $(x_1, \ldots, x_n)$ is distributed as a random walk of order 1, which simplifies model fitting because the second equation above can be rewritten as:

$$x_t - x_{t-1} = \omega_t, \ \omega_t \sim N(0, w), \ t = 2, \ldots, n$$

which is the definition of a first order random walk. Hence, model fitting here reduces to a model with a Gaussian response and random walk of order 1 in the linear predictor. However, we will describe the new approach developed in Ruiz-Cárdenas et al. (2012) as this provides a more general framework to fit space-state models.

The second line in the previous equation can be rewritten as follows:

$$0 = x_t - x_{t-1} - \omega_t, \ \omega_t \sim N(0, w), \ t = 2, \ldots, n$$

This can be regarded as a submodel with "faked zero observations" which depends on the vector of latent effects $\mathbf{x}$ and error terms ω.

Hence, this model can be fit using two likelihoods (as explained in Section 6.4): one to fit the model that explains $\mathbf{y}$ and the second one to fit the model that explains the "fake zero observations". Given that both submodels depend on the same latent effects $\mathbf{x}$, they can be shared between the two models using the `copy` feature described in Section 6.5.

8.5.1 Example: Alcohol consumption in Finland

As an example of the analysis of non-Gaussian data we will consider the analysis of alcohol related deaths in Finland in the period 1969-2013 in the age group between 30 and 39 years. This is available as dataset `alcohol` in package `KFAS` (Helske, 2017), which is a time series object.

TABLE 8.3: Variables in the `alcohol` dataset.

Variable	Description
`death at age 30-39`	Number of alcohol related deaths (age group 30-39).
`death at age 40-49`	Number of alcohol related deaths (age group 40-49).
`death at age 50-59`	Number of alcohol related deaths (age group 50-59).
`death at age 60-69`	Number of alcohol related deaths (age group 60-69).
`population by age 30-39`	Population (age group 30-39) divided by 100000.
`population by age 40-49`	Population (age group 40-49) divided by 100000.

Variable	Description
`population by age 50-59`	Population (age group 50-59) divided by 100000.
`population by age 60-69`	Population (age group 60-69) divided by 100000.

The `alcohol` dataset can be loaded with:

```
library("KFAS")
data(alcohol)
```

In order to fit a space-state model data need to be put in a two-column matrix as the model will contain two likelihoods, as explained in Section 6.4. In the first column, we will include the number of deaths in the age group 30-39, and in the second column the "fake zero" observations. Note that we have to remove the last row because it contains `NA`'s.

```
n <- nrow(alcohol) - 1 #There is an NA
Y <- matrix(NA, ncol = 2, nrow = n + (n - 1))
Y[1:n, 1] <- alcohol[1:n, 1]
Y[-c(1:n), 2] <- 0
```

The model will contain an offset with the population in the age group 30-39 for the data in the first column only:

```
#offset
oset <- c(alcohol[1:n, 5], rep(NA, n - 1))
```

Next, a number of indices and weights for the latent effect need to be created as well. These indices and weights are described in the formulation of the model above. Note that all indices have length $n + n + 1$ because the model will be made of two likelihoods. The first one is a Poisson likelihood to model the response, and the second one is a Gaussian likelihood to model the latent "fake zeroes" than define variable x_t. When an index only works on one likelihood, then the corresponding values for the other likelihood will be set to `NA`.

```
#x_t
i <- c(1:n, 2:n)
#x_(t-1) 2:n
j <- c(rep(NA, n), 1:(n - 1))
# Weight to have -1 * x_(t-1)
w1 <- c(rep(NA, n), rep(-1, n - 1))
#x_(t-1), 2:n
l <- c(rep(NA, n), 2:n)
# Weight to have  * omega_(t-1)
w2 <- c(rep(NA, n), rep(-1, n - 1))
```

The final model is fit as follows:

```
prec.prior <- list(prec = list(param = c(0.001, 0.001)))
alc.inla <- inla(Y ~ 0 + offset(log(oset)) +
```

```
       f(i, model = "iid",
         hyper = list(prec = list(initial = -10, fixed = TRUE))) +
       f(j, w1, copy = "i") + f(1, w2, model = "iid"),
     data = list(Y = Y, oset = oset), family = c("poisson", "gaussian"),
     control.family = list(list(),
       list(hyper = list(prec = list(initial = 10, fixed = TRUE)))),
     control.predictor = list(compute = TRUE)
   )
```

Note that the previous model does not impose any distribution of the values of **x** and they can take any values. For this reason, they have been included in the linear predictor using an `iid` model with a fixed tiny precision equal to $\exp(-10)$, which is equivalent to having a large variance of $\exp(10)$. That is, in practice effects in **x** can take any value. Furthermore, `control.family` takes a list of two values (because of the two likelihoods) but only the second one is set because the first likelihoods do not require any extra constraints. The second argument is to fix the precision of the Gaussian likelihood.

The estimates and model fitting are summarized here:

```
 summary(alc.inla)
```

```
##
## Call:
##    c("inla(formula = Y ~ 0 + offset(log(oset)) + f(i, model =
##    \"iid\", ", " hyper = list(prec = list(initial = -10, fixed =
##    TRUE))) + ", " f(j, w1, copy = \"i\") + f(1, w2, model = \"iid\"),
##    family = c(\"poisson\", ", " \"gaussian\"), data = list(Y = Y,
##    oset = oset), control.predictor = list(compute = TRUE), ", "
##    control.family = list(list(), list(hyper = list(prec =
##    list(initial = 10, ", " fixed = TRUE)))))")
## Time used:
##     Pre = 1.61, Running = 0.147, Post = 0.0723, Total = 1.83
## Random effects:
##   Name     Model
##     i IID model
##     1 IID model
##     j Copy
##
## Model hyperparameters:
##                    mean    sd 0.025quant 0.5quant 0.975quant  mode
## Precision for 1 111.05 53.27      43.37    99.61     245.82 81.25
##
## Expected number of effective parameters(stdev): 63.52(3.50)
## Number of equivalent replicates : 1.37
##
## Marginal log-Likelihood:  -457.34
## Posterior marginals for the linear predictor and
##   the fitted values are computed
```

Figure 8.6 shows the fitted values together with 95% credible intervals (shaded area). Note how the space-state model provides smoothed estimates.

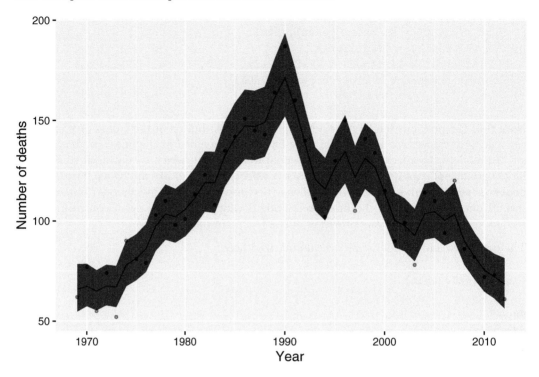

FIGURE 8.6 Space-state model fit to the `alcohol` dataset.

8.6 Spatio-temporal models

Spatial models have already been covered in Chapter 7. When time is also available, it is possible to build spatio-temporal models that include spatial and temporal random effects, as well as interaction effects between space and time.

A spatio-temporal model is said to be *separable* when the space-time covariance structure can be decomposed as a spatial and a temporal term. This often means that the spatio-temporal covariance can be written as a Kronecker product of a spatial and a temporal covariance (Fuentes et al., 2007) *Non-separable* covariance structures do not allow for a separate modeling of the spatial and temporal covariances (Wikle et al., 1998).

8.6.1 Separable models

Including separable spatial and temporal terms in the linear predictor can be done with ease by using the `f()` function to define two separate effects on space and time. Spatial effects are usually of the classes presented in Chapter 7, while temporal effects can be those presented in this chapter. However, latent effects used for spatial modeling can be used for temporal effects when the adjacency structure used reflects dependence between different temporal points.

The `brainNM` dataset from the `DClusterm` package (Gómez-Rubio et al., 2019) provides observed and expected counts of cases of brain cancer in the counties of New Mexico from 1973 to 1991 in a spatio-temporal `STFDF` object from the `spacetime` package (Pebesma, 2012). The original data have been analyzed in Kulldorff et al. (1998). See the Preface for more information about the original data sources.

Table 8.4 shows the variables in the dataset, that can be loaded as follows:

```
library("DClusterm")
data(brainNM)
```

TABLE 8.4: Variables in the `brainNM` dataset.

Variable	Description
Observed	Observed number of cases.
Expected	Expected number of cases.
SMR	Standardized Mortality Ratio.
Year	Year.
FIPS	County FIPS code.
ID	County ID (from 1 to 32).
IDLANL	Inverse distance to Los Alamos National Laboratory.
IDLANLre	Re-scaled value of IDLANL by dividing by its mean.

A simple estimate of risk is the standardized mortality ratio (SMR) which is a simple estimate of the relative risk which is equal to the observed number of cases divided by the expected cases. Figure 8.7 shows the SMR for each county and year.

Before fitting the spatio-temporal model the adjacency structure of the counties in New Mexico is computed using function `poly2nb()` on the spatial object of the `brainNM` dataset.

```
nm.adj <- poly2nb(brainst@sp)
adj.mat <- as(nb2mat(nm.adj, style = "B"), "Matrix")
```

Next, the model is fit considering a separable model. In particular, the spatial effect is modeled using an ICAR model and the temporal trend using a `rw1` latent effect. We will use vague priors (as in Chapter 3) to avoid overfitting.

```
# Prior of precision
prec.prior <- list(prec = list(param = c(0.001, 0.001)))

brain.st <- inla(Observed ~ 1 + f(Year, model = "rw1",
      hyper = prec.prior) +
    f(as.numeric(ID), model = "besag", graph = adj.mat,
      hyper = prec.prior),
  data = brainst@data, E = Expected, family = "poisson",
```

Standardized mortality ratio

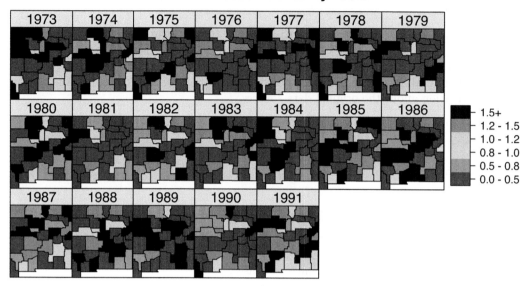

FIGURE 8.7 Standardized Mortality Ratio (SMR) of brain cancer in New Mexico from 1973 to 1991.

```
    control.predictor = list(compute = TRUE, link = 1))
  summary(brain.st)


##
## Call:
##    c("inla(formula = Observed ~ 1 + f(Year, model = \"rw1\", hyper =
##    prec.prior) + ", " f(as.numeric(ID), model = \"besag\", graph =
##    adj.mat, hyper = prec.prior), ", " family = \"poisson\", data =
##    brainst@data, E = Expected, control.predictor = list(compute =
##    TRUE, ", " link = 1))")
## Time used:
##     Pre = 1.46, Running = 0.6, Post = 0.0822, Total = 2.15
## Fixed effects:
##               mean    sd 0.025quant 0.5quant 0.975quant    mode kld
## (Intercept) -0.049 0.038     -0.127   -0.048      0.024 -0.046   0
##
## Random effects:
##   Name      Model
##     Year RW1 model
##     as.numeric(ID) Besags ICAR model
##
## Model hyperparameters:
##                               mean     sd 0.025quant 0.5quant 0.975quant
## Precision for Year          480.66 519.28      54.82   326.56    1849.12
## Precision for as.numeric(ID)  50.59  61.64       7.07    32.12     207.12
##                               mode
## Precision for Year          145.74
## Precision for as.numeric(ID)  16.18
```

```
##
## Expected number of effective parameters(stdev): 10.68(3.67)
## Number of equivalent replicates : 56.93
##
## Marginal log-Likelihood:  -824.62
## Posterior marginals for the linear predictor and
##  the fitted values are computed
```

Figure 8.8 shows the estimated relative risk. Note how several counties in the center of the state show an increased risk throughout the whole period.

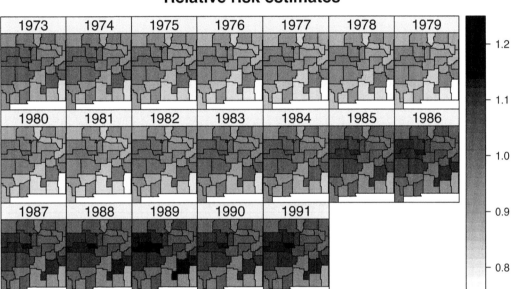

FIGURE 8.8 Posterior means of the relative risk estimate on the `brainNM` dataset.

This model assumes that the variation in each county is the sum of the spatial random effect and the overall temporal trend, i.e., there is no way to account for county-specific patterns. This may cause poor model fitting in some of the counties for certain years. Non-separable models may include space-time terms that account for this area-time interaction (Knorr-Held, 2000).

8.6.2   Separable models with the `group` option

The `f()` function provides the `group` argument to set an index for the temporal structure of the data. This index will be used to define different types of temporal dependence, whose definition will be done via the `control.group` argument in the `f()` function.

Available models are

```
names(inla.models()$group)
```

```
## [1] "exchangeable"    "exchangeablepos" "ar1"              "ar"
## [5] "rw1"             "rw2"             "besag"            "iid"
```

See Table 8.6 for a short summary of them. The options available to define the type of grouped effect and other required parameters is available in Table 8.5. Note that most of these options are only required if the latent effect defined in `model` needs them.

The resulting latent effect is a GMRF with zero mean and covariance matrix (Simpson, 2016):

$$\tau \Sigma_b \otimes \Sigma_w$$

where Σ_b is the structure of the covariance between the different groups and Σ_w the structure of the covariance matrix within each group.

The within-group effect is the one defined in the main `f()` function, while the between effect is the one defined using the `control.group` argument and it is of `exchangeable` type by default.

TABLE 8.5: Arguments available in `control.group` to define the temporal effect using the `group` argument.

Argument	Default	Description
model	"exchangeable"	Type of model.
order	NULL	Order of the model.
cyclic	FALSE	Whether this is a cyclic effect.
graph	NULL	Graph for spatial models.
scale.model	TRUE	Whether to scale the model.
adjust.for.con.comp	TRUE	Adjustment for non-connected components.
hyper	NULL	Definition of hyperprior.

TABLE 8.6: Types of latent effect in the `group` option.

Effect	Description
exchangeable	Exchangeable effect.
exchangeablepos	Exchangeable effect.
ar1	Autoregressive model of order 1.
ar	Autoregressive model of order p.
rw1	Random walk of order 1.
rw2	Random walk of order 2.
besag	Besag spatial model.
iid	Independent and identically distributed random effects.

A similar model can be fit using the `group` argument. In this case, variable `ID.Year` is created to index the year (from 1 to 19) used to define the `group`. Argument `control.group` takes a list with the model (`ar1`) and other arguments to define this effect could be added. Index ID2 is created as a copy of the ID index so that it can be used in another latent effect.

```
brainst@data$ID.Year <- brainst@data$Year - 1973 + 1
brainst@data$ID2 <- brainst@data$ID
```

The model is then defined as in the code below. Note that the model includes only the spatio-temporal random effects. Note that this and the previous models are not exactly the same and that estimates may differ.

```
brain.st2 <- inla(Observed ~ 1 +
    f(as.numeric(ID2), model = "besag", graph = adj.mat,
      group = ID.Year, control.group = list(model = "ar1"),
        hyper = prec.prior),
  data = brainst@data, E = Expected, family = "poisson",
  control.predictor = list(compute = TRUE, link = 1))
summary(brain.st2)
```

```
##
## Call:
##    c("inla(formula = Observed ~ 1 + f(as.numeric(ID2), model =
##    \"besag\", ", " graph = adj.mat, group = ID.Year, control.group =
##    list(model = \"ar1\"), ", " hyper = prec.prior), family =
##    \"poisson\", data = brainst@data, ", " E = Expected,
##    control.predictor = list(compute = TRUE, link = 1))" )
## Time used:
##    Pre = 1.18, Running = 14.8, Post = 0.0975, Total = 16
## Fixed effects:
##               mean    sd 0.025quant 0.5quant 0.975quant   mode kld
## (Intercept) -0.027 0.038     -0.105   -0.025      0.043 -0.022   0
##
## Random effects:
##   Name      Model
##     as.numeric(ID2) Besags ICAR model
##
## Model hyperparameters:
##                                mean     sd 0.025quant 0.5quant 0.975quant
## Precision for as.numeric(ID2) 42.282 51.433      6.056   26.867    172.118
## GroupRho for as.numeric(ID2)   0.794  0.261      0.005    0.894      0.995
##                                mode
## Precision for as.numeric(ID2) 13.69
## GroupRho for as.numeric(ID2)   0.99
##
## Expected number of effective parameters(stdev): 10.15(8.23)
## Number of equivalent replicates : 59.89
##
## Marginal log-Likelihood:  -1196.94
## Posterior marginals for the linear predictor and
##   the fitted values are computed
```

Figure 8.9 show the posterior means of the relative risk. Compared to the previous model this has a higher degree of smoothing. Note that this may be due to the fact that in the previous model the two effects were additive while now there is a single spatio-temporal effect. Furthermore, the estimate of the correlation of the `ar1` model is large, which means that the model is assuming a high correlation (i.e., similarities) between consecutive years and very similar estimates from year to another are obtained.

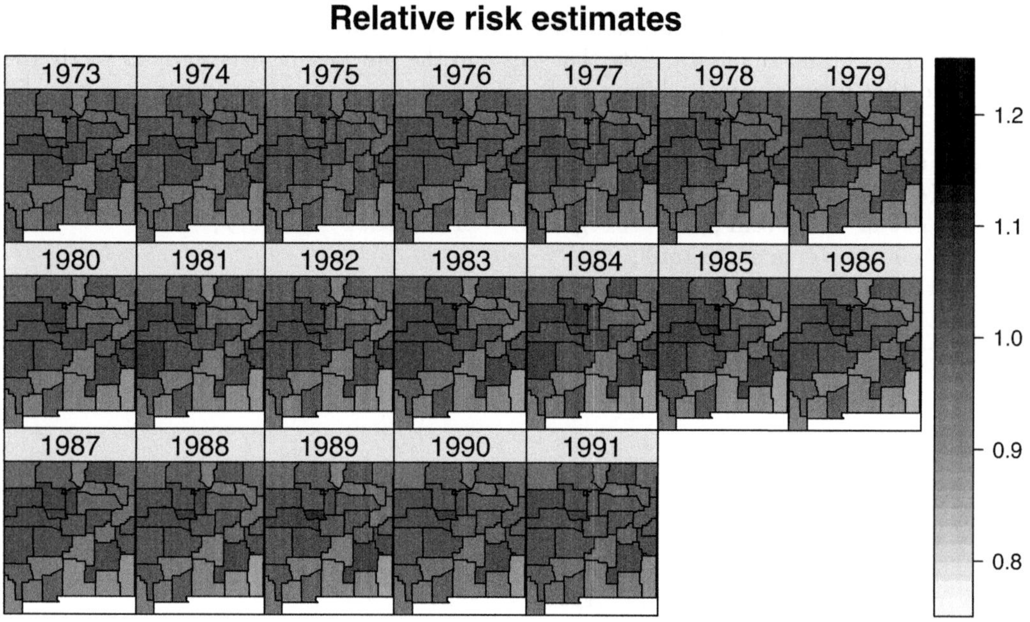

Relative risk estimates

FIGURE 8.9 Posterior means of the relative risks obtained from a model using the `group` option fit to the `brainNM` dataset.

Non-separable models include an interaction term between space and time that cannot be decomposed as the product of two terms. These models can be fit with INLA but are harder to define. The specification of these models is not straightforward as it often requires imposing additional constraints on the space-time random effects (Knorr-Held, 2000). Function `inla.knmodels()` can be used to fit these models with INLA. Goicoa et al. (2018) discuss the effect of imposing constraints on the space-time random effects and their impact on the estimates. Blangiardo and Cameletti (2015) cover some non-separable spatio-temporal models in Chapter 7.

8.7 Final remarks

Several types of spatial and spatio-temporal models that INLA can fit have been described in this chapter. Some of the latent effects mentioned here are also described in Chapter 3 and Chapter 9. For other models not implemented in INLA, the tools described in Chapter 11 can be used to implement new latent effects. Krainski et al. (2018) also propose a number of spatio-temporal models in the context of continuous processes and point processes.

Other spatio-temporal models that could be fit with `INLA` include those proposed in Knorr-Held (2000), which can be fit using function `inla.knmodels()`. Note that these models require imposing further constraints on the latent effects (see Section 6.6). Goicoa et al. (2018) discuss the effect of imposing constraints on the space-time random effects and their impact on the estimates.

Fitting non-separable spatio-temporal models with `INLA` is more difficult. Blangiardo and Cameletti (2015) cover some non-separable spatio-temporal models in Chapter 7. New models could be implemented using the methods described in Chapter 11 and, in particular, the `rgeneric` approach. Palmí-Perales et al. (2019) describe how to fit multivariate spatial latent effects with highly structured precision matrices that are implemented using `rgeneric`. This could be a guide on how to implement non-separable models because they often are based on specific parameterization of the spatio-temporal precision matrix.

9

Smoothing

9.1 Introduction

Many applications in statistics require that the model is flexible in a way that makes the relationship between the response and the covariates non-linear. For example, for Gaussian data observations y_i can be modeled as

$$y_i = f(x_i) + \epsilon_i \ i = 1, \ldots, n$$

Here, ϵ_i represent i.i.d. Gaussian errors with zero mean and precision τ. The shape of function $f()$ is typically not known and it is often estimated using semi-parametric or non-parametric methods, which are flexible enough to cope with non-linear effects. Ruppert et al. (2003) provide a nice introduction to semiparametric regression, and we will use some of the datasets in this book to illustrate some examples. Fahrmeir and Kneib (2011) give a thorough description of Bayesian smoothing methods. Finally, Wang et al. (2018), Chapter 7, cover smoothing with INLA in detail, including some approaches not mentioned here.

In this chapter we will introduce some non-parametric estimation methods that are useful to model complex relationships between the explanatory variables and the response. As described in Chapter 3, INLA implements some latent effects that can be used to smooth effects. The spatial models described in Chapter 7 can also be regarded as smoothers in two dimensions.

Splines are covered in Section 9.2. Other types of smooth terms with INLA are discussed in Section 9.3. Including smooth terms using SPDE's in one dimension is tackled in Section 9.4. Finally, smoothing in non-Gaussian models is described in Section 9.5.

9.2 Splines

In order to illustrate why smoothing may be required, we will consider the `lidar` dataset available in the package `SemiPar` (Wand, 2018). Original data have been analyzed in Holst et al. (1996) and Fahrmeir and Kneib (2011). LIDAR (LIght Detection And Ranging) is a remote-sensing technique widely used to obtain measurements of the distribution of atmospheric species.

```
library("SemiPar")
data(lidar)
```

Table 9.1 shows the variables in the `lidar` dataset, and Figure 9.1 displays the two variables in the dataset in a scatterplot. These measurements were obtained during a study on the concentration of atmospheric atomic mercury in an Italian geothermal field (see Holst et al., 1996, for details). There is a clear non-linear dependence between both variables, which shows the need for a smooth term in the linear predictor.

TABLE 9.1: Variables in the `lidar` dataset.

Variable	Description
range	Distance traveled before the light is reflected back to its source.
logratio	Logarithm of the ratio of received light from two laser sources.

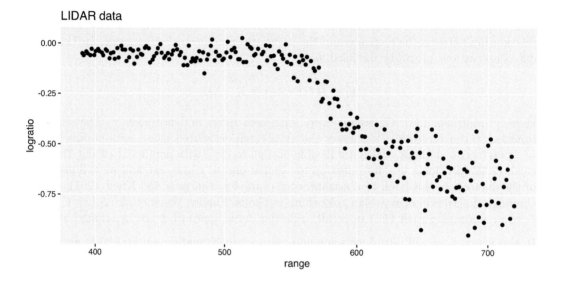

FIGURE 9.1 LIDAR measurements in the `lidar` dataset.

A first approach to developing a smooth function to fit the `lidar` dataset is by using linear combinations of smooth functions on the covariates. The set of functions is called a *basis* of functions. For example, polynomials up to a certain degree can be easily introduced into the linear predictor by using the `I()` function in the formula. Alternatively, the `poly()` function can be used to compute orthogonal polynomials on a covariate up to a certain degree.

Before fitting the model we will create a synthetic dataset with values of `range` between 390 and 720 (with a step of 5) and `NA` values, so that these are predicted with `INLA` (see Section 12.3 for details):

```
xx <- seq(390, 720, by = 5)
# Add data for prediction
new.data <- cbind(range = xx, logratio = NA)
new.data <- rbind(lidar, new.data)
```

This new dataset will allow us to obtain estimates of the fitted curve at regular intervals. Next, a model with a 3-degree polynomial on `range` will be fit:

```
m.poly <- inla(logratio ~ 1 + range +  I(range^2) + I(range^3),
   data = new.data, control.predictor = list(compute = TRUE))
```

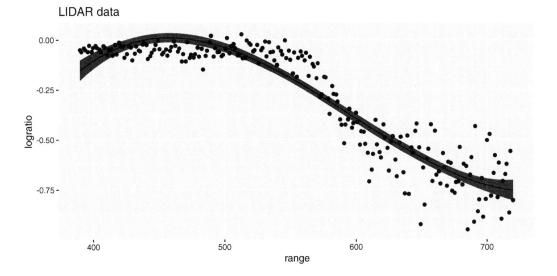

FIGURE 9.2 Posterior means and 95% credible intervals of the predictive distribution for different values of `range` using a polynomial of degree 3 fit to the `lidar` dataset.

The fitted values using these models are shown in Figure 9.2. Although the 3-degree polynomial does a good job of capturing the general variation of the curve, polynomials are not a good choice in general because they produce smooth terms that are fit using all the data because they lack a compact support. Hence, polynomials are too rigid to obtain good local smoothing and the smooth term produced will fit different parts of the dataset with different accuracy. This behavior can be observed in Figure 9.2 at the left edge of the plot where the polynomial does not follow the trend of the data but the polynomial itself.

A better fit could be achieved by using piece-wise functions that vary locally (Ruppert et al., 2003). A simple approach is to consider *broken stick* functions. These functions are defined on a number of points or *knots* so that they have two different slopes that join at the *knots*. For example, taking knot κ, a function can be defined such as

$$(x - \kappa)_+ = \left\{ \begin{array}{cc} 0 & x < \kappa \\ x - \kappa & x \geq \kappa \end{array} \right.$$

Note that given a set of knots this definition will produce a particular basis that can be used to model the LIDAR data. Note that $f(x)$ will be defined by a linear combination of the basis functions and that their coefficients will be estimated as part of the model. This basis is called a *linear spline basis*.

Hence, given a basis function $\{(x - \kappa_k)\}_{k=1}^{K}$ defined by a set of knots $\{\kappa_k\}_{k=1}^{K}$, the $f(\cdot)$ function can be represented as

$$f(x) = \beta_0 + \beta_1 x + \sum_{k=1}^{K} b_k (x - \kappa_k)_+$$

Note that the basis here is made of functions

$$\{1, x, (x - \kappa_1)_+, \ldots, (x - \kappa_K)_+\}$$

A *truncated power basis of degree p* can be obtained by taking the powers of degree p of functions $(x - \kappa_k)$, i.e., $(x - \kappa_k)_+^p$. This will produce smoother functions with continuous p derivatives in all the domain but κ_k. In this case, function $f(x)$ is defined as

$$f(x) = 1 + x + \ldots + x^p + \sum_{k=1}^{K} b_k (x - \kappa_k)_+^p$$

Although this is a first approach to producing local smoothing, broken stick functions may not be smooth enough and other type of functions may be required. For example, instead of piece-wise linear functions, other simple non-linear functions could be used.

In particular, splines (Ruppert et al., 2003) are a popular option when it comes to producing smooth terms with local smoothing. Splines are smooth functions that are defined using piece-wise functions that join at particular points called *knots*.

Local smoothing is determined by the number and location of the knots, and they must be chosen with care (Ruppert et al., 2003). Package `splines` (R Core Team, 2019a) includes several functions for the computation of different types of splines that can be easily combined with `INLA` to include smooth terms in the model.

For example, function `bs()` will return a B-spline basis matrix for a polynomial of a given degree. B-splines are preferred to splines because they are computationally more stable. B-splines have the property that they are equivalent to the truncated spline basis of the same degree, i.e., both bases are equivalent and produce the same values in the linear predictor. This means that they will produce the same values of $f(x)$ but with different coefficients, the B-splines coefficient estimation being more numerically stable (Ruppert et al., 2003).

In the next example, knots are placed between 400 and 700 at regular intervals using a step of 10. This ensures that the range of values of variable `range` is covered. The B-spline spline is of degree 3 (i.e., the default).

```
library("splines")

knots <- seq(400, 700, by = 10)
m.bs3 <- inla(logratio ~ 1 + bs(range, knots = knots),
  data = new.data, control.predictor = list(compute = TRUE))
```

Note that this model will estimate one coefficient per knot and that, in this case, there are 31 and the model summary is not shown here.

As an alternative to the knots, it is possible to specify the *degrees of freedom* (Ruppert et al., 2003) of the spline. Degrees of freedom are related to how flexible a smooth term is in order to capture the the variability in the data.

Natural cubic splines are implemented in function `ns()`. These types of splines are cubic splines with the added constraint that they are linear at the tail beyond the boundary knots by imposing that the second and third derivatives at the boundary knots (i.e., the ones at the extremes) are equal to zero. In the next example a natural cubic spline with 10 degrees of freedom is used to fit the data (by setting parameter `df` to 10).

```
m.ns3 <- inla(logratio ~ 1 + ns(range, df = 10),
  data = new.data, control.predictor = list(compute = TRUE))
summary(m.ns3)
```

```
##
## Call:
##    c("inla(formula = logratio ~ 1 + ns(range, df = 10), data =
##    new.data, ", " control.predictor = list(compute = TRUE))")
## Time used:
##     Pre = 1.34, Running = 0.183, Post = 0.0765, Total = 1.6
## Fixed effects:
##               mean    sd 0.025quant 0.5quant 0.975quant   mode kld
## (Intercept) -0.050 0.032     -0.113   -0.050      0.014 -0.050   0
## 1           -0.010 0.042     -0.093   -0.010      0.073 -0.010   0
## 2           -0.007 0.053     -0.111   -0.007      0.098 -0.007   0
## 3           -0.008 0.048     -0.102   -0.008      0.085 -0.008   0
## 4            0.026 0.051     -0.074    0.026      0.126  0.026   0
## 5           -0.326 0.049     -0.422   -0.326     -0.230 -0.326   0
## 6           -0.554 0.050     -0.652   -0.554     -0.456 -0.554   0
## 7           -0.537 0.049     -0.635   -0.537     -0.440 -0.537   0
## 8           -0.687 0.042     -0.769   -0.687     -0.605 -0.687   0
## 9           -0.656 0.083     -0.819   -0.656     -0.494 -0.656   0
## 10          -0.652 0.038     -0.726   -0.652     -0.578 -0.652   0
##
## Model hyperparameters:
##                                         mean    sd 0.025quant 0.5quant
## Precision for the Gaussian observations 159.78 15.51    130.83   159.27
##                                         0.975quant   mode
## Precision for the Gaussian observations    191.62 158.25
##
## Expected number of effective parameters(stdev): 11.21(0.021)
## Number of equivalent replicates : 19.72
##
## Marginal log-Likelihood:  173.09
## Posterior marginals for the linear predictor and
##  the fitted values are computed
```

In this case we have summarized the output because the number of coefficients is simply 10, in accordance with the degrees of freedom set in function ns() above. Note that there is an extra parameter in the linear predictor which is due to the presence of the intercept.

Figure 9.3 shows both smooth terms estimated using splines. It suggests that it may not be necessary to use as many as 31 when building the spline. The knots used by the second spline are computed using equally spaced quantiles by default:

```
attr(ns(lidar$range, df = 10), "knots")
```

```
## 10% 20% 30% 40% 50% 60% 70% 80% 90%
## 423 456 489 522 555 588 621 654 687
```

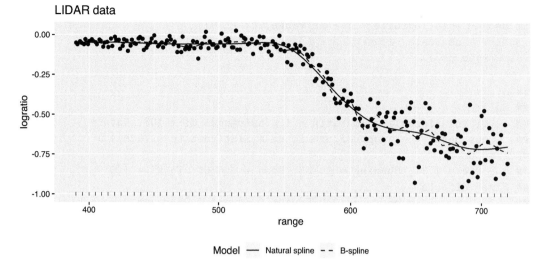

FIGURE 9.3 Smooth term fit to the `lidar` using splines of order 3. Knots are displayed at the bottom as tick marks.

Hence, it is clear that using too many knots will make the smooth term overfit the data, while using too few knots will most likely produce biased estimates (Ruppert et al., 2003).

The need for more or fewer knots can be assessed by looking at the estimates of the coefficients of the spline. Figure 9.4 shows the posterior means and 95% credible intervals on the 3-degree B-spline used above.

It is clear from that plot that most of the terms in the linear predictor can probably be removed without compromising model fitting. In addition, the values of the coefficients seem to follow the shape of the scatterplot of the data, with values close to zero in the regions where the data are more or less constant. Coefficients are away from zero in the regions where data change shape and show more variability.

Hence, it seems necessary to find a way to constrain or penalize the knots and coefficients of the spline so that it is not unnecessarily complex. This can be achieved by resorting to penalized splines or P-splines (Ruppert et al., 2003; Hastie et al., 2009), described in the next section.

9.3   Smooth terms with INLA

As seen above, splines provide a good way to include smooth terms in the linear predictor. However, splines have the problem of the selection of the number and position of the knots. Depending on the number and location, splines may overfit the data. As described in Ruppert et al. (2003), it may be necessary to constrain the influence of the knots by imposing further constraints on the spline coefficients.

Typically, this can be re-formulated as an optimization problem

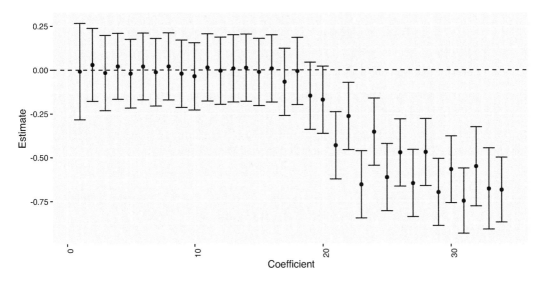

FIGURE 9.4 Estimates (posterior means and 95% credible intervals) of the coefficients of a 3-degree B-spline.

$$\min \sum_{i=1}^{n}(y_i - f(x_i))^2$$

subject to

$$\sum_{k=1}^{p} b_k^2 < C$$

with C being a positive constant that controls the degree of shrinkage of the coefficients. Small values of C will produce small estimates of the coefficients, while very large values will produce estimates that are close to the maximum likelihood estimates (Hastie et al., 2009; James et al., 2013). Note that only coefficients $\{b_k\}_{k=1}^{K}$ are used in the penalty term.

This is equivalent to minimizing the term

$$\min \sum_{i=1}^{n}(y_i - f(x_i))^2 + \lambda(\sum_{k=1}^{p} b_k^2)$$

for a fixed parameter $\lambda > 0$. This parameter can be set using cross-validation (Ruppert et al., 2003; Hastie et al., 2009; James et al., 2013).

In a Bayesian framework including the penalty term is equivalent to setting a specific prior on the coefficients of the covariates (see, for example, Fahrmeir and Kneib, 2011).

For equidistant knots $\{(\kappa_0, \ldots, \kappa_K)\}$ the prior is on the differences:

$$f(\kappa_{i+1}) - f(\kappa_i) \sim N(0, \tau), \ i = 1, \ldots, K-1$$

which is equivalent to setting a `rw1` prior on $f(\kappa_i)$.

Alternatively, when the prior is on the second order differences

$$f(\kappa_{i+1}) - 2f(\kappa_i) + f(\kappa_{i-1}) \sim N(0, \tau), \; i = 2, \ldots, K$$

This is equivalent to setting a `rw2` prior on the coefficients.

Hence, latent effects `rw1` and `rw2` can be used to include smooth terms on the covariates. The elements of the latent effect represent the values of the smooth term.

In the next example, a `rw1` latent effect is used. Note that `constr` is set to `FALSE` and that, for this reason, the intercept is not included in the linear predictor.

```
library("INLA")
m.rw1 <- inla(logratio ~ -1 + f(range, model = "rw1", constr = FALSE),
  data = lidar, control.predictor = list(compute = TRUE))
summary(m.rw1)
```

```
##
## Call:
##    c("inla(formula = logratio ~ -1 + f(range, model = \"rw1\", constr
##    = FALSE), ", " data = lidar, control.predictor = list(compute =
##    TRUE))" )
## Time used:
##     Pre = 0.985, Running = 0.58, Post = 0.0693, Total = 1.63
## Random effects:
##    Name     Model
##       range RW1 model
##
## Model hyperparameters:
##                                              mean       sd 0.025quant
## Precision for the Gaussian observations     166.64    17.21     134.99
## Precision for range                        4409.53 1356.52    2283.68
##                                            0.5quant 0.975quant     mode
## Precision for the Gaussian observations     165.90     202.68   164.60
## Precision for range                        4235.20    7551.69 3903.23
##
## Expected number of effective parameters(stdev): 27.74(4.65)
## Number of equivalent replicates : 7.97
##
## Marginal log-Likelihood:   251.75
## Posterior marginals for the linear predictor and
##   the fitted values are computed
```

Similarly, a `rw2` model can be used to fit a spline to the data:

```
m.rw2 <- inla(logratio ~ -1 + f(range, model = "rw2", constr = FALSE),
  data = lidar, control.predictor = list(compute = TRUE))
summary(m.rw2)
```

```
##
## Call:
##    c("inla(formula = logratio ~ -1 + f(range, model = \"rw2\", constr
##    = FALSE), ", " data = lidar, control.predictor = list(compute =
```

```
##     TRUE))" )
## Time used:
##     Pre = 1.07, Running = 0.629, Post = 0.0797, Total = 1.78
## Random effects:
##   Name      Model
##     range RW2 model
##
## Model hyperparameters:
##                                            mean        sd 0.025quant
## Precision for the Gaussian observations   159.30     15.79     130.09
## Precision for range                    166038.31  51798.38   84224.55
##                                         0.5quant 0.975quant       mode
## Precision for the Gaussian observations   158.68     192.20     157.65
## Precision for range                    159698.07 285932.26  147398.16
##
## Expected number of effective parameters(stdev): 20.30(1.68)
## Number of equivalent replicates : 10.89
##
## Marginal log-Likelihood:  319.01
## Posterior marginals for the linear predictor and
##   the fitted values are computed
```

Figure 9.5 shows the `lidar` dataset together with the fitted values under a `rw1` and `rw2` latent effects. Predictions seem very similar but, as expected, using a `rw2` smooth term provides a smoother function.

Note that this assumes that all the knots are regularly spaced. For the case of irregularly placed data, it is possible to use function `inla.group()` to bin data into groups according to the values of the covariate. The way in which values are grouped can be set with the `method` argument, that can be either `"cut"` (the default) or `"quantile"`. Option `"cut"` splits the data using equal length intervals, while option `"quantile"` uses equidistant quantiles in the probability space.

For example, to split the data into 20 groups using equally spaced quantiles the code is:

```
lidar$range.grp <- inla.group(lidar$range, n = 20, method = "quantile")
summary(lidar$range.grp)
```

```
##    Min. 1st Qu.  Median   Mean 3rd Qu.   Max.
##     394     477     546    555     633    716
```

The binned data can be see in Figure 9.6. Note that this does not guarantee that the new values of range are equally spaced, but it will help to reduce the number of knots used in the estimation of the smoothing effect.

The newly created variable `range.grp` can then be used to define the smooth term in the call to `inla()` inside the `f()` function. In the next models, this is employed to fit `rw1` and `rw2` models to the data:

```
m.grp.rw1 <- inla(logratio ~ -1 + f(range.grp, model = "rw1", constr = FALSE),
  data = lidar, control.predictor = list(compute = TRUE))
summary(m.grp.rw1)
```

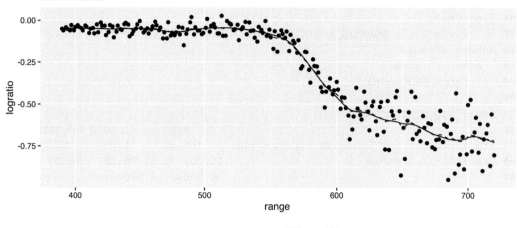

FIGURE 9.5 LIDAR data together with two smooth estimates (e.g., posterior means) based on **rw1** and **rw2** effects.

```
## 
## Call:
##    c("inla(formula = logratio ~ -1 + f(range.grp, model = \"rw1\",
##    constr = FALSE), ", " data = lidar, control.predictor =
##    list(compute = TRUE))" )
## Time used:
##      Pre = 0.966, Running = 0.369, Post = 0.0666, Total = 1.4
## Random effects:
##   Name       Model
##      range.grp RW1 model
## 
## Model hyperparameters:
##                                           mean       sd 0.025quant
## Precision for the Gaussian observations 155.65    15.27     127.38
## Precision for range.grp                4222.56  1401.73    2041.90
##                                        0.5quant 0.975quant     mode
## Precision for the Gaussian observations  155.07     187.45   154.09
## Precision for range.grp                 4040.57    7494.70  3684.20
## 
## Expected number of effective parameters(stdev): 16.31(0.979)
## Number of equivalent replicates : 13.55
## 
## Marginal log-Likelihood:   238.10
## Posterior marginals for the linear predictor and
##   the fitted values are computed
```

```
m.grp.rw2 <- inla(logratio ~ -1 + f(range.grp, model = "rw2", constr = FALSE),
  data = lidar, control.predictor = list(compute = TRUE))
summary(m.grp.rw2)
```

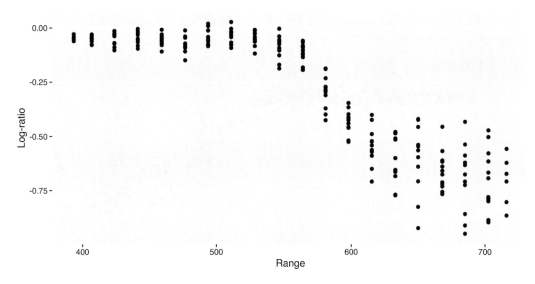

FIGURE 9.6 Observations of the LIDAR dataset binned according to variable `range`.

```
##
## Call:
##    c("inla(formula = logratio ~ -1 + f(range.grp, model = \"rw2\",
##    constr = FALSE), ", " data = lidar, control.predictor =
##    list(compute = TRUE))" )
## Time used:
##     Pre = 0.99, Running = 0.379, Post = 0.0723, Total = 1.44
## Random effects:
##   Name      Model
##     range.grp RW2 model
##
## Model hyperparameters:
##                                             mean        sd 0.025quant
## Precision for the Gaussian observations    154.60     15.25      126.37
## Precision for range.grp                 170350.19  54718.10    83873.88
##                                          0.5quant 0.975quant        mode
## Precision for the Gaussian observations    154.01     186.35      153.04
## Precision for range.grp                 163716.84  296980.19  150590.45
##
## Expected number of effective parameters(stdev): 18.45(0.498)
## Number of equivalent replicates : 11.98
##
## Marginal log-Likelihood:   273.05
## Posterior marginals for the linear predictor and
##   the fitted values are computed
```

Figure 9.7 shows the smooth terms estimated with the previous two models. They give very similar fits. The plot has also included the original data (in black) and the binned data (in gray). As compared to the previous models seen in Figure 9.5, the models fit to the binned data seem to be less smooth than the previous ones.

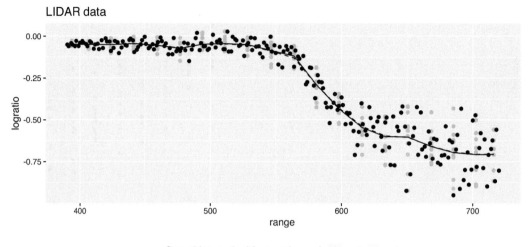

FIGURE 9.7 Smooth curve fit to the binned dataset on the actual dataset. Original data are shown in black and binned data in gray.

9.4 Smoothing with SPDE

For the case of irregularly spaced data or knots, it is possible to build smooth terms using other latent effects in `INLA`. In particular, the `spde` latent effect described in Chapter 7 can also be used in one dimension. In this case, the effect models a Matérn process in one dimension with correlation matrix

$$Cov(d_{ij}) = \frac{1}{\tau} \frac{2^{1-\nu}}{\Gamma(\nu)} (\kappa d_{ij})^\nu K_\nu(\kappa d_{ij})$$

Here, d_{ij} is the distance between observations i and j, $\nu > 0$ a smoothness parameter, $\kappa > 0$ a scale parameter, $\Gamma(\cdot)$ is the Gamma function and $K_\nu(\cdot)$ is the modified Bessel function of the second kind.

This is described in detail in Krainski et al. (2018), Chapter 2. Usually, the smoothness parameter is fixed and only the precision and the effective range, which is $\sqrt{8\nu}/\kappa$, are estimated. We describe now how to fit this model, for which we will rely on some of the contents described in Chapter 7 to define the model. Note that the focus now is in modeling in one dimension instead of in spatial models (that are defined in two dimensions). Furthermore, being familiar with Krainski et al. (2018) will be helpful now.

First of all, a set of knots to define the `spde` model is defined to create a mesh in one dimension and compute the projector matrix:

```
mesh1d <- inla.mesh.1d(seq(390, 720, by = 20))
A1 <- inla.spde.make.A(mesh1d, lidar$range)
```

Next, the `spde` model is defined.

```
spde1 <- inla.spde2.matern(mesh1d, constr = FALSE)
spde1.idx <- inla.spde.make.index("x", n.spde = spde1$n.spde)
```

In order to fit the model and predict the curve at some points, two data stacks (see Section 7.3) need to be created. The first one includes the data to fit the model:

```
stack <- inla.stack(data = list(y = lidar$logratio),
  A = list(1, A1),
  effects = list(Intercept = rep(1, nrow(lidar)), spde1.idx),
  tag = "est")
```

The second stack refers to the points at which the function needs to be estimated. In this case, the points span the values of **range** with a step of 5 units between each two consecutive values:

```
# Predict at a finer grid
xx <- seq(390, 720, by = 5)
A.xx <- inla.spde.make.A(mesh1d, xx)
stack.pred <- inla.stack(data = list(y = NA),
  A = list(1, A.xx),
  effects = list(Intercept = rep(1, length(xx)), spde1.idx),
  tag = "pred")
```

Both data stacks must be put together using function `inla.stack()`.

```
joint.stack <- inla.stack(stack, stack.pred)
```

The model is defined now. The formula does not include an intercept because it has been included within the data stack in order to make prediction easier to compute:

```
formula <- y ~ -1 + f(x, model = spde1)
```

Then, the `inla()` function is called to fit the model:

```
m.spde <- inla(formula, data = inla.stack.data(joint.stack),
  control.predictor = list(A = inla.stack.A(joint.stack), compute = TRUE)
)
```

Figure 9.8 shows the smooth term fitted to the data using the SPDE model. The fitted curve seems very similar to the ones obtained with **rw1** and **rw2** models. However, 95% credible intervals seem to be narrower. This shows that the hypothesis of constant variance does not hold for this data. Hence, a family that does not assume a constant variance could also be used to model this data.

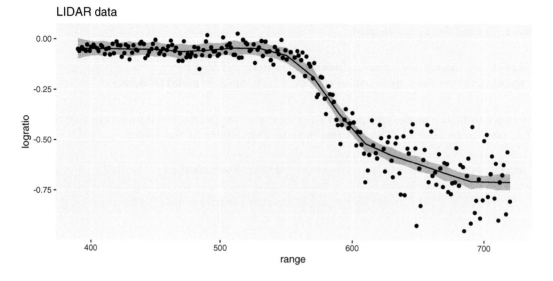

FIGURE 9.8 Smoothing of LIDAR data using a SPDE in one dimension. The solid line represents the posterior mean and the shaded area is the 95% credible interval of the predictive distribution on `range`.

9.5 Non-Gaussian models

So far, models for a Gaussian response have been considered. However, the models presented in this chapter can be easily extended to consider the non-Gaussian case. In particular, generalized linear models with smooth terms can be considered. This means that the mean of the non-Gaussian distribution is linked to the linear predictor using an appropriate function. As an example, we will consider an example based on a binomial likelihood using dose-response data.

Dose-response data are a typical example in which the use of a smooth term to explain the relationship between the dose and the number of events is required. Hence, non-parametric methods may be useful to learn the shape of the function that governs this relationship.

The `H.virescens` dataset (Venables and Ripley, 2002) in the `drc` package (Ritz et al., 2015) contains data from a dose-response experiment in which moths of the tobacco budworm (*Heliothis virescens*) were exposed for three days to different doses of the pyrethroid trans-cypermethrin (an insecticide). Table 9.2 describes the variables in the dataset.

TABLE 9.2: Variables in the `H.virescens` dataset.

Variable	Description
dose	Dose values (in μg).
numdead	Number of dead or knock-down moths.

Variable	Description
total	Total number of moths.
sex	Sex (M for male, F for female).

Data can be loaded and summarized as follows:

```
library("drc")

data(H.virescens)
levels(H.virescens$sex) <- c("Female", "Male")
summary(H.virescens)
```

```
##      dose          numdead          total        sex
## Min.    : 1.0   Min.   : 0.00   Min.    :20   Female:6
## 1st Qu.: 2.0   1st Qu.: 3.50   1st Qu.:20   Male  :6
## Median : 6.0   Median : 9.50   Median :20
## Mean    :10.5   Mean   : 9.25   Mean    :20
## 3rd Qu.:16.0   3rd Qu.:13.75   3rd Qu.:20
## Max.    :32.0   Max.   :20.00   Max.    :20
```

Dose-response data are typically non-linear because of the effect of the drug administered to the subjects in the study. Furthermore, this data are typically analyzed using a binomial distribution. In the next model, sex is included as control variable and sex is modeled using a rw1 latent effect:

```
vir.rw1 <- inla(numdead ~ -1 + f(dose, model = "rw1", constr = FALSE) + sex,
  data = H.virescens, family ="binomial", Ntrial = total,
  control.predictor = list(compute = TRUE))
summary(vir.rw1)
```

```
##
## Call:
##    c("inla(formula = numdead ~ -1 + f(dose, model = \"rw1\", constr =
##    FALSE) + ", " sex, family = \"binomial\", data = H.virescens,
##    Ntrials = total, ", " control.predictor = list(compute = TRUE))")
## Time used:
##     Pre = 1.17, Running = 0.128, Post = 0.0886, Total = 1.39
## Fixed effects:
##               mean    sd 0.025quant 0.5quant 0.975quant    mode kld
## sexFemale -0.532 22.36     -44.44   -0.533     43.33 -0.532   0
## sexMale    0.532 22.36     -43.37    0.532     44.40  0.532   0
##
## Random effects:
##   Name     Model
##     dose RW1 model
##
## Model hyperparameters:
##                    mean    sd 0.025quant 0.5quant 0.975quant mode
## Precision for dose 4.06 3.04      0.644     3.27      12.07 1.96
##
```

```
## Expected number of effective parameters(stdev): 5.75(0.444)
## Number of equivalent replicates : 2.09
##
## Marginal log-Likelihood:  -36.48
## Posterior marginals for the linear predictor and
##   the fitted values are computed
```

Another model using a `rw2` model is fit:

```
vir.rw2 <- inla(numdead ~ -1 + f(dose, model = "rw2", constr = FALSE) + sex,
   data = H.virescens, family = "binomial", Ntrial = total,
   control.predictor = list(compute = TRUE))
 summary(vir.rw2)
```

```
##
## Call:
##    c("inla(formula = numdead ~ -1 + f(dose, model = \"rw2\", constr =
##    FALSE) + ", " sex, family = \"binomial\", data = H.virescens,
##    Ntrials = total, ", " control.predictor = list(compute = TRUE))")
## Time used:
##     Pre = 1.1, Running = 0.0995, Post = 0.0688, Total = 1.27
## Fixed effects:
##              mean    sd 0.025quant 0.5quant 0.975quant    mode kld
## sexFemale -0.527 22.36    -44.43   -0.528      43.34 -0.527   0
## sexMale    0.527 22.36    -43.38    0.527      44.39  0.527   0
##
## Random effects:
##    Name     Model
##      dose RW2 model
##
## Model hyperparameters:
##                        mean       sd 0.025quant 0.5quant 0.975quant   mode
## Precision for dose 3608.23 8982.04      39.97   783.37    28952.37  81.62
##
## Expected number of effective parameters(stdev): 4.19(0.646)
## Number of equivalent replicates : 2.87
##
## Marginal log-Likelihood:  -25.38
## Posterior marginals for the linear predictor and
##   the fitted values are computed
```

The models fit to the data are displayed in Figure 9.9. Both models provide very similar estimates of the dose-response effect. Note that the fitted values are shown in Figure 9.10.

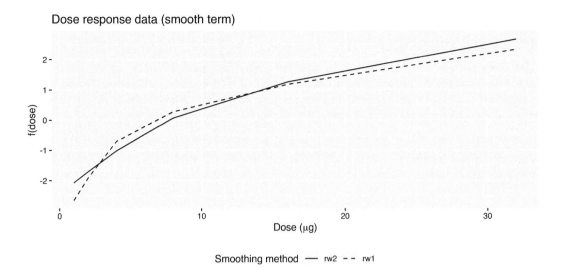

FIGURE 9.9 Posterior means of the random effects (`rw1` or `rw2`) of the models fit to the dose-response dataset.

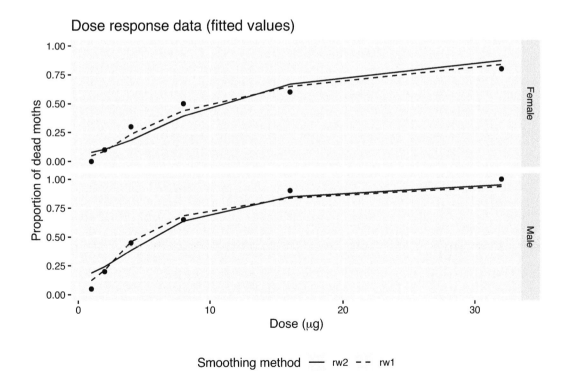

FIGURE 9.10 Posterior means of the random effects of the models fit to the dose-response dataset.

9.6   Final remarks

This chapter has covered different models for including smooth terms on the covariates in the linear predictor. Smoothing in two dimensions is described in Chapter 7, and some space-time models are also covered in Chapter 8. Wang et al. (2018) describe in detail other types of smoothing functions not covered here, such as thin plate splines.

`INLA` is flexible enough regarding the types of latent effects that can be included. Other types of smooth functions can be implemented using the different frameworks to extend the latent effects implemented in `INLA` described in Chapter 11.

10

Survival Models

10.1   Introduction

Survival data analysis tackles the problem of modeling observations of time to event. In this context, the interest is the time until a certain event happens. This can be death (e.g., survival time since diagnosis) or failure (e.g., time until a piece breaks down). We will give a brief overview of survival analysis now, in order to introduce the main concepts and define our notation. A more comprehensive treatment of Bayesian survival analysis can be found in Ibrahim et al. (2001). Moore (2016) also provides a nice introduction to survival analysis with R.

Considering T as the random variable that measures time to event, the *survival function* $S(t)$ can be defined as the probability that T is higher than a given time t, i.e., $S(t) = P(T > t)$. For example, this could be the probability that a patient will survive at least until time t since diagnosis. In survival analysis there are the implicit assumptions that $S(0) = 1$, i.e., all patients are alive at the beginning of the study, and that $\lim_{t \to +\infty} S(t) = 0$, i.e., all patients will eventually die (*Valar Morghullis*).

When considering a survival function, it will be related to a distribution function $F(t) = P(T < t) = 1 - S(t)$ with density function $f(t)$. This can be a parametric distribution, as we will see below.

The *hazard function* $h(t)$ measures the probability that the event occurs at a small instant given that the patient has survived until time t. More precisely,

$$h(t) = \lim_{\Delta t \to 0} \frac{P(T < t + \Delta t \mid T > t)}{\Delta t}$$

The *cumulative hazard* $H(t)$ is defined as

$$H(t) = \int_0^t h(u)du$$

Hence, the hazard function can be expressed as $h(t) = f(t)/S(t)$. Furthermore, the survival function can be expressed in terms of the cumulative hazard function as

$$S(t) = \exp(-H(t))$$

Survival data are often censored. For example, patients may experience the event during the study period, in which case the time to event is observed, or after the study has been finished, in which case the event time is unobserved. For this reason, each observation is accompanied by a status variable δ_i to indicate whether the event was observed or not.

In addition, a vector of covariates may be available for each patient. Hence, the data will be made of $\{(t_i, \delta_i, \mathbf{x}_i\}_{i=1}^n$, where t_i is time of patient i, δ_i the associated censoring status variable and $\mathbf{x}_i$ the covariates associated to patient i.

The likelihood of this model can be expressed as:

$$\prod_{i=1}^n f(t_i)^{\delta_i} S(t_i)^{1-\delta_i}$$

Note how depending on whether an observation has been censored its contribution to the likelihood will be either $f(t_i)$ or $S(t_i)$.

10.2   Non-parametric estimation of the survival curve

The Kaplan-Meier estimator provides a non-parametric estimate of the survival curve. It is based on the conditional probability of surviving until time t given that the patient has survived until time t_i and it is defined as

$$\hat{S}(t) = \prod_{t_i \leq t} (1 - \frac{d_i}{n_i})$$

Here, n_i is the number of subjects at risk at time i and d_i the number of individuals that fail at that time. Note that at a given time t_i, $(1 - d_i/n_i)$ is the proportion of individuals at risk at time t_i that do not experience any event. Hence, the Kaplan-Meier estimate is the product of all conditional probabilities of not experiencing the event up to time t.

The `survival` package (Terry M. Therneau and Patricia M. Grambsch, 2000; Therneau, 2015) implements a number of functions for the analysis of survival data, including the Kaplan-Meier estimator, and includes various datasets. We will be using the `veteran` dataset (Kalbfleisch and Prentice, 1980), which contains data from the Veteran's Administration Lung Cancer Trial. This dataset records time to death of 137 male patients with advanced inoperable lung cancer. Patients were assigned at random a standard treatment or a test treatment. Only 9 patients left the trial before they experienced death. In addition to the time to death and the treatment received, there are other covariates measured and they have been summarized in Table 10.1.

TABLE 10.1: Variables in the `veteran` dataset.

Variable	Description
trt	Treatment (1 for standard, 2 for test treatment)
celltype	Histological type of tumor (1=squamous, 2=smallcell, 3=adeno, 4=large).
time	Survival time (in days).
status	Censoring status (1 for death, 0 for censored).
karno	Karnofsky performance score (100 means good).
diagtime	Months from diagnosis to randomization.
age	Age in years.
prior	Prior therapy (0 for no, 10 for prior treatment).

First of all, we will load the data and recode some of the variables in the study as factors:

```
library("survival")
data(veteran)

veteran$trt <- as.factor(veteran$trt)
levels(veteran$trt) <- c("standard", "test")
veteran$prior <- as.factor(veteran$prior)
levels(veteran$prior) <- c("No", "Yes")
```

As stated in the INLA documentation, some likelihoods for survival data may be affected by numerical overflow when observed times are large. For this reason, we will re-scale time before fitting any model and express time as 30-day months.

```
veteran$time.m <- round(veteran$time / 30, 3)
```

We will use the Surv() function to create a data structure with the required format for data analysis using the survival/censoring times and the censoring indicator. This is illustrated in the next lines where the first 20 values in the survival data structure are shown:

```
surv.vet <- Surv(veteran$time.m, veteran$status)
surv.vet[1:20]
```

```
##  [1]  2.400  13.700   7.600   4.200   3.933   0.333   2.733   3.667
##  [9] 10.467   3.333+  1.400   0.267   4.800   0.833+  0.367   1.000
## [17] 12.800   0.133   1.800   0.433
```

Note how censored observations are marked with a + to indicate that the time to event has been censored and it is larger than the value shown.

The Kaplan-Meier estimator can be used to obtain an estimate of the survival function as follows:

```
km.vet <- survfit(surv.vet ~ 1)
```

Figure 10.2 (left plot) shows a Kaplan-Meier estimate of the survival time for the veteran dataset. The plot includes confidence intervals as well as point estimates of the survival time. Note that the plot on the right corresponds to a parametric estimate discussed later in Section 10.3. They have been put side by side so that the different estimates can be compared.

Furthermore, four different survival curves can be estimated by splitting the data according to the different types of tumors:

```
km.vet.cell <- survfit(surv.vet ~ -1 + celltype, data = veteran)
```

Figure 10.1 shows estimates of the survival times for each of the four groups of patients defined by the covariate. Here, function autoplot() (in package ggpot2, Wickham, 2016) has been used to produce the plot. Survival seems to be worst for those patients with tumors with a histological classification of adeno or smallcell.

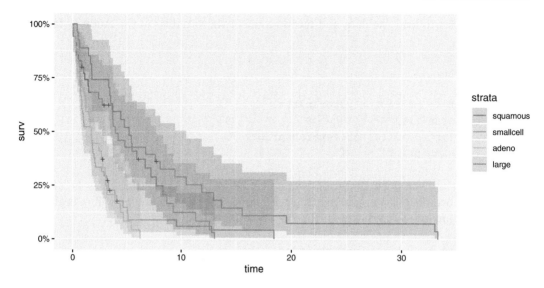

FIGURE 10.1 Survival estimates of patients according to histological type of tumor (i.e., cell type).

10.3   Parametric modeling of the survival function

INLA provides a number of distributions that can be used to model the survival function, as seen in Table 10.2.

For this first example we will fit a survival model to the the `veteran` dataset. INLA provides a similar function to `Surv`, called `inla.surv`, to create the necessary data structure to conduct a survival analysis, which is used as follows:

```
library("INLA")
sinla.vet <- inla.surv(veteran$time.m, veteran$status)
```

The model fitted to the `veteran` dataset in this first example is an exponential model. This corresponds to a model with constant hazard, i.e., $h(t) = \lambda$, where λ is the rate parameter of the exponential distribution (see Table 10.2).

```
exp.vet <- inla(sinla.vet ~ 1, data = veteran, family = "exponential.surv")
summary(exp.vet)
```

```
##
## Call:
##    "inla(formula = sinla.vet ~ 1, family = \"exponential.surv\", data
##    = veteran)"
## Time used:
##    Pre = 1.04, Running = 0.0956, Post = 0.0628, Total = 1.2
## Fixed effects:
```

```
##                 mean    sd 0.025quant 0.5quant 0.975quant    mode kld
## (Intercept) -1.468 0.088    -1.646   -1.466     -1.298 -1.463   0
##
## Expected number of effective parameters(stdev): 1.00(0.00)
## Number of equivalent replicates : 136.89
##
## Marginal log-Likelihood:  -317.37
```

TABLE 10.2: Summary of some likelihoods available in `INLA` for survival analysis.

Likelihood	$h(t)$	$H(t)$	$S(t)$	family
Exponential	λ	λt	$\exp(-\lambda t)$	exponential.surv
Weibull	$\alpha\lambda(\lambda t)^{\alpha-1}$	$(\lambda t)^{\alpha}$	$\exp(-(\lambda t)^{\alpha})$	weibull.surv
Loglogistic	$\frac{(\beta/\alpha)(t/\alpha)^{\beta-1}}{1+(t/\alpha)^{\beta}}$	-	$(1+(t/\alpha)^{\beta})^{-1}$	loglogistic.surv
Lognormal	-	-	-	lognormal.surv

In the previous model, a log link is used. Hence, $\lambda = \exp(\alpha)$, where α is the model intercept. In this particular case, the survival function is

$$S(t) = \exp(-H(t)) = \exp\left(-\int_0^t \lambda du\right) = \exp(-\lambda t)$$

We can use function `inla.tmarginal()` to transform the posterior marginal of α into the marginal of $S(t)$ for a given time and compute 95% credible intervals. Note that this is required because the intercept α reported by `INLA` is actually $\log(\lambda)$. Hence, for each time t, the marginal of α is transformed into the posterior marginal of $S(t)$ and summary statistics are computed with function `inla.zmarginal()`:

```
library("parallel")
# Set number of cores to use
options(mc.cores = 4)
# Grid of times
times <- seq(0.01, 35, by = 1)
# Marginal of alpha
alpha.marg <- exp.vet$marginals.fixed[["(Intercept)"]]
# Compute post. marg. of survival function
S.inla <- mclapply(times, function(t){
  S.marg <- inla.tmarginal(function(x) {exp(- exp(x) * t)}, alpha.marg)
  S.stats <- inla.zmarginal(S.marg, silent = TRUE)
  return(unlist(S.stats[c("quant0.025", "mean", "quant0.975")]))
})

S.inla <- as.data.frame(do.call(rbind, S.inla))
```

Figure 10.2 shows the survival function obtained with an exponential model. Median survival time is about 4 months, similar to the value obtained with the non-parametric Kaplan-Meier estimator. Furthermore, uncertainty is very similar between both estimates, with the credible intervals of the Bayesian parametric estimate narrower in the sides.

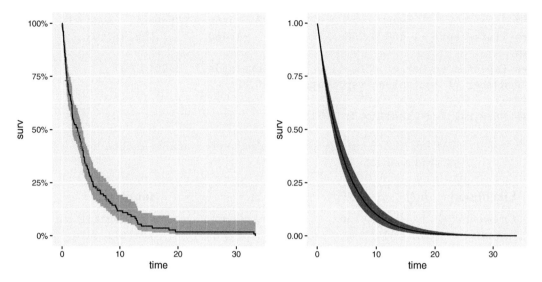

FIGURE 10.2 Kaplan-Meier estimate (left) and survival function using an exponential model (right) for the `veteran` dataset.

10.4   Semi-parametric estimation: Cox proportional hazards

Cox (1972) proposed a model in which the hazard function is the product of a baseline hazard $h_0(t)$ and a term that depends on a number of covariates $\mathbf{x}$. The baseline hazard can be estimated using non-parametric methods, while the term on the covariates is a function on a linear predictor on the covariates. In particular, a Cox proportional hazards models can be written down as:

$$h(t) = h_0(t) \exp(\beta \mathbf{x})$$

Hence, the hazard function is *modulated* by the covariates and their associated influence (as measured by coeffients β).

`INLA` implements a likelihood for a Cox proportional hazards model as follows:

$$h(t) = h_0(t) \exp(\eta)$$

Here, $h_0(t)$ is the baseline hazard function and η is a linear predictor on some covariates and, possibly, other effects. Furthermore, the baseline hazard $h_0(t)$ is modeled as:

$$h_0(t) = \exp(b_k); t \in (s_{k-1}, s_k], k = 1, \ldots, K$$

Hence, the baseline hazard is a piecewise constant function. Variables $\mathbf{b} = (b_1, \ldots, b_K)$ are assigned a prior which is a random walk of order 1 (default) or 2.

As described earlier, the `veteran` dataset includes a covariate that measures whether the patient received a standard treatment or a test treatment. We will use a Cox model to model survival time on this covariate and the type of tumor in order to assess the effect of the test treatment. Control option `control.hazard` (see Section 2.5) can be used to define a number of options on how the baseline hazard function is computed. Below, we only set the prior of the random effect to a vague prior (as seen in Chapter 3).

```
coxinla.vet <- inla(sinla.vet ~ 1  + celltype + trt, data = veteran,
  family = "coxph",
  control.hazard = list(hyper = list(prec = list(param = c(0.001, 0.001)))))
summary(coxinla.vet)
```

```
##
## Call:
##    c("inla(formula = cph$formula, family = cph$family, contrasts =
##    contrasts, ", " data = c(as.list(cph$data), cph$data.list),
##    quantiles = quantiles, ", " E = cph$E, offset = offset, scale =
##    scale, weights = weights, ", " Ntrials = NULL, strata = NULL,
##    verbose = verbose, lincomb = lincomb, ", " control.compute =
##    control.compute, control.predictor = control.predictor, ", "
##    control.family = control.family, control.inla = control.inla, ", "
##    control.results = control.results, control.fixed = control.fixed,
##    ", " control.mode = control.mode, control.expert = control.expert,
##    ", " control.hazard = control.hazard, control.lincomb =
##    control.lincomb, ", " control.update = control.update,
##    only.hyperparam = only.hyperparam, ", " inla.call = inla.call,
##    inla.arg = inla.arg, num.threads = num.threads, ", "
##    blas.num.threads = blas.num.threads, keep = keep,
##    working.directory = working.directory, ", " silent = silent, debug
##    = debug)")
## Time used:
##     Pre = 1.16, Running = 0.164, Post = 0.0637, Total = 1.38
## Fixed effects:
##                       mean    sd 0.025quant 0.5quant 0.975quant    mode kld
## (Intercept)         -2.157 0.235     -2.633   -2.152     -1.709  -2.141   0
## celltypesmallcell    1.167 0.253      0.676    1.166      1.668   1.163   0
## celltypeadeno        1.240 0.268      0.711    1.241      1.762   1.244   0
## celltypelarge        0.334 0.276     -0.212    0.335      0.873   0.338   0
## trttest              0.171 0.194     -0.211    0.171      0.551   0.171   0
##
## Random effects:
##   Name        Model
##     baseline.hazard RW1 model
##
## Model hyperparameters:
##                                   mean       sd 0.025quant 0.5quant
## Precision for baseline.hazard 20406.74 19866.92     719.48 14282.41
##                                0.975quant     mode
## Precision for baseline.hazard   73795.12 1340.76
##
## Expected number of effective parameters(stdev): 5.07(0.15)
## Number of equivalent replicates : 64.37
##
## Marginal log-Likelihood:  -359.33
```

The summary of the model indicates that survival depends on the type of tumor and that the test treatment does not seem to be better than the standard treatment.

The summary shows an estimate of the precision of the baseline hazard, which is modeled as a random walk of order 1 (in the log-scale). Because the estimate of the baseline risk is in the log-scale, we need to back-transform it and re-compute the summary statistics from the marginals:

```
#Transform baseline hazard
h0 <- lapply(coxinla.vet$marginals.random[["baseline.hazard"]],
  function(X) {inla.tmarginal(exp, X)}
)
#Compute summary statistics for plotting
h0.stats <- lapply(h0, inla.zmarginal)
```

Next, we have included the times and summary statistics of the baseline hazard together into a single data frame for plotting:

```
h0.df <- data.frame(t = coxinla.vet$summary.random[["baseline.hazard"]]$ID)
h0.df <- cbind(h0.df, do.call(rbind, lapply(h0.stats, unlist)))
```

Finally, Figure 10.3 shows the posterior means and 95% credible intervals of the baseline hazard function. We have added a red line to mark a hazard of 1. The estimated baseline hazard function seems to be constant about 1. This may occur because the covariates included in the model explain most of the variability in the data.

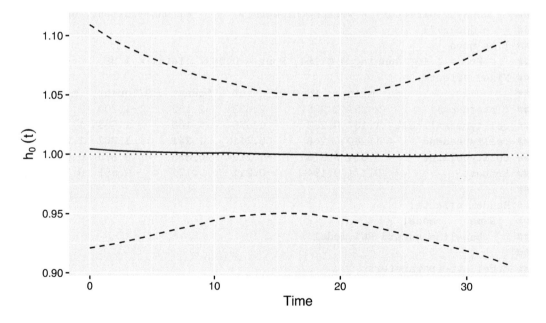

FIGURE 10.3 Posterior mean (solid line) and 95% credible interval (dashed lines) of baseline hazard function estimate using a Cox model on the `veteran` dataset.

10.5 Accelerated failure time models

Accelerated failure time (AFT) models are log-linear regression models that are widely applied in survival analysis. They take the following general form:

$$\log(T) = \beta \mathbf{x} + \sigma \varepsilon$$

Here, $\mathbf{x}$ is a vector of covariates with associated coefficients β, σ is a precision parameter and ε is an error term. This error term can take different density distributions f_ε that will eventually define the survival and hazard functions.

TABLE 10.3: Summary of distributions used in accelerated time failure models.

Distribution of T	Distribution of error term (f_ε)
Log-normal	Standard normal
Log-logistic	Logistic
Exponential	Extreme Value
Weibull	Extreme Value

Table 10.3 shows the distributions for the error term ε and the corresponding distribution of T.

10.5.1 Log-normal model

The way to specify the AFT model to use with INLA is via the `family` option. In the next lines, a log-normal likelihood is used to fit a survival model to the `veteran` dataset:

```
logninla.vet <- inla(sinla.vet ~ -1 + celltype + trt, data = veteran,
   family = "lognormal.surv")
```

Note that the log-survival likelihood used in the model (i.e., `lognormal.surv`) is different from the typical log-normal distribution (i.e., `lognormal`), which does not takes censoring status into account.

The effects of the covariates on hazard can be assessed by checking the posterior summary statistics:

```
summary(logninla.vet)
```

```
##
## Call:
##    c("inla(formula = sinla.vet ~ -1 + celltype + trt, family =
##    \"lognormal.surv\", ", " data = veteran)")
## Time used:
##    Pre = 1, Running = 0.107, Post = 0.0654, Total = 1.17
## Fixed effects:
```

```
##                      mean    sd 0.025quant 0.5quant 0.975quant    mode kld
## celltypesquamous    1.254 0.266      0.734    1.254      1.779   1.252   0
## celltypesmallcell   0.420 0.211      0.005    0.419      0.835   0.419   0
## celltypeadeno       0.507 0.299     -0.080    0.506      1.094   0.506   0
## celltypelarge       1.495 0.276      0.953    1.495      2.038   1.494   0
## trttest            -0.214 0.234     -0.674   -0.214      0.245  -0.214   0
##
## Model hyperparameters:
##                                                      mean    sd 0.025quant
## Precision for the lognormalsurv observations        0.584 0.074      0.448
##                                                  0.5quant 0.975quant  mode
## Precision for the lognormalsurv observations        0.581      0.738 0.574
##
## Expected number of effective parameters(stdev): 5.00(0.00)
## Number of equivalent replicates : 27.40
##
## Marginal log-Likelihood:  -342.10
```

Given this model's survival time, positive coefficients indicate a longer survival. For example, the effect of having an histological tumor of type large seems to provide the best survival among all patients.

In order to assess what risk factors increase survival time (and reduce hazard), the posterior probability of the coefficients of the fixed effects being positive can be computed with function inla.pmarginal():

```
lapply(logninla.vet$marginals.fixed, function(X){1 - inla.pmarginal(0, X)})
```

```
## $celltypesquamous
## [1] 1
##
## $celltypesmallcell
## [1] 0.9764
##
## $celltypeadeno
## [1] 0.955
##
## $celltypelarge
## [1] 1
##
## $trttest
## [1] 0.1779
```

Note that logninla.vet$marginals.fixed is a list with all the posterior marginals of the fixed effects. In order to compute the posterior probability of being lower than one, one minus the probability of being lower than zero is computed with 1 - inla.pmarginal(0, X) (where X represents a given posterior marginal).

10.5.2   Weibull model

Next, a Weibull survival model will be fitted to the veteran dataset:

```
weibinla.vet <- inla(sinla.vet ~ -1 + celltype + trt,
  data = veteran, family = "weibull.surv",
  control.family = list(variant=0))
```

The option `control.family = list(variant=0)` is used to use the following parameterisation for the distribution of time t:

$$f(t) = \alpha t^{\alpha-1} \lambda \exp\{-\lambda t^{\alpha}\}$$

Then, the linear predictor η is linked to λ as $\log(\lambda) = \eta$.

```
summary(weibinla.vet)
```

```
##
## Call:
##    c("inla(formula = sinla.vet ~ -1 + celltype + trt, family =
##    \"weibull.surv\", ", " data = veteran, control.family =
##    list(variant = 0))")
## Time used:
##    Pre = 0.996, Running = 0.144, Post = 0.0599, Total = 1.2
## Fixed effects:
##                      mean    sd 0.025quant 0.5quant 0.975quant    mode kld
## celltypesquamous   -2.104 0.273     -2.656   -2.099     -1.583  -2.089   0
## celltypesmallcell  -0.958 0.175     -1.313   -0.955     -0.624  -0.947   0
## celltypeadeno      -0.891 0.242     -1.384   -0.884     -0.433  -0.872   0
## celltypelarge      -1.779 0.237     -2.261   -1.774     -1.332  -1.762   0
## trttest             0.167 0.194     -0.214    0.167      0.548   0.167   0
##
## Model hyperparameters:
##                                   mean    sd 0.025quant 0.5quant 0.975quant
## alpha parameter for weibullsurv   0.98 0.057      0.867    0.981       1.09
##                                   mode
## alpha parameter for weibullsurv  0.993
##
## Expected number of effective parameters(stdev): 5.00(0.00)
## Number of equivalent replicates : 27.40
##
## Marginal log-Likelihood:  -322.42
```

Because of the parametcrisation of this model, negative coefficients will increase survival time (and reduce hazard). Hence, the posterior probability of the coefficients being lower than zero can be computed to assess increased hazard:

```
lapply(weibinla.vet$marginals.fixed, function(X){inla.pmarginal(0, X)})
```

```
## $celltypesquamous
## [1] 1
##
## $celltypesmallcell
## [1] 1
##
## $celltypeadeno
```

```
## [1] 1
##
## $celltypelarge
## [1] 1
##
## $trttest
## [1] 0.1954
```

10.6   Frailty models

Under some circumstances, survival may be similar for certain patients. For example, members of a family may be resistant to certain types of cancer or pieces manufactured at a particular factory may have a lower quality that decreases survival time. This dependence means that observations are no longer independent within groups. This correlation is often modeled by means of random effects or frailties, in the survival argot.

Frailty models are essentially mixed-effects models for survival data. Sometimes survival data are clustered or grouped (i.e., families, schools, etc.) and observations are not independent. For this reason, random effects may be included in the survival model to account for correlation between subjects within groups. In the next examples we will show how to use INLA to fit these types of models.

The `retinopathy` dataset (Blair et al., 1976, Huster et al. (1989)) in the `survival` package records data from a trial on laser coagulation treatment to delay diabetic retinopathy. This trial enrolled 197 patients with high-risk diabetic retinopathy and the event of interest was the time of loss of vision (measured as having a score below 5/200 in two consecutive visits). Each patient had one eye treated and the other eye was used as a control. Variables in this dataset are summarized in Table 10.4. In this case, between patient variation will be modeled using random effects in the frailty model.

TABLE 10.4: Variables in the `retinopathy` dataset.

Variable	Description
id	Patient identification number.
laser	Type of laser used ('xenon' or 'argon').
eye	Eye that was treated ('right' or 'left').
age	Age at the diagnosis of diabetes.
type	Type of diabetes ('juvenile' or 'adult').
trt	Treatment (0 for control eye, 1 for treated eye).
futime	Time to loss of vision or last follow-up (in months).
status	Censoring status (0 for censored, 1 for loss of vision).
risk	Risk score for the eye (values of 6 or greater indicate high risk).

First of all, the data will be loaded and the treatment variables converted into a factor:

```
data(retinopathy)

#Recode some covariates as factors
retinopathy$trt <- as.factor(c("control", "treated")[retinopathy$trt + 1])

#Summary
summary(retinopathy)
```

```
##        id            laser           eye             age             type
##  Min.   :   5    xenon:200    right:178    Min.   : 1.0    juvenile:228
##  1st Qu.: 480    argon:194    left :216    1st Qu.:10.0    adult   :166
##  Median : 834                              Median :16.0
##  Mean   : 873                              Mean   :20.8
##  3rd Qu.:1296                              3rd Qu.:30.0
##  Max.   :1749                              Max.   :58.0
##       trt           futime          status          risk
##  control:197    Min.   : 0.3    Min.   :0.000    Min.   : 6.0
##  treated:197    1st Qu.:14.0    1st Qu.:0.000    1st Qu.: 9.0
##                 Median :38.8    Median :0.000    Median :10.0
##                 Mean   :35.6    Mean   :0.393    Mean   : 9.7
##                 3rd Qu.:54.2    3rd Qu.:1.000    3rd Qu.:11.0
##                 Max.   :75.0    Max.   :1.000    Max.   :12.0
```

In order to avoid numerical problems, the time to event has been converted into years:

```
retinopathy$futime <- retinopathy$futime / 12
```

A Kaplan-Meier estimate of the survival function can be obtained as:

```
surv.ret <- Surv(retinopathy$futime, retinopathy$status)

km.ret <- survfit(surv.ret ~ 1)
```

Figure 10.4 shows the Kaplan-Meier estimate. The large amount of censored observations above 70 months can be seen, which makes it difficult to estimate median survival time and survival for large periods of time.

In this example we will consider a frailty model defined on patient (variable `id`) and a vague prior is used on the precision of the frailty effect:

```
# Model formula
form <- inla.surv(futime, status) ~ 1 + trt + risk + f(id, model = "iid",
  hyper = list(prec = list(param = c(0.001, 0.001))))

# Model fitting
fr.ret <- inla(form, data = retinopathy,
  family = "weibullsurv")
```

Note that in the previous model the random effects are defined using a Gaussian distribution. A summary of the model is.

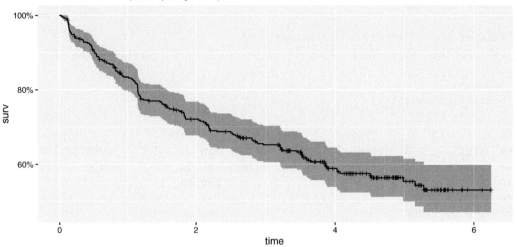

FIGURE 10.4 Survival function of the `retinopathy` dataset.

```
summary(fr.ret)
```

```
##
## Call:
##    "inla(formula = form, family = \"weibullsurv\", data =
##    retinopathy)"
## Time used:
##     Pre = 1.11, Running = 0.838, Post = 0.0652, Total = 2.02
## Fixed effects:
##                mean    sd 0.025quant 0.5quant 0.975quant    mode kld
## (Intercept) -3.363 0.704     -4.778   -3.351     -2.013  -3.328   0
## trttreated  -0.947 0.182     -1.309   -0.945     -0.596  -0.940   0
## risk         0.171 0.069      0.038    0.171      0.308   0.170   0
##
## Random effects:
##   Name      Model
##     id IID model
##
## Model hyperparameters:
##                                  mean    sd 0.025quant 0.5quant 0.975quant
## alpha parameter for weibullsurv 0.975 0.058      0.857    0.977       1.08
## Precision for id                1.100 0.386      0.556    1.029       2.05
##                                  mode
## alpha parameter for weibullsurv 0.987
## Precision for id                0.903
##
## Expected number of effective parameters(stdev): 79.08(16.40)
## Number of equivalent replicates : 4.98
##
## Marginal log-Likelihood:  -458.17
```

The large precision of the frailties suggests that there is a small between patient variation given the other factors accounted for. Figure 10.5 shows 95% credible intervals of the frailties for each patient. These suggest that none of the patients have an intrinsic effect not accounted for by the covariates included in the model.

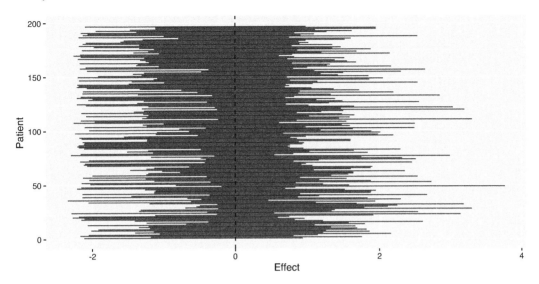

FIGURE 10.5 95% credible intervals of the frailties in the retinopathy dataset analysis.

10.7 Joint modeling

So far, censorship and time to event have been assumed to be independent. However, these two variables may be correlated and relevant covariates may be available to explain this dependence. For example, patients may drop out from a clinical trial for a worsening in their clinical state. When clinical state can be modeled on several covariates using longitudinal data, censoring itself will also depend on these covariates. Hence, it is important to model clinical state (as measured by a convenient variable) and survival time.

This model will require a joint model with two components: a longitudinal model and a survival model. In practice, we will use a model with two likelihoods (see Section 6.4 for details) that share some latent effects. As an example, we will fit a joint model to a data set about 488 patients with liver cirrhosis in a randomized trial (Andersen et al., 1993). Prothrombin measurements were taken at irregular times as a measure of liver function. Furthermore, time to death (which can be censored) was also recorded for each patient. In addition, the randomized treatment for each patient (placebo or prednisone) is also available for all patients.

This dataset is available in package JMbayes (Rizopoulos, 2016). The longitudinal and survival parts of the data set is available as prothro, while the survival part alone is prothros. In order to introduce the joint model step by step, we will fit a longitudinal model first, followed by a purely survival model and then the joint model.

10.7.1   Survival analysis

As stated before, the variables for the survival analysis are available in dataset `prothros` in package `JMbayes`. Table 10.5 shows a description of the variables in the dataset.

TABLE 10.5: Variables in the `prothros` dataset.

Variable	Description
id	Patient id number.
Time	Time to event or censoring time.
death	Indicator of whether the patient died (1) or not (0).
treat	Treatment (placebo or prednisone).

A summary of the variables in this dataset is shown below:

```
library("JMbayes")
data(prothros)
summary(prothros)
```

```
##       id             Time              death            treat
##  Min.   :  1   Min.   : 0.011   Min.   :0.000   placebo   :251
##  1st Qu.:167   1st Qu.: 0.632   1st Qu.:0.000   prednisone:237
##  Median :302   Median : 2.616   Median :1.000
##  Mean   :295   Mean   : 3.643   Mean   :0.598
##  3rd Qu.:431   3rd Qu.: 6.236   3rd Qu.:1.000
##  Max.   :561   Max.   :13.394   Max.   :1.000
```

A survival model of the patients with treatment as a covariate can be fit to the data in order to assess the effect of the treatment and account for the variability between the patients. Note that for survival models time to event may be required to be re-scaled , e.g., to be in the $(0, 1)$ interval, to avoid numerical problems with INLA. In this case, no re-scaling is done.

```
#prothros$Time <- prothros$Time  / max(prothros$Time) # Re-scaling
pro.surv <- inla.surv(prothros$Time, prothros$death)

form.pro.surv <- pro.surv ~ 1 + treat

pro.surv.inla <- inla(form.pro.surv, data = prothros,
  family = "weibull.surv")

summary(pro.surv.inla)
```

```
##
## Call:
##    "inla(formula = form.pro.surv, family = \"weibull.surv\", data =
##    prothros)"
## Time used:
##    Pre = 0.874, Running = 0.159, Post = 0.0577, Total = 1.09
## Fixed effects:
```

```
##                      mean     sd 0.025quant 0.5quant 0.975quant    mode kld
## (Intercept)        -1.561 0.106     -1.774   -1.560     -1.357 -1.557   0
## treatprednisone     0.093 0.117     -0.137    0.093      0.323  0.093   0
##
## Model hyperparameters:
##                                      mean    sd 0.025quant 0.5quant 0.975quant
## alpha parameter for weibullsurv 0.825 0.04      0.748    0.824      0.905
##                                      mode
## alpha parameter for weibullsurv 0.823
##
## Expected number of effective parameters(stdev): 2.00(0.00)
## Number of equivalent replicates : 243.78
##
## Marginal log-Likelihood:  -815.53
```

The results show that prednisone has a positive coefficient but its effect does not seem to be significant, i.e., it does not increase survival time compared to the placebo.

10.7.2 Longitudinal analysis

Next, we will carry out a longitudinal analysis of the data to model how prothrombin measurements change over time. The longitudinal model will also consider the effect of treatment, which can be a placebo or prednisone.

TABLE 10.6: Variables in the `prothro` dataset.

Variable	Description
id	Patient id number.
pro	Prothrombin measurement.
time	Time of prothrombin measurement.
treat	Treatment (placebo or prednisone).
Time	Time to event or censoring time.
start	Time of prothrombin measurement.
stop	Time of next prothrombin measurement or to event or censoring time.
death	Indicator of whether the patient died (1) or not (0).
event	Indicator of whether the event was observed in this time interval (1) or not (0).

As stated earlier, the longitudinal data is available in dataset `prothro` in package `JMbayes`. Table 10.6 describes the variables in the longitudinal part of the dataset. Data is loaded and summarized below:

```
data(prothro)
summary(prothro)
```

```
##        id           pro            time           treat
## Min.   :  1   Min.   :  6   Min.   : 0.000   placebo   :1498
## 1st Qu.:138   1st Qu.: 60   1st Qu.: 0.274   prednisone:1470
## Median :277   Median : 79   Median : 1.010
```

```
## Mean   :277   Mean   : 79   Mean   : 2.039
## 3rd Qu.:418   3rd Qu.:100   3rd Qu.: 3.158
## Max.   :561   Max.   :176   Max.   :11.108
##      Time             start             stop            death
## Min.   : 0.011   Min.   : 0.000   Min.   : 0.011   Min.   :0.00
## 1st Qu.: 2.467   1st Qu.: 0.274   1st Qu.: 0.539   1st Qu.:0.00
## Median : 5.632   Median : 1.010   Median : 1.851   Median :1.00
## Mean   : 5.410   Mean   : 2.039   Mean   : 2.638   Mean   :0.55
## 3rd Qu.: 8.145   3rd Qu.: 3.158   3rd Qu.: 4.082   3rd Qu.:1.00
## Max.   :13.394   Max.   :11.108   Max.   :13.394   Max.   :1.00
##      event
## Min.   :0.0000
## 1st Qu.:0.0000
## Median :0.0000
## Mean   :0.0984
## 3rd Qu.:0.0000
## Max.   :1.0000
```

In this case, a longitudinal model is built to explain how prothrombin measurements change with time and according to treatment (as a fixed effect) or patient (included as a random effect). A log-normal likelihood is used in this case given that the response variable can only be positive:

```
form.pro.long <- pro ~ 1 + time + f(id, model = "iid") + treat
pro.long.inla <- inla(form.pro.long, data = prothro, family = "lognormal")
summary(pro.long.inla)
```

```
##
## Call:
##    "inla(formula = form.pro.long, family = \"lognormal\", data =
##    prothro)"
## Time used:
##    Pre = 1.14, Running = 1.72, Post = 0.0667, Total = 2.92
## Fixed effects:
##                   mean    sd 0.025quant 0.5quant 0.975quant    mode kld
## (Intercept)      4.264 0.021      4.223    4.264      4.306   4.264   0
## time             0.018 0.003      0.013    0.018      0.023   0.018   0
## treatprednisone -0.093 0.030     -0.151   -0.093     -0.034  -0.093   0
##
## Random effects:
##   Name      Model
##     id IID model
##
## Model hyperparameters:
##                                         mean    sd 0.025quant 0.5quant
## Precision for the lognormal observations 12.24 0.349      11.57    12.24
## Precision for id                         11.39 0.918       9.69    11.36
##                                         0.975quant  mode
## Precision for the lognormal observations     12.94 12.23
## Precision for id                             13.30 11.29
##
```

```
## Expected number of effective parameters(stdev): 400.65(5.89)
## Number of equivalent replicates : 7.41
##
## Marginal log-Likelihood:  -13745.94
```

In this case, prothrombin increases with time but now patients treated with prednisone had lower values of prothrombin than patients treated with the placebo.

10.7.3   Joint model

For the joint model, we will be using a model with two likelihoods (see Section 6.4 for details), for the longitudinal and survival parts, respectively. First of all, we need to prepare the data. Using joint models with INLA is a bit tricky and requires extra preparation of the data.

First, we will create some auxiliary variables that we will use later. Essentially, these variables will help us fill the *empty* spaces of the variables used in the joint models with NA or zero.

```
#Number of observations in each dataset
n.l <- nrow(prothro)
n.s <- nrow(prothros)

#Vector of NA's
NAs.l <- rep(NA, n.l)
NAs.s <- rep(NA, n.s)
#Vector of zeros
zeros.l <- rep(0, n.l)
zeros.s <- rep(0, n.s)
```

The longitudinal and survival responses, now called `Y.long` and `Y.surv`, need to be *expanded* with NAs so that both variables have the same length and then put together in a list:

```
#Long. and survival responses
Y.long <- c(prothro$pro, NAs.s)
Y.surv <- inla.surv(time = c(NAs.l, prothros$Time),
  event = c(NAs.l, prothros$death))

Y.joint <- list(Y.long, Y.surv)
```

Covariates need to be *expanded* in a similar way:

```
#Covariates
covariates <- data.frame(
  #Intercepts (as factor with 2 levels)
  inter = as.factor(c(rep("b.l", n.l), rep("b.s", n.s))),
  #Time
  time.l = c(prothro$time, NAs.s),
  time.s = c(NAs.l, prothros$Time),
  #Treatment (longitudinal)
  treat.l = c(as.integer(prothro$treat =="prednisone"), NAs.s),
  #Treat.s
```

```
    treat.s = c(NAs.l, as.integer(prothros$treat =="prednisone"))
)


#Indices for random effects
r.effects <- list(
  #Patiend id (long.)
  id.l = c(prothro$id, NAs.s),
  #Patient id (surv.)
  id.s = c(NAs.l, prothros$id)
)
```

The last step in the data preparation step is to create a new object, `joint.data`, with the covariates, the indices of the random effects and the response variables:

```
joint.data  <- c(covariates, r.effects)
joint.data$Y <- Y.joint
```

10.7.4   Model with no shared terms

Once we have the data ready, we can proceed with model fitting. Firstly, we will fit a model with no shared terms between the longitudinal and the survival parts. Estimates from this model should match those obtained with the previous models:

```
pro.joint.inla <- inla(Y ~ -1 + inter +
    # Longitudinal part
    f(id.l) +
    time.l + treat.l +
    #Survival part
    treat.s,
  data = joint.data, family = c("lognormal", "weibull.surv")
)

summary(pro.joint.inla)
```

```
##
## Call:
##    c("inla(formula = Y ~ -1 + inter + f(id.l) + time.l + treat.l + ",
##    " treat.s, family = c(\"lognormal\", \"weibull.surv\"), data = ",
##    joint.data)" )
## Time used:
##     Pre = 1.35, Running = 1.53, Post = 0.0746, Total = 2.95
## Fixed effects:
##             mean    sd 0.025quant 0.5quant 0.975quant   mode kld
## interb.l  4.264 0.021      4.223    4.264      4.306  4.264   0
## interb.s -1.560 0.107     -1.772   -1.559     -1.356 -1.555   0
## time.l    0.018 0.003      0.013    0.018      0.023  0.018   0
## treat.l  -0.093 0.030     -0.151   -0.093     -0.034 -0.093   0
## treat.s   0.093 0.117     -0.137    0.093      0.323  0.093   0
##
```

```
## Random effects:
##   Name      Model
##     id.1 IID model
##
## Model hyperparameters:
##                                           mean     sd 0.025quant 0.5quant
## Precision for the lognormal observations 12.245 0.349     11.570   12.240
## alpha parameter for weibullsurv[2]        0.824 0.040      0.749    0.823
## Precision for id.1                       11.387 0.919      9.695   11.347
##                                         0.975quant   mode
## Precision for the lognormal observations    12.945 12.233
## alpha parameter for weibullsurv[2]           0.906  0.819
## Precision for id.1                          13.303 11.267
##
## Expected number of effective parameters(stdev): 402.69(5.79)
## Number of equivalent replicates : 8.58
##
## Marginal log-Likelihood:  -14570.25
```

Note how the point estimates of this model are very close to the one obtained for the independent survival and longitudinal models fit earlier in this section.

10.7.5 Joint model with correlated terms

Next, we will fit a joint model where some effects are shared between both parts of the model. In particular, a patient specific intercept and coefficient on time is considered in the longitudinal model with a different intercept and coefficient per patient, and these are copied into the survival model multiplied by a scaling coefficient (which is the same for all patients, but different from the intercepts and coefficient on time).

The longitudinal model that we are trying to fit includes fixed effects on time of measurement (time) and treatment (trt), a random intercept and random coefficient on time for each patient:

$$y_j \sim lognorm(\mu_j, \tau), \; j = 1, \ldots, 2968$$

$$\mu_j = \beta_{l,0} + \beta_{l,t} \cdot t_j + \beta_{l,trt} \cdot trt_j + \beta_{1,i(j)} + \beta_{2,i(j)} t_j$$

Note that index j indicates the row of the table in the prothros dataset (which included repeated observations per patient) and that index $i(j)$ is used to identify the patient to which data in row j belongs.

Similarly, the survival part of the model contains a fixed effect on treatment plus copied effects of the random intercept and coefficient:

$$t_i \sim Weib(\lambda_i, \alpha), \; i = 1, \ldots, 488$$

$$\log(\lambda_i) = \beta_{s,0} + \beta_{s,trt} \cdot trt_i + \beta_1 \cdot \beta_{1,i} + \beta_2 \cdot \beta_{2,i} \cdot t_i$$

This model requires a bit of data preparation before it can be fit. First of all, unique ids of the patients are obtained to be used in both parts of the model. This is done by collecting the list of unique ids and matching variable `id` in the longitudinal and survival datasets:

```
#Unique index for patient from 1 to n.patients
unique.id <- unique(prothro$id)
n.id <- length(unique.id)
idx <- 1:n.id

#Unique indices for long. and survival data
idx.l <- match(prothro$id, unique.id )
idx.s <- match(prothros$id, unique.id )
```

Then, indices are created to indicate the patients in the longitudinal and survival part of the model:

```
#Indices for random intercept
joint.data$idx.sh.1 <- c(idx.l, NAs.s)
joint.data$idx.sh.12 <- c(idx.l, NAs.s)

#Indices for coefficient of time
joint.data$idx.sh.s <- c(NAs.l, idx.s)
joint.data$idx.sh.s2 <- c(NAs.l, idx.s)
```

Note that these indices will be used to identify (using the patient's id) the random intercept and coefficient of time in order to be able to copy the effects of $\beta_{1,i}$ and $\beta_{2,i}$. Given that we are copying two effects, two sets of indices are required.

Now, we can display the estimates of the shared random effects that have been 'copied' from the longitudinal part of the model to the survival part. Shared components are defined in INLA using the `copy` feature:

```
pro.joint.inla2 <- inla(Y ~ -1 +
    #Intercepts
    inter +
    #Longitudinal model
    time.l + treat.l +
    f(idx.sh.1, model = "iid") +
    f(idx.sh.12, time.l, model = "iid") +
    #Survival model
    treat.s +
    f(idx.sh.s, copy = "idx.sh.1", fixed = FALSE) +
    f(idx.sh.s2, time.s, copy = "idx.sh.1", fixed = FALSE),
  data = joint.data,
  family = c("lognormal", "weibull.surv")
)

summary(pro.joint.inla2)

##
## Call:
```

```
##      c("inla(formula = Y ~ -1 + inter + time.l + treat.l + f(idx.sh.l,
##      ", " model = \"iid\") + f(idx.sh.l2, time.l, model = \"iid\") +
##      treat.s + ", " f(idx.sh.s, copy = \"idx.sh.l\", fixed = FALSE) +
##      f(idx.sh.s2, ", " time.s, copy = \"idx.sh.l\", fixed = FALSE),
##      family = c(\"lognormal\", ", " \"weibull.surv\"), data =
##      joint.data)")
## Time used:
##     Pre = 2.12, Running = 11, Post = 0.303, Total = 13.5
## Fixed effects:
##             mean    sd 0.025quant 0.5quant 0.975quant   mode kld
## interb.l  4.239 0.024      4.191    4.239      4.286  4.239   0
## interb.s -1.482 0.114     -1.708   -1.481     -1.261 -1.478   0
## time.l    0.007 0.005     -0.003    0.007      0.016  0.007   0
## treat.l  -0.100 0.030     -0.159   -0.100     -0.041 -0.100   0
## treat.s   0.082 0.127     -0.167    0.082      0.330  0.082   0
##
## Random effects:
##   Name       Model
##     idx.sh.l IID model
##     idx.sh.l2 IID model
##     idx.sh.s Copy
##     idx.sh.s2 Copy
##
## Model hyperparameters:
##                                                 mean      sd 0.025quant
## Precision for the lognormal observations      14.192   0.454     13.317
## alpha parameter for weibullsurv[2]             0.866   0.042      0.787
## Precision for idx.sh.l                         11.034   0.907      9.379
## Precision for idx.sh.l2                       313.465  71.037    203.518
## Beta for idx.sh.s                             -0.454   0.316     -1.079
## Beta for idx.sh.s2                            -0.191   0.071     -0.330
##                                             0.5quant 0.975quant    mode
## Precision for the lognormal observations      14.186     15.104  14.175
## alpha parameter for weibullsurv[2]             0.865      0.953   0.861
## Precision for idx.sh.l                         10.990     12.933  10.894
## Precision for idx.sh.l2                       303.100    480.029 282.287
## Beta for idx.sh.s                             -0.453      0.163  -0.447
## Beta for idx.sh.s2                            -0.191     -0.051  -0.190
##
## Expected number of effective parameters(stdev): 554.49(13.70)
## Number of equivalent replicates : 6.23
##
## Marginal log-Likelihood:  -14513.30
```

The effect on the *copied* effects is measured by hyperparameters Beta. Beta for idx.sh.s is the one that multiplies the patient specific intercept in the longitudinal model to add it to the linear predictor of the survival model, while Beta for idx.sh.s2 is the one that multiplies the shared effect on time.

Figure 10.6 displays the patient specific intercepts and their respective copied values into the survival model. There is a linear dependence between them because the random effects in the survival part are the random effects in the longitudinal part multiplied by a constant scaling factor. The red line is a line with slope the posterior mean of the scaling factor.

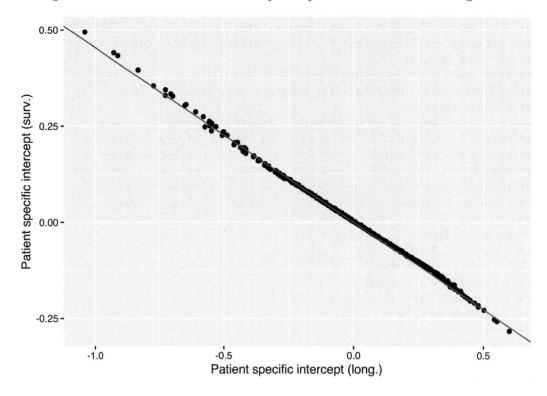

FIGURE 10.6 Patient specific intercept in the longitudinal models versus their copied values into the survival model. The red line represents a line with slope equal to the posterior mean of the scaling factor β_1.

11

Implementing New Latent Models

11.1 Introduction

In previous chapters we have covered several latent effects implemented in the INLA package. These include a number of important and popular latent effects that are widely used. However, it may be the case that an unimplemented latent effect is required in our model. Given that most of the latent effects are implemented in a mix of C and R code, it is difficult to add new latent effects to the INLA package directly.

The INLA methodology can handle many more latent effects than those included in the INLA package. For this reason, we will describe now how to add new latent effects. In particular, the spatial autoregressive model described in Section 11.2 will be considered. The implementation of this new latent effect will be done considering three different approaches. In Section 11.3 we will cover the `rgeneric` latent effect that allows new latent effects implemented in R code. In Section 11.4 we describe a novel approach to fit unimplemented latent effects by means of Bayesian model averaging (BMA, Hoeting et al., 1999; Gómez-Rubio et al., 2019). Finally, in Section 11.5 we describe how to combine INLA and MCMC (Gómez-Rubio and Rue, 2018) to increase the number of models that can be fitted using INLA.

11.2 Spatial latent effects

As a case study, we will show how to implement a spatial model. In particular, we will consider the conditionally autoregressive (CAR) specification (Banerjee et al., 2014). Now, the latent effects have a Gaussian distribution with zero mean and precision matrix

$$\Sigma = \tau(I - \rho W)$$

Here, τ is a precision hyperparameter, ρ is a spatial autocorrelation parameter and W is a binary adjacency matrix. Σ is a very sparse matrix given that both I and W are very sparse matrices.

Note that matrix W must be provided. This can be easily obtained by loading some spatial data from R. For example, we will consider the North Carolina SIDS dataset that was analyzed in Section 2.3.2. However, a spatial analysis will be considered now. First of all, a shapefile with the data will be loaded and the expected number of cases, standardized mortality ratios and proportion of non-white births per county in the period will be computed:

```
library("spdep")
library("rgdal")

SIDS <- readOGR(system.file("shapes/sids.shp", package="spData")[1])
proj4string(SIDS) <- CRS("+proj=longlat +ellps=clrk66")

#Expected cases
SIDS$EXP74 <- SIDS$BIR74 * sum(SIDS$SID74) / sum(SIDS$BIR74)
#Standardised Mortality Ratio
SIDS$SMR74 <- SIDS$SID74 / SIDS$EXP74
#Proportion of non-white births
SIDS$PNWB74 <- SIDS$NWBIR74 / SIDS$BIR74
```

Figure 11.1 shows the standardized mortality ratio (i.e., observed divided by expected cases) in each county in North Carolina.

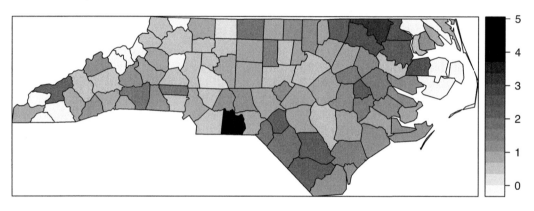

FIGURE 11.1 Standardised mortality ratio of the North Carolina SIDS dataset for the period 1971-1974.

Next, a binary adjacency matrix needs to be computed using function poly2nb:

```
#Adjacency matrix
adj <- poly2nb(SIDS)
W <- as(nb2mat(adj, style = "B"), "sparseMatrix")
```

This model is well defined when ρ is in the range $(1/\lambda_{min}, 1/\lambda_{max})$, where λ_{min} and λ_{max} are the minimum and maximum eigenvalues of W, respectively. Hence, we will compute this first:

```
e.values <- eigen(W)$values
rho.min <- min(e.values)
rho.max <- max(e.values)
```

In order to have the spatial autocorrelation parameter constrained to be lower than 1 (see, for example, Haining, 2003, for details), the adjacency matrix will be re-scaled by dividing by λ_{max}:

```
#Re-scale adjacency matrix
W <- W / rho.max
```

Usually, the range of the spatial autocorrelation parameter will be considered to be $(0, 1)$, so that it can be interpreted similarly as a correlation parameter.

11.3   R implementation with `rgeneric`

The `rgeneric` latent effect is a mechanism implemented in the `INLA` package to allow users to implement latent effects in R. This is possible because R can be embedded into other front-end programs in a way that allows R code to be run from C (R Core Team, 2019b). A detailed description of this feature can be accessed by typing `inla.doc('rgeneric')`.

The definition of a new latent effect requires the definition of the latent effect as a GMRF. This means that the mean and precision matrix of the GRMF need to be defined, as well as the hyperparameters $\boldsymbol{\theta}$ involved and their prior distributions.

Specifying the latent effect as a GMRF also requires a binary representation of the precision matrix to exploit conditional independence properties. i.e., a 'graph'. This is simply a matrix of the same dimension as the precision matrix with entries equal to zero where the precision matrix is zero and 1 otherwise. When passing this graph matrix to define an `rgeneric` latent effect, the precision matrix can be used as well regardless of whether it is binary or not.

To sum up, in order to define a new latent effect, the following need to be defined using several R functions:

- The mean of the latent effects $\mu(\theta)$.

- The precision of the latent effects $Q(\theta)$.

- A 'graph', with a binary representation of the precision matrix.

- The initial values of θ.

- A log-normalizing constant.

- The log-prior of θ.

Before starting coding all this, it is important to provide an internal representation of the hyperparameters that make numerical optimization easier. As a rule, it is good to have a reparameterization of the parameters so that the internal parameters are not bounded as this will simplify computations. In particular, we will use $\theta_1 = \log(\tau)$ and $\theta_2 = logit(\rho)$.

`INLA` will internally work with parameters (θ_1, θ_2). For this reason, we will need first to define the following function to convert the hyperparameters from the internal scale to the model scale, i.e, to obtain parameters (τ, ρ) from (θ_1, θ_2):

$$\tau = \exp(\theta_1)$$

$$\rho = \frac{1}{1 + \exp(-\theta_2)}$$

A variable `theta` is defined by `INLA` in the code to store $\theta = (\theta_1, \theta_2)$. So, the following function `interpret.theta` will take the parameters in the internal scale and return the precision and spatial autocorrelation parameters:

```
interpret.theta <- function() {
  return(
    list(prec = exp(theta[1L]),
    rho = 1 / (1 + exp(-theta[2L]))))
  )
}
```

Next, we will define the 'graph', which essentially defines what entries of the precision matrix are non-zero. Note that this is a matrix of the same size as the precision matrix and that W must be passed as a sparse matrix (as defined in package `Matrix`) and the returned matrix must be sparse too.

```
graph <- function(){
  require(Matrix)

  return(Diagonal(nrow(W), x = 1) + W)
}
```

The precision matrix is defined in a similar way:

```
Q <- function() {
  require(Matrix)

  param <- interpret.theta()

  return(param$prec * (Diagonal(nrow(W), x = 1) - param$rho * W) )
}
```

The mean can be defined very easily now because it is zero:

```
mu = function()
{
  return(numeric(0))
}
```

The logarithm of the normalizing constant in this case is the typical normalizing constant of a multivariate Gaussian distribution:

```
log.norm.const <- function() {
  param <- interpret.theta()
  n <- nrow(W)

  Q <- param$prec * (Diagonal(nrow(W), x = 1) - param$rho * W)

  res <- n * (-0.5 * log(2 * pi)) +
```

```
    0.5 * Matrix::determinant(Q, logarithm = TRUE)

  return(res)
}
```

Note that `INLA` will compute this normalizing constant if `numeric(0)` is returned, so this can be omitted.

The log-prior must be specified in another function. For precision τ, we will be using a gamma distribution with parameters 1 and 0.00005, and for ρ a uniform distribution on $(0, 1)$:

```
log.prior <- function() {
  param = interpret.theta()

  res <- dgamma(param$prec, 1, 5e-05, log = TRUE) + log(param$prec) +
      log(1) + log(param$rho) + log(1 - param$rho)

  return(res)
}
```

Note that the extra terms that appear in the definition of the log-density of the prior are due to the change of variable involved. `INLA` works with (θ_1, θ_2) internally, but the prior is set on (τ, ρ). See Chapter 5 for details on how to set the prior properly.

Finally, a function to set the initial values of the parameters in the internal scale must be provided:

```
initial <- function() {
  return(rep(0, 0))
}
```

This implies that the initial values of τ and ρ are 1 and 0.5, respectively.

A `quit()` function is called when all computations are finished before exiting the `C` code. In this case, we will simply return nothing.

```
quit <- function() {
  return(invisible())
}
```

The actual definition of the latent effect is done via function `inla.rgeneric.define`. This function takes as first argument the functions defined before and some extra arguments needed to evaluate the different functions:

```
'inla.rgeneric.CAR.model' <- function(
  cmd = c("graph", "Q", "mu", "initial", "log.norm.const",
    "log.prior", "quit"),
  theta = NULL) {
```

```r
#Internal function
interpret.theta <- function() {
  return(
    list(prec = exp(theta[1L]),
    rho = 1 / (1 + exp(-theta[2L])))
  )
}

graph <- function(){
  require(Matrix)

  return(Diagonal(nrow(W), x = 1) + W)
}

Q <- function() {
  require(Matrix)

  param <- interpret.theta()

  return(param$prec * (Diagonal(nrow(W), x = 1) - param$rho * W) )
}

mu <- function()
{
  return(numeric(0))
}

log.norm.const <- function() {
  return(numeric(0))

}

log.prior <- function() {
  param = interpret.theta()

  res <- dgamma(param$prec, 1, 5e-05, log = TRUE) + log(param$prec) +
    log(1) + log(param$rho) + log(1 - param$rho)

  return(res)
}

initial <- function() {
  return(c(0, 0))
}

quit <- function() {
  return(invisible())
}

res <- do.call(match.arg(cmd), args = list())
```

```
    return(res)
}
```

Then, the model is defined to be used by INLA using function `inla.rgeneric.define` as follows:

```
library("INLA")

CAR.model <- inla.rgeneric.define(inla.rgeneric.CAR.model, W = W)
```

Note that `inla.rgeneric.define()` takes as first argument the function that defines the latent effect followed by a sequence of named arguments with variables that are required in the computation of the latent effect. In this case, matrix `W` is the adjacency matrix required by the CAR latent effect but more arguments could follow when needed.

The model can now be fitted as follows:

```
SIDS$idx <- 1:nrow(SIDS)

f.car <- SID74 ~ 1 + f(idx, model = CAR.model)

m.car <- inla(f.car, data = as.data.frame(SIDS), family = "poisson",
  E = SIDS$EXP74)#, control.inla = list(tolerance = 1e-20, h = 1e-4))
```

A summary of the model can be obtained as usual:

```
summary(m.car)
```

```
##
## Call:
##    c("inla(formula = f.car, family = \"poisson\", data =
##    as.data.frame(SIDS), ", " E = SIDS$EXP74)")
## Time used:
##    Pre = 1.14, Running = 2.63, Post = 0.0687, Total = 3.85
## Fixed effects:
##               mean    sd 0.025quant 0.5quant 0.975quant  mode kld
## (Intercept) 0.035 0.109     -0.172    0.031      0.261 0.022   0
##
## Random effects:
##   Name     Model
##     idx RGeneric2
##
## Model hyperparameters:
##                  mean    sd 0.025quant 0.5quant 0.975quant mode
## Theta1 for idx 2.20 0.347      1.534     2.19       2.90 2.17
## Theta2 for idx 2.29 1.132      0.134     2.26       4.58 2.16
##
## Expected number of effective parameters(stdev): 36.77(6.22)
## Number of equivalent replicates : 2.72
```

```
##
## Marginal log-Likelihood:  -241.15
```

The marginals of the hyperparameters are in the internal scale and they need to be transformed:

```
marg.prec <- inla.tmarginal(exp, m.car$marginals.hyperpar[[1]])
marg.rho <- inla.tmarginal(function(x) { 1/(1 + exp(-x))},
  m.car$marginals.hyperpar[[2]])
```

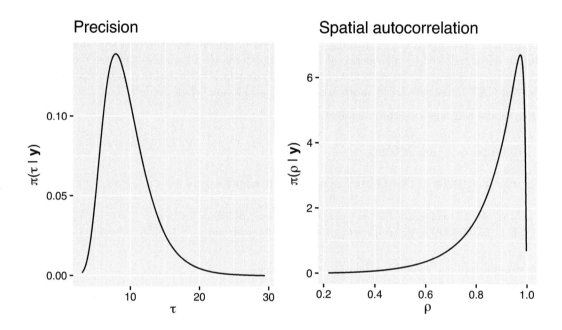

FIGURE 11.2 Posterior marginals of parameters τ and ρ of the proper CAR latent model for the SIDS dataset.

Figure 11.2 shows the posterior marginals of τ and ρ. These show a strong spatial autocorrelation. Finally, summary statistics on these parameters can be obtained with `inla.zmarginal` (see Section 2.6):

```
inla.zmarginal(marg.prec, FALSE)
```

```
## Mean              9.57826
## Stdev             3.44714
## Quantile  0.025 4.64991
## Quantile  0.25  7.11261
## Quantile  0.5   8.95156
## Quantile  0.75  11.3598
## Quantile  0.975 18.0326
```

```
inla.zmarginal(marg.rho, FALSE)
```

```
## Mean              0.867613
## Stdev             0.120107
## Quantile  0.025 0.53626
## Quantile  0.25  0.81936
## Quantile  0.5   0.905226
## Quantile  0.75  0.954126
## Quantile  0.975 0.989483
```

Posterior means of the random effects have been plotted in a map in Figure 11.3. It shows the underlying spatial pattern of the risk from SIDS. It should be mentioned that the spatial pattern of the proportion of non-white births is very similar to the one shown in Figure 11.3 and that is why when this covariate is included in the model (as discussed in Section 2.3.2) it accounts for most of the overdispersion in the data and random effects are not required any more.

```
SIDS$CAR <- m.car$summary.random$idx[, "mean"]
spplot(SIDS, "CAR",  col.regions = rev(inferno(16)))
```

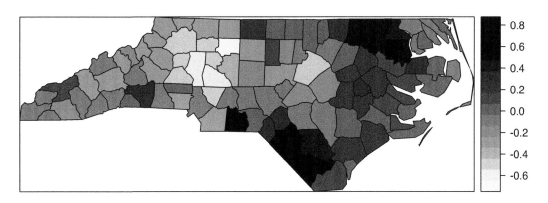

FIGURE 11.3 Posterior means of the CAR random effects.

11.4 Bayesian model averaging

Bivand et al. (2014) describe a novel approach to fit new models with INLA. Their approach is based on conditioning on one of the hyperparameters in the model and fit conditional models on several values of this parameter. Then, all models are combined using Bayesian model averaging (BMA, Hoeting et al., 1999) to obtain the posterior marginals of all the parameters in the model. Bivand et al. (2014) use this approach to fit a number of spatial econometrics models, which are available in package INLABMA (Bivand et al., 2015). Recently, Gómez-Rubio et al. (2019) have extended the work in Bivand et al. (2014) to consider a wider family of spatial econometrics models.

In the case of the CAR specification, it is worth noting that, given ρ, the resulting model can be implemented using a `generic0` latent effect because the structure of the precision matrix is known and only hyperparameter τ needs to be estimated. By giving values to ρ in a bounded interval the posterior marginal of ρ can be computed as well by Bayesian model averaging.

First of all, we will create a function that will take a value of ρ and the adjacency matrix W and fit the CAR model conditional on ρ:

```
car.inla <- function(formula, d, rho, W, ...) {

  #Create structure of precision matrix I - rho * W
  IrhoW <- Matrix::Diagonal(nrow(W), x = 1) - rho * W

  #Add CAR index
  d$CARidx <- 1:nrow(d)

  formula <- update(formula, . ~ . + f(CARidx, model = "generic0",
          Cmatrix = IrhoW))
  res <- inla(formula, data = d, ..., control.compute = list(mlik = TRUE),
    control.inla = list(tolerance = 1e-20, h = 1e-4))

  #Update mlik
  logdet <- determinant(IrhoW)$modulus
  res$mlik <- res$mlik + logdet / 2

  return(res)
}
```

Note that the log-marginal likelihood needs to be corrected to account for the structure of the precision matrix and this is why term `logdet / 2` is added to the value of the marginal likelihood. By default, INLA will not compute it in this case because it assumes that the structure of the precision matrix is known. Hence, its determinant is constant and does not need to be computed and only the precision hyperparameter τ is accounted for when computing the marginal likelihood. Furthermore, `control.inla` has been used to set the values of `tolerance` and `h` to obtain accurate estimates of the marginal likelihood.

Next, a regular grid of points in the domain of ρ where to evaluate the model is required. In this case, the domain is the interval $(0, 1)$ and the grid points will be denoted by $\{\rho^{(i)}\}_{i=1}^{N}$, where N is the number of points. For this particular case, as we already know that the region of high probability of the posterior marginal of ρ is very close to one, the grid will be made of 100 points from 0.5 to 1:

```
rho.val <- seq(0.5, 1, length.out = 100)
```

It should be noted that values very close to 1 may cause computational problems because the precision matrix becomes almost singular.

Next, we evaluate the model at all these points. Although this involves fitting a large number of models, these can be fitted in parallel using function `mclapply`. In the next lines, the `parallel` library will be loaded and set up to use 4 cores before fitting the conditional models:

```
library("parallel")
options(mc.cores = 4)
```

Model fitting will be in parallel and we set each parallel `INLA` process to use a single core (by setting `num.threads` to 1):

```
car.models <- mclapply (rho.val, function(rho) {
    car.inla(SID74 ~ 1, as.data.frame(SIDS), rho, W,
      family = "poisson", E = SIDS$EXP74,
      num.threads = 1)
})
```

When `INLA` is used to fit several models in parallel on the same machine it is convenient to set the number of threads used by each `INLA` process to a value that ensures that no more cores than available are used. For example, in the previous example, the `mclapply` loop will be using 4 cores (as set in `mc.cores`), which means that 4 `INLA` processes will be run. Each one of these processes will be using 1 core at a time (as set in `num.threads`), so that altogether 4 cores are used. Similarly, if the total number of cores is 8, then `num.threads` could be set to 2 so that each `INLA` process takes 2 cores and the total number of cores used is 8.

Then, we have a number of conditional models on ρ that we can combine to obtain the desired model. These models will be combined using Bayesian model averaging, which is the appropriate way of combining models.

Note that, given any particular value of ρ, the fitted conditional model with `INLA` will provide the conditional marginals of the parameters, $\pi(\cdot \mid \rho)$, and the conditional marginal likelihood $\pi(\mathbf{y} \mid \rho)$. The posterior marginal of ρ can be obtained as:

$$\pi(\rho \mid \mathbf{y}) = \frac{\pi(\mathbf{y} \mid \rho)\pi(\rho)}{\pi(\mathbf{y})} \propto \pi(\mathbf{y} \mid \rho)\pi(\rho)$$

This can be computed from the previous output because $\pi(\mathbf{y} \mid \rho)$ is the conditional marginal likelihood for a conditional model on ρ and $\pi(\rho)$ is the value of the prior on ρ (which is known and equal to 1 in this case). $\pi(\mathbf{y})$ is a constant that can be ignored as the posterior marginal can be re-scaled to integrate 1.

In practice, we will estimate the value of the posterior marginals at the points of the grid, fit a smooth function and then re-scale the resulting function to integrate 1, so that we have a proper density function. Here, this is done by function `INLABMA` but function `inla.merge()` could have also been used (as shown in the next section):

```
library("INLABMA")
car.bma <- INLABMA(car.models, rho.val, log(1))
```

The posterior marginal of ρ estimated with this method can be seen in Figure 11.5, which also includes two other estimates using different approaches explained below.

If required, the log-marginal likelihoods (conditional on ρ) from the fit models can be easily obtained with:

```
#Obtain log-marginal likelihoods
mliks <- unlist(lapply(car.models, function(X){X$mlik[1, 1]}))
```

The posterior marginals for the remainder of latent effects and hyperparameters in the model can be computed by integrating ρ out. For example, for a hyperparameter θ_t (and similarly for any latent effect) this would mean:

$$\pi(\theta_t \mid \mathbf{y}) = \int \pi(\theta_t, \rho \mid \mathbf{y})d\rho = \int \pi(\theta_t \mid \mathbf{y}, \rho)\pi(\rho \mid \mathbf{y})d\rho$$

Taking a set of values of ρ in a grid $\{\rho^{(i)}\}_{i=1}^N$, this can be approximated by the following expression (Bivand et al., 2014):

$$\pi(\theta_t \mid \mathbf{y}) \simeq \sum_{i=1}^N \pi(\theta_t \mid \mathbf{y}, \rho^{(i)})w_i$$

with weights w_i equal to

$$w_i = \frac{\pi(\mathbf{y} \mid \rho^{(i)})\pi(\rho^{(i)})}{\sum_{i=1}^N \pi(\mathbf{y} \mid \rho^{(i)})\pi(\rho^{(i)})}$$

Note the approximation to $\pi(\theta_t \mid \mathbf{y})$ can be regarded as Bayesian model averaging (Hoeting et al., 1999), as it is a weighted sum of conditional posterior marginals from different models.

Function INLAMH() computes this model average to obtain the marginals of the other hyperparameters and latent effects in the model. See Bivand et al. (2015) for details. The summaries of the coefficients of the fixed effects and the hyperparameters can be obtained as follows:

```
# Fixed effects
car.bma$summary.fixed
```

```
##                 mean     sd 0.025quant 0.5quant 0.975quant    mode        kld
## (Intercept) 0.0336 0.1011    -0.1717  0.03573      0.227 0.03983 6.082e-12
```

It is worth mentioning that function inla.merge() can also compute the average of the posterior marginals from different models (see next section). In this case, each model has a different weight w_i that must be passed to the inla.merge() function in order to obtain the right model.

11.5   INLA within MCMC

Finally, the third approach that will be discussed to use INLA to fit models with unimplemented latent effects is based on Gómez-Rubio and Rue (2018). They point out that the approach in Bivand et al. (2014) is useful for a very small number of hyperparameters with bounded support. However, when the hyperparameters do not have a bounded support or there are many of them, simple numerical approximations will be difficult to implement.

For this reason, Gómez-Rubio and Rue (2018) propose the use of INLA within the Metropolis-Hastings algorithm so that the hyperparameter space is conveniently explored. The main idea is to split the set of hyperparameters into two groups, so that conditional on one of the subsets the resulting model can be easily fitted with INLA. This is essentially what we have done in Section 11.4 when fitting models conditional on ρ.

Function INLAMH, in package INLABMA, implements the INLA within Metropolis-Hastings algorithm. It requires a function to fit the model conditional on some of the hyperparameters, two functions (that implement the proposal distribution) to sample new values of the hyperparameters and compute its density, and the prior of the hyperparameters.

Similarly as in Section 11.4, the models fitted with INLA will be conditional on ρ, and the marginal distribution of ρ will be obtained from the samples from the Metropolis-Hastings algorithm.

The function to fit a model conditional on ρ is the following:

```
fit.inla <- function(d, x){
  #Rho
  rho <- x

  res <- car.inla(SID74 ~ 1, d, rho, W,
    family = "poisson", E = d$EXP74)

  return(list(model.sim = res, mlik = res$mlik[1, 1]))
}
```

This function returns a list with the fit model (model.sim) and the estimate of the marginal likelihood (mlik).

The function used to propose new values of ρ, in the logit-scale, will be a Gaussian centered at the current value with a small precision. For this, function rlogitnorm from package logitnorm(Wutzler, 2018) will be used. By using this function we avoid dealing with changes in the scale of the parameters (see Chapter 5 for details).

```
library("logitnorm")
#Sample values of rho
rq.rho <- function(x, sigma = 0.15) {
  rlogitnorm(1, mu = logit(x), sigma = sigma)
}

#Log-density of proposal distribution
dq.rho <- function(x, y, sigma = 0.15, log = TRUE) {
  dlogitnorm(y, mu = logit(x), sigma = sigma, log = log)
}
```

Here, x represents the current value of ρ, y the proposed value and sigma is the standard deviation of the proposal distribution. Note also that the density is returned in the log-scale.

Finally, we need to set the prior on ρ:

```
#Log-density of prior
prior.rho <- function(rho, log = TRUE) {
  return(dunif(rho, log = log))
}
```

Once all the required functions have been defined, the `INLAMH` function can be called to run the INLA with MCMC algorithm. In the next lines, the starting point for ρ is set to 0.95:

```
inlamh.res <- INLAMH(as.data.frame(SIDS), fit.inla, 0.95, rq.rho, dq.rho,
  prior.rho,
  n.sim = 100, n.burnin = 100, n.thin = 5, verbose = TRUE)
```

The resulting object `inlamh.res` is a list with three elements:

- `acc.sim`, indicates whether the proposed value of ρ was accepted or not, and it is useful to compute the acceptance rate.

- `model.sim` is a list with the conditional models fitted with `INLA`.

- `b.sim` is a list with the values of ρ. In this case, each element in the list is a vector of length one, but this can take many other forms.

A simple way to put all the samples from ρ together is the following:

```
rho.sim <- unlist(inlamh.res$b.sim)
```

Figure 11.4 displays the samples from the posterior of ρ drawn by INLA within MCMC and a kernel density estimate of the posterior marginal.

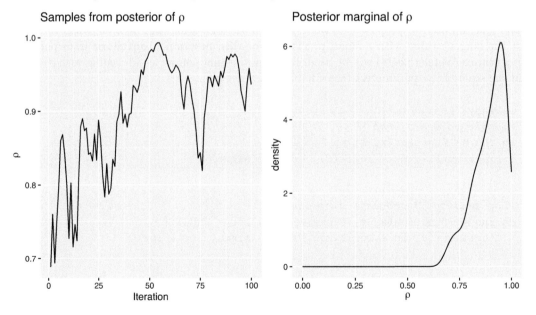

FIGURE 11.4 Samples from the posterior distribuion (left) and kernel density estimate of the posterior marginal of the spatial autocorrelation parameter.

In addition, summary statistics can be obtained from these samples:

```
#Posterior mean
mean(rho.sim)
```

[1] 0.8956

```
#Posterior st. dev.
sd(rho.sim)
```

[1] 0.07529

```
#Quantiles
quantile(rho.sim)
```

```
##      0%    25%    50%    75%   100%
## 0.6886 0.8432 0.9157 0.9560 0.9930
```

Finally, the posterior marginals of all the other parameters of interest can be obtained from the output generated by the INLA within MCMC algorithm. Bayesian model averaging can be used on the conditional marginals and all fitted models are assumed to have the same weight, as these are associated with independent samples from the posterior distribution of ρ.

11.6   Comparison of results

In the previous sections three different methods to implement new latent effects have been described. Figure 11.5 displays the different posterior marginals of ρ computed using these three different approaches. Marginals obtained with **rgeneric** and INLA within MCMC are very close, and the one obtained by BMA is not far from those. In all cases, marginals seem to favor values of ρ very close to the upper bound of its support. This is a well known behavior for the proper CAR model when data have a strong spatial pattern that is not accounted for by the covariates.

Having estimates close to the boundaries of the support of the parameter can be problematic. In particular, BMA may struggle. The reason may be that when the parameter is close to the boundary of its support INLA finds it difficult to obtain accurate estimates of the marginal likelihood required to combine all the conditional models together.

11.7   Final remarks

In this chapter we have considered three different options to use **INLA** to fit models with unimplemented latent effects. The **rgeneric** latent effect provides an adequate way of making computations completely within the **INLA** package. The other two options, based on BMA and MCMC, are alternative approaches that can be more flexible as to the types of variables that they can handle.

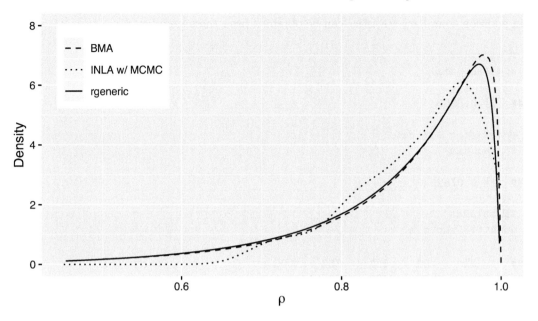

FIGURE 11.5 Comparison of posterior marginals of the spatial autocorrelation parameter obtained with three different methods.

For example, INLA assumes that all hyperparameters are continuous in some interval. BMA and INLA within MCMC can be used to fit models in which the hyperparameters are discrete. This is discussed, for example, in Chapter 13 where fitting mixture models with INLA is considered and Chapter 12, where the imputation of missing covariates is discussed.

In addition, INLA within MCMC can be regarded as a novel way of implementing MCMC algorithms. As seen in the previous sections, it makes implementing MCMC algorithms easy as it focuses in on a small number of hyperparameters and all the others are integrated out by INLA.

Finally, the rgeneric framework can be used to develop multivariate latent random effects. This requires a model with different likelihoods and a definition of the latent effect that works on data in more than one likelihood of the model. Palmí-Perales et al. (2019) show how to implement multivariate latent spatial effects for multivariate spatial data and provide different applications in disease mapping. Similarly, Gómez-Rubio et al. (2019) describe how to implement new latent effects to deal with missing values in the covariates and impute them.

12

Missing Values and Imputation

12.1 Introduction

Missing observations are common in real life datasets. Values may not be recorded for a number of reasons. For example, environmental data is often not recorded due to failures in measurement devices or instruments. In clinical trials, survival times and other covariates may be missing because of patient's drop-out.

The literature on missing values is ample. To mention a few, Little and Rubin (2002) provides a nice overview of missing values and imputation. van Buuren (2018) gives a more recent description of the area, which includes examples using R code. A curated list of R packages for missing data is available in the *Missing data* CRAN Task View available at `https://cran.r-project.org/web/views/MissingData.html`.

In general, missing values can seldom be ignored. Models that include a way to account for missing data should be preferred to simply ignoring the missing observations. When missing values can be modeled from the observed data, imputation models can be used to provide estimates of the missing observations. Models can be extended to incorporate a sub-model for the imputation.

The different mechanisms that lead to missing observations in the data are introduced in Section 12.2. `INLA` can fit models with missing observations in the response by computing their predictive distribution, as discussed in Section 12.3. In principle, `INLA` cannot directly handle missing observations in the covariates, as they are part of the latent field, but imputation of missing covariates using different methods is discussed in Section 12.4. Multiple imputation of missing observations in the covariates using INLA within MCMC is described in Section 12.5.

12.2 Missingness mechanism

Dealing with missing observations usually requires prior reflection on how the data went missing and the missingness mechanism. Depending on the reasons why the data has missing observations the statistical analysis needs to be conducted in one way or another. Little and Rubin (2002) describe the different mechanisms for missing data.

Missing completely at random (MCAR) occurs when the missing data are independent from the observed or unobserved data. This means that the missing values can be ignored and the analysis can be conducted as usual. *Missing at random (MAR)* occurs when the missing data depends on the observed data. In this case, this can be introduced into the model so that missing observations are imputed as part of the model fitting. Finally, *Missing not at random (MNAR)* occurs when the missingness mechanism depends on both the observed and missing data. This scenario is difficult to tackle since there is no information about the missingness mechanism and the missing data.

Furthermore, a distinction between missing observations in the response variable or the covariates can be done. The missing observations in the response variable can naturally be predicted as the distribution of the response values is determined by the statistical model to be fit. On the other hand, missing values in the covariates are explanatory variables in the model and it is not always clear how they can be estimated. Similarly, missing indices in the definition of the latent random effects are difficult to handle as it is not always obvious how their values can be filled-in. However, different imputation mechanisms can be considered.

INLA does not allow missing values in the definition of the effects in the latent field, and this is a practical problem for model fitting. In general, INLA will not include the fixed or random term in the linear predictor of an observation if the associate covariate has a value of NA. See Gómez-Rubio et al. (2019) and the FAQ at the INLA website (http://www.r-inla.org/faq) for details.

12.3   Missing values in the response

First of all, handling missing observations in the response will be considered. Given that the distribution of the response variable is part of the model, it is possible to predict the missing values by computing their *predictive* distribution. Given a missing response y_m its predictive distribution is

$$\pi(y_m \mid \mathbf{y}_{obs}) = \int \pi(y_m, \boldsymbol{\theta} \mid \mathbf{y}_{obs})d\boldsymbol{\theta} = \int \pi(y_m \mid \mathbf{y}_{obs}, \boldsymbol{\theta})\pi(\boldsymbol{\theta} \mid \mathbf{y}_{obs})d\boldsymbol{\theta}.$$

INLA will automatically compute the predictive distributions for all missing values in the response, which should be assigned a NA value when defining the data.

To illustrate the computation of the predictive distribution of the missing values in the response the fdgs dataset (in package mice, van Buuren and Groothuis-Oudshoorn, 2011) will be used. This dataset records information of 10030 children measured within the Fifth Dutch Growth Study 2009 (Schonbeck et al., 2011, 2013). Table 12.1 shows the different variables in the dataset.

TABLE 12.1: Variables in the fdgs dataset on children measured in the Fifth Dutch Growth Study 2009, including the number of missing values.

Variable	Description	# missing
id	Child unique id number.	0
reg	Region (a factor with 5 levels).	0
age	Age (in year).	0
sex	Sex (boy or girl).	0
hgt	Height (in cm).	23
wgt	Weight (in kg).	20
hgt.z	Re-scaled height (as a Z-score).	23
wgt.z	Re-scaled weight (as a Z-score).	20

Data can be loaded and summarized as follows:

```
library("mice")
data(fdgs)
summary(fdgs)
```

```
##       id              reg          age         sex
## Min.   :100001   North: 732   Min.   : 0.008   boy :4829
## 1st Qu.:106352   East :2528   1st Qu.: 1.619   girl:5201
## Median :203855   South:2931   Median : 8.085
## Mean   :180091   West :2578   Mean   : 8.158
## 3rd Qu.:210591   City :1261   3rd Qu.:13.548
## Max.   :401955                Max.   :21.993
##
##       hgt              wgt            hgt.z            wgt.z
## Min.   : 46.0    Min.   :  2.58   Min.   :-4.470   Min.   :-5.040
## 1st Qu.: 83.8    1st Qu.: 11.60   1st Qu.:-0.678   1st Qu.:-0.625
## Median :131.5    Median : 27.50   Median :-0.019   Median : 0.026
## Mean   :123.9    Mean   : 32.38   Mean   :-0.006   Mean   : 0.046
## 3rd Qu.:162.3    3rd Qu.: 51.10   3rd Qu.: 0.677   3rd Qu.: 0.707
## Max.   :208.0    Max.   :135.30   Max.   : 3.900   Max.   : 4.741
## NA's   :23       NA's   :20       NA's   :23       NA's   :20
```

Note that several variables in the dataset have missing observations. In particular, height (`hgt`) and weight (`wgt`), which are common variables used as response or predictors in models.

In order to provide a smaller dataset to speed up computations, only the children with missing values (in height and weight) and another 1000 ones taken at random will be used in the analysis:

```
# Subset for speed-up and testing
# Subsect 1, observations with NA's
subset1 <- which(is.na(fdgs$wgt) | is.na(fdgs$hgt))

#Subset 2, random sample of 500 individuals
set.seed(1)
subset2 <- sample((1:nrow(fdgs))[-subset1], 1000)
# Subset 1 + subset 2
fdgs.sub <- fdgs[c(subset1, subset2), ]
summary(fdgs.sub)
```

```
##       id              reg         age         sex          hgt
## Min.   :100098   North: 78   Min.   : 0.071   boy :493   Min.   : 46.0
## 1st Qu.:106293   East :275   1st Qu.: 1.743   girl:550   1st Qu.: 86.3
## Median :204306   South:298   Median : 8.594              Median :136.1
## Mean   :183214   West :250   Mean   : 8.565              Mean   :127.0
## 3rd Qu.:211388   City :142   3rd Qu.:14.164              3rd Qu.:165.1
## Max.   :401949               Max.   :21.884              Max.   :199.0
##                                                          NA's   :23
##       wgt            hgt.z            wgt.z
## Min.   :  2.58   Min.   :-4.263   Min.   :-4.075
## 1st Qu.: 11.96   1st Qu.:-0.668   1st Qu.:-0.652
```

```
## Median : 29.00    Median :-0.046    Median :-0.007
## Mean    : 33.61    Mean    :-0.023    Mean    : 0.020
## 3rd Qu.: 53.10    3rd Qu.: 0.646    3rd Qu.: 0.696
## Max.    :117.30    Max.    : 3.200    Max.    : 3.630
## NA's    :20        NA's    :23        NA's    :20
```

Next, a model to predict height based on age and sex is fit to the subset data set fdgs.sub with INLA. This model includes the options to compute the predictive distributions of the missing observations in the response by setting compute = TRUE in argument control.predictor.

```
library("INLA")
hgt.inla <- inla(hgt ~ age + sex, data = fdgs.sub,
control.predictor = list(compute = TRUE))
summary(hgt.inla)
```

```
##
## Call:
##     "inla(formula = hgt ~ age + sex, data = fdgs.sub,
##     control.predictor = list(compute = TRUE))"
## Time used:
##     Pre = 1.1, Running = 0.286, Post = 0.243, Total = 1.63
## Fixed effects:
##                 mean    sd 0.025quant 0.5quant 0.975quant    mode kld
## (Intercept) 77.148 0.720     75.735   77.148     78.560 77.148   0
## age           6.023 0.055      5.914    6.023      6.131  6.023   0
## sexgirl      -4.716 0.730     -6.149   -4.716     -3.284 -4.716   0
##
## Model hyperparameters:
##                                           mean    sd 0.025quant 0.5quant
## Precision for the Gaussian observations 0.007 0.00      0.007    0.007
##                                           0.975quant   mode
## Precision for the Gaussian observations      0.008 0.007
##
## Expected number of effective parameters(stdev): 3.00(0.00)
## Number of equivalent replicates : 340.06
##
## Marginal log-Likelihood:   -3976.34
## Posterior marginals for the linear predictor and
##   the fitted values are computed
```

In order to show the predictive distribution, we will obtain first the indices of the first two children with missing values of height in the reduced dataset and show the row names in the original dataset.

```
hgt.na <- which(is.na(fdgs.sub$hgt))[1:2]
rownames(fdgs.sub)[hgt.na]
```

```
## [1] "273"   "2034"
```

Next, the summary statistics of the fitted values can be shown using index hgt.na:

```
hgt.inla$summary.fitted.values[hgt.na, c("mean", "sd")]
```

```
##                          mean     sd
## fitted.Predictor.0001 122.25 0.5354
## fitted.Predictor.0005  83.25 0.6831
```

Similarly, a model can be fit to explain weight based on age and sex and to compute the predictive distribution of the missing observations:

```
wgt.inla <- inla(wgt ~ age + sex, data = fdgs.sub,
 control.predictor = list(compute = TRUE),
 control.compute = list(config = TRUE))
 summary(wgt.inla)
```

```
##
## Call:
##    c("inla(formula = wgt ~ age + sex, data = fdgs.sub,
##    control.compute = list(config = TRUE), ", " control.predictor =
##    list(compute = TRUE))")
## Time used:
##     Pre = 0.905, Running = 0.296, Post = 0.105, Total = 1.31
## Fixed effects:
##               mean    sd 0.025quant 0.5quant 0.975quant   mode kld
## (Intercept)  6.259 0.436      5.403    6.259      7.115  6.259   0
## age          3.331 0.034      3.265    3.331      3.397  3.331   0
## sexgirl     -2.379 0.446     -3.255   -2.379     -1.503 -2.379   0
##
## Model hyperparameters:
##                                            mean     sd 0.025quant 0.5quant
## Precision for the Gaussian observations 0.02 0.001      0.018     0.02
##                                            0.975quant mode
## Precision for the Gaussian observations      0.021 0.02
##
## Expected number of effective parameters(stdev): 3.00(0.00)
## Number of equivalent replicates : 341.01
##
## Marginal log-Likelihood:  -3486.82
## Posterior marginals for the linear predictor and
##  the fitted values are computed
```

This model could be used as a simple imputation mechanism for the missing values of weight, so that the complete dataset could be used to fit, for example, another model to explain height based on age, sex, and weight. Here, we check the posterior means of the predictive distribution of weight for the first two children with missing values of the variable `wgt`:

```
wgt.na <- which(is.na(fdgs.sub$wgt))
 wgt.inla$summary.fitted.values[wgt.na[1:2], c("mean", "sd")]
```

```
##                         mean     sd
## fitted.Predictor.0002 23.07 0.3204
## fitted.Predictor.0003 27.62 0.3332
```

12.3.1   Joint model with height and weight

The two previous models consider height and weight separately, but it is clear that there is a high correlation between height and weight, which is caused by the age and sex of the child. For this reason, a joint model for height and weight could be proposed to exploit a correlated effect between the coefficients of age in both models.

This can be easily implemented with `INLA` by using a model with two Gaussian likelihoods (for height and weight, respectively) and the latent effect `iid2d` to include two correlated coefficients in the two parts of the model. Hence, the model will be the following:

$$hgt_i = \alpha_h + \beta_h age_i + \beta_{h,1} sex_i + \epsilon_{h,i}$$

$$wgt_i = \alpha_w + \beta_w age_i + \beta_{w,1} sex_i + \epsilon_{w,i}$$

Here, α_h and α_w are model intercepts, β_h and β_w coefficients on `age` (which will be correlated), $\beta_{h,1}$ and $\beta_{w,1}$ coefficients on `sex`, and $\epsilon_{h,i}$ and $\epsilon_{w,i}$ two error terms.

Vector $(\beta_h, \beta_w)^\top$ is modeled using a multivariate Gaussian distribution with mean $c(0,0)^\top$ and covariance matrix

$$\begin{bmatrix} 1/\tau_h & \rho/\sqrt{(\tau_h \tau_w)} \\ \rho/\sqrt{(\tau_h \tau_w)} & 1/\tau_w \end{bmatrix}$$

Here, τ_h and τ_w are the precisions of the coefficients and ρ is the correlation parameter, which is between 0 and 1. This model is implemented in `INLA` as the `iid2d` latent effect (see Section 3.3 for more details). Note that the covariate `age` will be introduced as a weight of this latent effect (see below for details) when it is defined with function `f()`.

First of all, the bivariate response variable needs to be put in a two-column matrix given that the model will be made of two likelihoods (see Section 6.4 for details).

```
n <- nrow(fdgs.sub)
y <- matrix(NA, nrow = 2 * n, ncol = 2)
y[1:n, 1] <- fdgs.sub$hgt
y[n + 1:n, 2] <- fdgs.sub$wgt
```

Similarly, given that the model will include two intercepts, these need to be defined explicitly as covariates with all values equal to one. The structure must also be a two-column matrix to have two different intercepts, one for each likelihood.

```
I <- matrix(NA, nrow = 2 * n, ncol = 2)
I[1:n, 1] <- 1
I[n + 1:n, 2] <- 1
```

Variable `sex` needs to be put in a similar format so that the model includes two separate coefficients in each of the two parts of the model.

```
SEX <- matrix(NA, nrow = 2 * n, ncol = 2)
SEX[1:n, 1] <- fdgs.sub$sex
SEX[n + 1:n, 2] <- fdgs.sub$sex
```

Variable `age` also needs to be put in a different format, but given that it will be a weight in the `iid2d` latent effect, it must be passed as a vector of replicated values:

```
age.joint <- rep(fdgs.sub$age, 2)
```

Finally, an index vector to indicate which coefficient to use from the `iid2d` model is required. This index will be 1 for the first half of observations (to indicate that the coefficient is β_h) and 2 for the second half (to indicate that the coefficient is β_w).

```
idx.age = rep(1:2, each = n)
```

The model is fit and summarized as seen below. Note how the estimates of the intercepts and the coefficients for `sex` are very similar to those from the univariate models.

```
# Model formula
joint.f <- y ~ -1 + I + f(idx.age, age, model = "iid2d", n = 2) + SEX
# Model fit
fdgs.joint <- inla(joint.f,
  data = list(y = y, I = I, SEX = SEX, age = age.joint, idx.age = idx.age),
  family = rep("gaussian", 2),
  control.predictor = list(compute = TRUE))
# Summary
summary(fdgs.joint)
```

```
##
## Call:
##    c("inla(formula = joint.f, family = rep(\"gaussian\", 2), data =
##    list(y = y, ", " I = I, SEX = SEX, age = age.joint, idx.age =
##    idx.age), control.predictor = list(compute = TRUE))" )
## Time used:
##     Pre = 1.34, Running = 1.7, Post = 0.139, Total = 3.17
## Fixed effects:
##        mean    sd 0.025quant 0.5quant 0.975quant   mode kld
## I1    81.758 1.265     79.274   81.758     84.240 81.758   0
## I2     8.633 0.778      7.104    8.633     10.160  8.633   0
## SEX1 -4.650 0.725     -6.074   -4.651     -3.228 -4.651   0
## SEX2 -2.376 0.448     -3.255   -2.376     -1.498 -2.376   0
##
## Random effects:
##   Name      Model
##     idx.age IID2D model
##
## Model hyperparameters:
##                                              mean    sd 0.025quant 0.5quant
## Precision for the Gaussian observations      0.007 0.000      0.007    0.007
## Precision for the Gaussian observations[2]   0.020 0.001      0.018    0.020
## Precision for idx.age (component 1)          0.125 0.073      0.032    0.110
```

```
## Precision for idx.age (component 2)        0.378 0.224     0.100     0.329
## Rho1:2 for idx.age                         0.947 0.050     0.812     0.961
##                                            0.975quant  mode
## Precision for the Gaussian observations       0.008 0.008
## Precision for the Gaussian observations[2]    0.022 0.019
## Precision for idx.age (component 1)           0.309 0.079
## Precision for idx.age (component 2)           0.946 0.238
## Rho1:2 for idx.age                            0.993 0.982
##
## Expected number of effective parameters(stdev): 5.99(0.006)
## Number of equivalent replicates : 341.18
##
## Marginal log-Likelihood:  -7478.33
## Posterior marginals for the linear predictor and
##  the fitted values are computed
```

The coefficients for age are part of the random effects of the model. The estimates are very similar to the ones obtained in the univariate models. Note how the standard deviations seem to be slightly smaller.

```
fdgs.joint$summary.random$idx.age
```

```
##   ID  mean       sd 0.025quant 0.5quant 0.975quant  mode       kld
## 1  1 6.022 0.05504      5.914    6.022      6.130 6.022 2.125e-06
## 2  2 3.331 0.03381      3.265    3.331      3.397 3.331 1.308e-06
```

The estimates of height of the children that had missing values are these now:

```
fdgs.joint$summary.fitted.values[hgt.na, c("mean", "sd")]
```

```
##                          mean      sd
## fitted.Predictor.0001 122.20 0.5318
## fitted.Predictor.0005  83.21 0.6785
```

In a similar way, the estimates of weight of the children with missing values explored above can also be checked:

```
fdgs.joint$summary.fitted.values[n + wgt.na[1:2], c("mean", "sd")]
```

```
##                         mean     sd
## fitted.Predictor.1045 23.07 0.3214
## fitted.Predictor.1046 27.62 0.3342
```

12.4   Imputation of missing covariates

As seen in the previous section, the missing values in the response can be handled by computing their predictive distribution and this is possible because the data generating process is specified in the model likelihood. Missing values in the covariates pose a different problem as covariates are supposed to be explanatory variables and the model does not provide any information about the generating process of the covariates. However, imputation models can be proposed by exploiting the correlation among the different observed variables.

A simple approach to tackle missing observations in the covariates is to build a regression model to explain the covariate with the missing observations and plug-in the obtained estimates (e.g., posterior means) from their predictive distributions (Little and Rubin, 2002). This approach is simple and easy to implement in most cases, but it ignores the uncertainty about the imputed values.

A better approach would be to include a sub-model for the imputation of missing values within the main model to be fit. This will propagate the uncertainty from the imputed values throughout the model. However, this means than an extra level is required in the model and INLA is not designed to include this (see, for example, Gómez-Rubio et al., 2019).

In order to develop an example of the approaches mentioned above to fit models with missing observations in the covariates, we will build a model to explain height based on age, sex and weight. Note that now the missing observations in height are part of the response (and their predictive distributions can be computed) but the missing observations in weight are part of the latent effect.

First of all, a model is fit to the reduced dataset `fdgs.sub`. Note that this `data.frame` contains missing observations of variable `wgt`, which is in the linear predictor. Hence, `INLA` will not remove the rows with the missing observations in `wgt` before fitting the model, which means that some observations are actually not used to estimate the coefficient of `wgt`. This model will provide a baseline to compare to other approaches.

```
hgt.noimp <- inla(hgt ~ 1 +  age + sex + wgt, data = fdgs.sub)
summary(hgt.noimp)
```

```
##
## Call:
##    "inla(formula = hgt ~ 1 + age + sex + wgt, data = fdgs.sub)"
## Time used:
##     Pre = 0.949, Running = 0.201, Post = 0.0592, Total = 1.21
## Fixed effects:
##               mean    sd 0.025quant 0.5quant 0.975quant   mode kld
## (Intercept) 75.308 0.740     73.856   75.308     76.760 75.308   0
## age          4.971 0.147      4.681    4.971      5.260  4.971   0
## sexgirl     -4.012 0.715     -5.416   -4.012     -2.608 -4.012   0
## wgt          0.318 0.041      0.236    0.318      0.399  0.318   0
##
## Model hyperparameters:
##                                          mean   sd 0.025quant 0.5quant
## Precision for the Gaussian observations 0.008 0.00      0.007    0.008
```

```
##                                                    0.975quant  mode
## Precision for the Gaussian observations        0.009 0.008
##
## Expected number of effective parameters(stdev): 4.00(0.00)
## Number of equivalent replicates : 255.03
##
## Marginal log-Likelihood:  -3954.26
```

Next, we take the previous model fit to `wgt` to plug-in the posterior means of the missing observations into a new imputed data set called `fdgs.imp`:

```
fdgs.plg <- fdgs.sub
fdgs.plg$wgt[wgt.na] <- wgt.inla$summary.fitted.values[wgt.na, "mean"]
```

Note how the values of `wgt` in the new dataset `fdgs.plg` do not contain any NA's:

```
summary(fdgs.plg$wgt)
```

```
##    Min. 1st Qu.  Median    Mean 3rd Qu.    Max.
##    2.58   12.00   29.00   33.54   52.90  117.30
```

This new dataset is used to fit a new model where there are only missing observations in the response:

```
hgt.plg <- inla(hgt ~ 1 +  age + sex + wgt, data = fdgs.plg,
control.predictor = list(compute = TRUE))
summary(hgt.plg)
```

```
##
## Call:
##    "inla(formula = hgt ~ 1 + age + sex + wgt, data = fdgs.plg,
##    control.predictor = list(compute = TRUE))"
## Time used:
##    Pre = 0.954, Running = 0.297, Post = 0.0939, Total = 1.34
## Fixed effects:
##              mean    sd 0.025quant 0.5quant 0.975quant   mode kld
## (Intercept) 73.982 0.750     72.508   73.982     75.454 73.982   0
## age          4.348 0.171      4.013    4.348      4.683  4.348   0
## sexgirl     -3.490 0.704     -4.873   -3.490     -2.108 -3.490   0
## wgt          0.503 0.049      0.407    0.503      0.598  0.503   0
##
## Model hyperparameters:
##                                       mean   sd 0.025quant 0.5quant
## Precision for the Gaussian observations 0.008 0.00      0.007    0.008
##                                       0.975quant  mode
## Precision for the Gaussian observations    0.009 0.008
##
## Expected number of effective parameters(stdev): 4.00(0.00)
## Number of equivalent replicates : 255.03
##
```

```
## Marginal log-Likelihood:  -3932.14
## Posterior marginals for the linear predictor and
##  the fitted values are computed
```

The estimates of height for the two first children with missing observations is:

```
hgt.plg$summary.fitted.values[hgt.na[1:2], ]
```

```
##                            mean     sd 0.025quant 0.5quant 0.975quant   mode
## fitted.Predictor.0001 118.20 0.6426     116.94   118.20     119.46 118.20
## fitted.Predictor.0005  82.63 0.6525      81.35    82.63      83.91  82.63
```

Note how the estimates of the model effects have changed. It is worth mentioning that the last model has included the subjects that had missing observations of the weight to estimate its coefficient because they have now been imputed.

Including the full imputation mechanism in the model will require a sub-model within the main model. This is not currently implemented in INLA but this can be easily implemented as a new latent effect with the methods described in Section 11 (Gómez-Rubio et al., 2019). Alternatively, Cameletti et al. (2019) propose sampling from the predictive distribution of the imputation model, fitting models conditional on this imputed values and then using Bayesian model average on all the models fit to estimate a final model. The resulting model will account for the uncertainty of the imputation mechanism. In the next sections we provide different solutions to this problem by using a sample from the imputation model and by implementing an imputation mechanism using INLA within MCMC (Gómez-Rubio and Rue, 2018).

12.4.1 Sampling from the imputation model

When imputed values are plugged-into the data the actual model fit is conditional on these values and therefore, ignores the uncertainty about the imputation process. The marginals resulting from this model can be represented as

$$\pi(\theta_t \mid \mathbf{y}_{obs}, \mathbf{x}_{mis} = x^*_{mis})$$

where x^*_{mis} are the plugged-in values of the missing covariates and θ_t represents a latent effect or hyperparameter in the model.

Note that the imputation model will produce predictive distributions $\pi_I(\mathbf{x}_{mis} \mid \mathbf{y}_{imp})$, where $\mathbf{y}_{imp}$ are the observed data used in the imputation model. This model may have further parameters $\boldsymbol{\theta}_I$, for which posterior marginals can be obtained (but these are not really of interest now).

The posterior distribution of the parameters in the model can be obtained by integrating out the missing observations with regard to the imputation model, i.e.,

$$\pi(\theta_t \mid \mathbf{y}_{obs}) = \int \pi(\theta_t, \mathbf{x}_{mis} \mid \mathbf{y}_{obs}) d\mathbf{x}_{mis} = \int \pi(\theta_t \mid \mathbf{x}_{mis}, \mathbf{y}_{obs}) \pi(\mathbf{x}_{mis} \mid \mathbf{y}_{obs}) d\mathbf{x}_{mis}$$

Note that now $\mathbf{y}_{obs}$ refers to the observed data for the main model and the imputation model, i.e., $\mathbf{y}_{obs} = (\mathbf{y}, \mathbf{y}_{imp})$. $\mathbf{y}$ now includes the response variables plus any other fully observed covariates in the main model. The previous equation makes it clear that the predictive distribution of the missing observations is informed by the observed data in the general model and the data used in the imputation model.

As $\pi(\mathbf{x}_{mis} \mid \mathbf{y}_{obs})$ is seldom available, it can be replaced by the predictive distribution of $\mathbf{x}_{mis}$ obtained with the imputation model, i.e., $\pi_I(\mathbf{x}_{mis} \mid \mathbf{y}_{imp})$. This assumes that $\mathbf{x}_{mis}$ is only informed by the observed data in the imputation model ($\mathbf{y}_{imp}$) and ignores any dependence on the response variable and the main model. Then, the approximation is

$$\pi(\theta_t \mid \mathbf{y}_{obs}) \simeq \int \pi(\theta_t \mid \mathbf{x}_{mis}, \mathbf{y}_{obs}) \pi_I(\mathbf{x}_{mis} \mid \mathbf{y}_{imp}) d\mathbf{x}_{mis}$$

Hence, the the posterior marginal of θ_t can be approximated by sampling n_{imp} values of $\mathbf{x}_{mis}$ from their predictive distribution $\{\mathbf{x}_{mis}^{(i)}\}_{i=1}^{n_m}$ (see discussion in Cameletti et al., 2019):

$$\pi(\theta_t \mid \mathbf{y}_{obs}) \simeq \frac{1}{n_i} \sum_{i=1}^{n_{imp}} \pi(\theta_t \mid \mathbf{y}_{obs}, \mathbf{x}_{mis} = \mathbf{x}_{mis}^{(i)})$$

Note that $\pi(\theta_t \mid \mathbf{y}_{obs}, \mathbf{x}_{mis} = \mathbf{x}_{mis}^{(i)})$ is obtained by fitting a model with INLA in which the missing observations have been set to $\mathbf{x}_{mis}^{(i)}$.

The following code obtains 50 samples from the posterior distribution of the imputation model obtained using function `inla.posterior.sample()` (see Section 2.7):

```
n.imp <- 50
wgt.pred <- inla.posterior.sample(n.imp, wgt.inla)
```

The samples include the linear predictor. For the first set of samples, the values of the imputed weights (i.e., the linear predictor) are:

```
wgt.pred[[1]]$latent[wgt.na,]
```

```
##  Predictor:2  Predictor:3  Predictor:4  Predictor:6  Predictor:9
##       22.477       27.522       52.876       13.306        7.518
## Predictor:11 Predictor:14 Predictor:15 Predictor:21 Predictor:22
##       11.746       12.493        6.210       17.201       70.037
## Predictor:28 Predictor:29 Predictor:34 Predictor:35 Predictor:36
##       44.484       12.355       23.686       26.014       55.913
## Predictor:37 Predictor:38 Predictor:39 Predictor:40 Predictor:42
##       34.227       37.247       33.164       36.284       37.637
```

The original dataset can be completed with each of the 50 sets of imputed values and the the model can be fit with INLA:

```
imp.models <- lapply(1:n.imp, function(i) {
  fdgs.plg$wgt[wgt.na] <- wgt.pred[[i]]$latent[wgt.na, ]
  inla(hgt ~ 1 +  age + sex + wgt, data = fdgs.plg,
    control.predictor = list(compute = TRUE))
})
```

The fit models can be put together by computing the *average* model using Bayesian model averaging (Hoeting et al., 1999). For this, function `inla.merge()` is used with equal weights ($1/n_{imp}$):

```
model.imp <- inla.merge(imp.models, rep(1 / n.imp, n.imp))
```

The marginals for the fixed effects and hyperparameters are then extracted to be used later:

```
marg.fixed <- model.imp$marginals.fixed
marg.hyperpar <- model.imp$marginals.hyperpar
```

Summary statistics of the marginals of the fixed effects can be obtained as usual:

```
summary(model.imp)
```

```
##
## Call:
##    "inla(formula = hgt ~ 1 + age + sex + wgt, data = fdgs.plg,
##    control.predictor = list(compute = TRUE))"
## Time used:
##    Pre = 80.8, Running = 11.2, Post = 5.92, Total = 97.8
## Fixed effects:
##               mean    sd
## (Intercept) 75.712 2.702
## age          3.722 0.641
## sexgirl     -1.869 2.343
## wgt          0.654 0.185
##
## Model hyperparameters:
##                                        mean    sd
## Precision for the Gaussian observations 0.013 0.002
##
## Marginal log-Likelihood:  -278.21
## Posterior marginals for the linear predictor and
##   the fitted values are computed
```

Similarly, summary statistics of the predictive distribution for the first two children with missing values of height can be obtained using the estimates of the linear predictor:

```
model.imp$summary.linear.predictor[hgt.na[1:2], ]
```

```
##               mean    sd
## Predictor.01 118.7 2.412
## Predictor.05  85.0 2.193
```

Note that if the likelihood is not Gaussian in order to get the estimates of the fitted values the linear predictor needs to be conveniently transformed.

In order to assess the impact of the imputed values of weight in the model, the averaged predictive distribution for a given child with a missing value of height can be compared to the predictive distribution obtained from fitting the models to the 50 imputed values. Figure 12.1 shows the averaged predictive distribution (in black) as well as the different 50 predictive distributions. In this particular case, all of them are very similar.

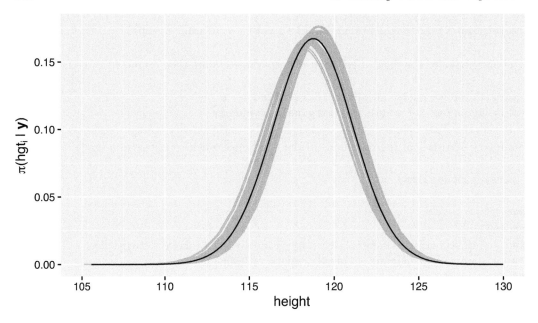

FIGURE 12.1 Predictive distribution of a missing observation of height in the `fdgs` dataset in the final average model (black) and predictive distributions from the 50 different models fit to the imputed datasets (gray).

12.5   Multiple imputation of missing values

Gómez-Rubio and Rue (2018) discuss the use of INLA within MCMC to fit models with missing observations. In a Bayesian framework, missing observations can be treated as any other parameter in the model, which means that they need to be assigned a prior distribution (if an imputation model is not provided).

This example will be illustrated using the `nhanes2` (Schafer, 1997), available in the `mice` package (van Buuren and Groothuis-Oudshoorn, 2011). The R code reproduced here is taken from the example in Gómez-Rubio and Rue (2018) and it is available from GitHub (see Preface for details).

The `nhanes2` dataset is a subset of 25 observations from the National Health and Nutrition Examination Survey (NHANES). Table 12.2 shows the different variables in this dataset, which can be loaded and summarized as:

```
library("mice")

data(nhanes2)
summary(nhanes2)
```

```
##      age           bmi           hyp          chl
##   20-39:12   Min.   :20.4   no  :13   Min.   :113
##   40-59: 7   1st Qu.:22.6   yes : 4   1st Qu.:185
```

```
## 60-99: 6    Median :26.8   NA's: 8   Median :187
##             Mean   :26.6             Mean   :191
##             3rd Qu.:28.9             3rd Qu.:212
##             Max.   :35.3             Max.   :284
##             NA's   :9               NA's   :10
```

TABLE 12.2: Variables in the **nhanes2** dataset.

Variable	Description
age	Age group (numeric, with 1=20-39, 2=40-59 and 3=60+).
bmi	Body mass index (in kg / m^2).
hyp	Hypertensive (numeric, with 1=no and 2=yes).
chl	Cholesterol level (mg/dL).

Note how there are missing observations of the body mass index and the cholesterol level. The interest now is to build a model to explain the cholesterol level based on the other variables in the dataset:

$$chl_i = \alpha + \beta_1 bmi_i + \beta_2 age_i^{40-59} + \beta_3 age_i^{60+} + \epsilon_i, \ i = 1, \ldots, 25$$

Here, age_i^{40-59} and age_i^{60+} are indicator variables derived from **age** to indicate whether a patient is in age group 40-59 or 60+, respectively. In addition, α is the model intercept, β_j, $j = 1, \ldots, 3$ are coefficients and ϵ_i an error term.

This model can be fit to the original dataset as follows (but bear in mind that **INLA** will not remove the rows in the dataset with missing observations of the covariates):

```
m1 <- inla(chl ~ 1 + bmi + age, data = nhanes2)
summary(m1)
```

```
##
## Call:
##    "inla(formula = chl ~ 1 + bmi + age, data = nhanes2)"
## Time used:
##     Pre = 0.973, Running = 0.0941, Post = 0.06, Total = 1.13
## Fixed effects:
##               mean     sd 0.025quant 0.5quant 0.975quant    mode kld
## (Intercept) 150.543 29.845     93.325  149.815    212.003 148.493   0
## bmi           1.243  1.128     -1.042    1.256      3.453   1.279   0
## age40-59     15.689 18.938    -22.853   16.100     51.952  16.909   0
## age60-99     35.180 22.200    -10.495   35.900     76.868  37.359   0
##
## Model hyperparameters:
##                                        mean   sd 0.025quant 0.5quant
## Precision for the Gaussian observations 0.001 0.00       0.00    0.001
##                                        0.975quant  mode
## Precision for the Gaussian observations     0.001 0.001
##
## Expected number of effective parameters(stdev): 3.20(0.198)
## Number of equivalent replicates : 4.69
```

```
##
## Marginal log-Likelihood:   -94.77
```

In order to consider the imputation of the missing observations together with model fitting, INLA within MCMC will be used as described in Section 11.5. This means that the Metropolis-Hastings will be used to sample new values of the missing observations of `bmi` and a new model will be fit on the imputed dataset at every step of the Metropolis-Hastings algorithm.

Before starting with the implementation of this method, a copy of the original dataset is created (`d.mis`) required by the general implementation of the algorithm in function `INLAMH()`, and then the indices of the missing values of `bmi` (`idx.mis`) and their number (`n.mis`) are obtained. This will be used in the implementation of the functions required in the Metropolis-Hastings algorithm.

```
#Generic variables for model fitting
d.mis <- nhanes2
idx.mis <- which(is.na(d.mis$bmi))
n.mis <- length(idx.mis)
```

Thr first function to be defined (`fit.inla()`) is the one to fit the model with INLA given the imputed values of `bmi`:

```
#Fit linear model with R-INLA with a fixed beta
#d.mis: Dataset
#x.mis: Imputed values
fit.inla <- function(data, x.mis) {

   data$bmi[idx.mis] <- x.mis

   res <- inla(chl ~ 1 + bmi + age, data = data)

   return(list(mlik = res$mlik[1,1], model = res))
}
```

Next, the proposal distribution is defined. In this case, a Gaussian distribution centered at the current imputed values of `bmi` with variance 10 is used. Two functions to compute the density, `dq.beta()`, and to obtain random values, `rq.beta()`, are created:

```
#Proposal x -> y
#density
dq.beta <- function(x, y, sigma = sqrt(10), log =TRUE) {
    res <- dnorm(y, mean = x, sd = sigma, log = log)

    if(log) {
        return(sum(res))
    } else {
        return(prod(res))
    }
}
#random
```

```
rq.beta <- function(x, sigma = sqrt(10) ) {
    rnorm(length(x), mean = x, sd = sigma)
}
```

Next, the prior on the missing values is set, in this case, a Gaussian distribution with mean that of the observed values and standard deviation twice that of the observed values. This will provide an informative prior but with ample variability:

```
#Prior for beta
prior.beta <- function(x, mu = mean(d.mis$bmi, na.rm = TRUE),
    sigma = 2*sd(d.mis$bmi, na.rm = TRUE), log = TRUE) {
    res <- dnorm(x, mean = mu, sd= sigma, log = log)

    if(log) {
        return(sum(res))
    } else {
        return(prod(res))
    }
}
```

The implementation of the Metropolis-Hastings is available in function `INLAMH()`. A total of 100 simulations will be used for inference, after 50 burn-in iterations and thinning one in 10 from 1000 iterations.

```
library("INLABMA")
# Set initial values to mean of bmi
d.init <- rep(mean(d.mis$bmi, na.rm = TRUE), n.mis)
#Run MCMC simulations
inlamh.res <- INLAMH(d.mis, fit.inla, d.init,
  rq.beta, dq.beta, prior.beta,
  n.sim = 100, n.burnin = 50, n.thin = 10)
```

The simulated values of the missing values of `bmi` can be put together and summarized as follows:

```
#Show results
x.sim <- do.call(rbind, inlamh.res$b.sim)
summary(x.sim)
```

```
##       V1               V2               V3               V4
## Min.   : 9.69   Min.   : 8.97   Min.   : 3.75   Min.   :10.7
## 1st Qu.:21.06   1st Qu.:24.90   1st Qu.:23.57   1st Qu.:18.6
## Median :25.31   Median :28.50   Median :30.20   Median :21.6
## Mean   :24.96   Mean   :27.28   Mean   :29.68   Mean   :22.4
## 3rd Qu.:29.20   3rd Qu.:30.95   3rd Qu.:35.47   3rd Qu.:25.3
## Max.   :38.02   Max.   :38.68   Max.   :53.45   Max.   :38.6
##       V5               V6               V7               V8
## Min.   : 8.02   Min.   : 0.83   Min.   : 8.99   Min.   : 8.85
## 1st Qu.:21.97   1st Qu.:20.26   1st Qu.:22.82   1st Qu.:23.37
```

```
## Median :28.73    Median :25.71    Median :27.51    Median :28.14
## Mean   :27.77    Mean   :25.88    Mean   :27.50    Mean   :28.17
## 3rd Qu.:33.18    3rd Qu.:30.40    3rd Qu.:32.29    3rd Qu.:32.53
## Max.   :41.76    Max.   :49.38    Max.   :44.75    Max.   :53.56
##         V9
## Min.   :12.7
## 1st Qu.:21.4
## Median :26.4
## Mean   :27.7
## 3rd Qu.:33.1
## Max.   :52.4
```

Figure 12.2 shows density estimates of the posterior distributions of the nine imputed values of `bmi`. As can be seen, there is ample variability in the posterior distributions. This may be due to the vague prior assigned to the missing values of `bmi` and the small sample size of the dataset with full observations, which makes it difficult to obtain accurate estimates of the missing values. Hence, a more informative prior or an imputation model that exploits the available information better (e.g., a linear regression) may be required to produce more accurate estimates.

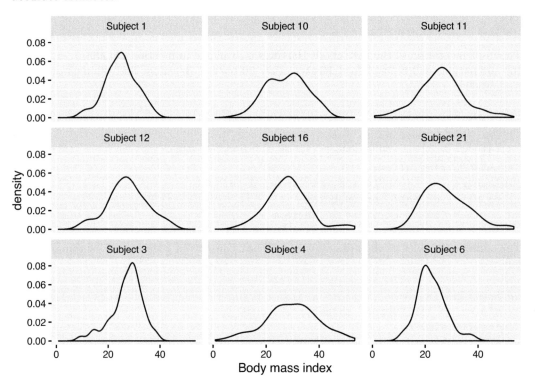

FIGURE 12.2 Posterior distribution of the missing observations of body mass index in the `nhanes2` dataset.

This example has shown how to fit models that can include a simple imputation mechanism for missing values in the covariates. In order to obtain estimates of the parameters of the full model, the fit models obtained in the INLA within MCMC run must be put together with function `inla.merge()`.

```
nhanes2.models <- lapply(inlamh.res$model.sim, function(X) { X$model })
nhanes2.imp <- inla.merge(nhanes2.models, rep(1, length(nhanes2.models)))
summary(nhanes2.imp)
```

```
##
## Call:
##    "inla(formula = chl ~ 1 + bmi + age, data = data)"
## Time used:
##     Pre = 86.5, Running = 8.23, Post = 5.34, Total = 100
## Fixed effects:
##               mean     sd
## (Intercept) 41.953 63.724
## bmi          4.929  2.238
## age40-59    29.421 17.994
## age60-99    49.389 23.081
##
## Model hyperparameters:
##                                          mean    sd
## Precision for the Gaussian observations 0.001 0.001
##
## Marginal log-Likelihood:  -90.54
```

As compared to the model fit to the observations without missing values of `bmi`, the posterior means of all the fixed effects change. The uncertainty about the intercept and coefficient of `bmi` also increases (i.e., they have a larger posterior standard deviation). Note that this may be due to the vague prior given to the missing values of `bmi`. However, the uncertainty about the estimates of `age` are very close to those obtained with the previous model.

12.6   Final remarks

Although the analysis of data with missing observations is feasible with `INLA` it is computationally very expensive when missing values are in the covariates. Computing the predictive distribution of missing observations in the response is still reasonable because it is implemented inside the `INLA` package, but when different models need to be fit to impute missing observations in the covariate computational times increase. This may be alleviated by the use of parallel computing methods and hardware. Finally, Gómez-Rubio et al. (2019) describe a promising approach to include new latent effects in the model to impute missing observations in the covariates.

13

Mixture models

13.1 Introduction

Multimodal data are not uncommon in statistics and they often appear when observations come from two or more underlying groups or populations. The analysis of these types of data is often undertaken with mixture models, which make use of different components that can model the different groups or populations in the data. Essentially, a mixture model is a convex combination of several statistical distributions that represent the different underlying populations. For a recent review on the topic see, for example, Frühwirth-Schnatter et al. (2018).

Mixture models do not follow the paradigm of Gaussian Markov random fields. A simple way to see this is that data generated from mixture models is often multimodal. However, Gómez-Rubio and Rue (2018) provide a way to fit mixture models with INLA by combining INLA and MCMC. Gómez-Rubio (2017) also explore the use of other algorithms to fit mixture models with INLA. In general, the analysis of mixture models is complex and the aim of this chapter is to provide a short link between INLA and these models. Furthermore, we will show how to fit these models with INLA.

This chapter starts with an introduction to mixture models in Section 13.2. Fitting a mixture model with INLA using the Metropolis-Hastings algorithm will be discussed next in Section 13.3. Section 13.4 will follow with a discussion of how the marginal likelihood of a mixture model can be approximated with INLA for model selection. Finally, Section 13.5 focuses on fitting cure rate models, which are mixture models in survival analysis, with INLA. Finally, Section 13.6 ends the chapter with a short discussion.

13.2 Bayesian analysis of mixture models

Mixture models are often represented as follows:

$$y_i \sim \sum_{k=1}^{K} w_k f_k(y_i \mid \theta_k)$$

Here, $\{f_k(\cdot \mid \theta_k)\}_{k=1}^{K}$ is a set of (parametric) distributions and $\mathbf{w} = (w_1, \ldots, w_K)$ associated weights They are defined so that they sum up to one, i.e., $\sum_{k=1}^{K} w_k = 1$, and they can be regarded the proportion of observations from each group expected in the data.

A common approach to fit mixture models is to consider the *augmented* data (Dempster et al., 1977) which considers an auxiliary variable $\mathbf{z} = (z_1, \ldots, z_n)$ to assign each observation to a group. For this reason, variables $z_i, i = 1, \ldots, n$ take values in the set $\{1, \ldots, K\}$. Hence, the mixture model can also be represented as follows:

$$y_i \mid z_i \sim f_{z_i}(y_i \mid \theta_{z_i}), \; z_i \in \{1, \ldots, K\}$$

The distribution of the auxiliary variables $\mathbf{z}$ can be stated as:

$$\pi(z_i = k \mid \mathbf{w}) = w_k, \; k = 1, \ldots, K$$

This representation is quite convenient in practice as it simplifies the representation of the model. Considering the complete data $(\mathbf{y}, \mathbf{z})$, the model likelihood becomes

$$\pi(\mathbf{y}, \mathbf{z} \mid \boldsymbol{\theta}, \mathbf{w}) = \left(\prod_{i=1}^{n} f_{z_i}(y_i \mid \theta_{z_i}) \right) w_k^{n_k}$$

Here, $n_k, k = 1, \ldots, K$, is the number of observations in group k.

It is worth noting that, if exchangeable priors are used, given $\mathbf{z}$ the different groups are independent. This means that, conditional on $\mathbf{z}$, mixture models can be fit with INLA using a model with several likelihoods. This can be exploited to fit mixture models with INLA in a number of ways, as described below.

Mixture models are not identifiable because the way in which the different groups are labeled is somewhat arbitrary and a different labeling may lead to exactly the same model. For example, in a mixture with two groups, given a value of $\mathbf{z}$, if the labels are reversed (i.e., 1 is set to 2 and vice versa) then exactly the same model is obtained. This is the well known problem of *label switching* (Celeux et al., 2000; Stephens, 2000). For this reason, additional constraints on the priors of $\boldsymbol{\theta}$ are often imposed and improper priors should not be used (Frühwirth-Schnatter et al., 2018, Chapter 4). A simple way to deal with this problem is to assign informative priors (Carlin and Chib, 1995) or ordering constraints on the means of the different groups (Diebolt and Robert, 1994; Richardson and Green, 1997).

13.2.1 Eruption times analysis

The `geyser` dataset (Azzalini and Bowman, 1990) in the `MASS` package describes duration times of the Old Faithful geyser in Yellowstone National Park as well as time between eruptions, as described in Table 13.1.

TABLE 13.1: Variables in the `geyser` dataset.

Variable	Description
`duration`	Duration of the eruption (in minutes).
`waiting`	Waiting time for this eruption (in minutes)

The following code shows how to load the data and a summary of the variables in the dataset:

```
library("MASS")
data(geyser)
summary(geyser)
```

```
##      waiting            duration
##   Min.    : 43.0    Min.    :0.833
##   1st Qu.: 59.0    1st Qu.:2.000
##   Median : 76.0    Median :4.000
##   Mean    : 72.3    Mean    :3.461
##   3rd Qu.: 83.0    3rd Qu.:4.383
##   Max.    :108.0    Max.    :5.450
```

Furthermore, Figure 13.1 shows a scatter plot of both variables as well as a histogram and kernel density estimate of duration times. The distribution of the eruption times is clearly multimodal and fitting a typical linear regression may not be appropriate.

The bivariate plot also shows a high correlation between the time that precedes an eruption and its duration. In fact, NPS rangers are able to predict when the next eruption will happen based on the duration of the previous eruption.

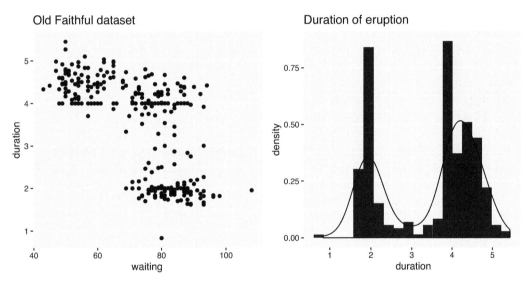

FIGURE 13.1 Variables in the `geyser` dataset.

The question of interest now is to quantify how many groups there are in the dataset and, at the same time, being able to characterize each group of duration times. A visual inspection of the right plot in Figure 13.1 suggests that there are (at least) two different groups in the data, with means roughly at about 2 and 4, and similar standard deviations between the two groups. Note that several authors have suggested a larger number of components in this dataset (Zucchini et al., 2016), but we will only consider the analysis with two groups for simplicity.

A simple approach is to simply split the data in two groups and fit a model with two likelihoods. For example, we can assign all eruption times with a duration lower than or equal to three to group 1 and the other observations to group 2. Alternatively, the K-means algorithm can be used to obtain an initial rough classification of the data. In this particular case, both approaches will create the same initial classification of the data. Note that the response needs to be put into a 2-column matrix because two different likelihoods will be used, as described in Chapter 6.

```
#Index of group 1
idx1 <- geyser$duration <=3
```

This index will be used later to create the dataset, but it can be used now to show the number of observations assigned to each group:

```
table(idx1)
```

```
## idx1
## FALSE  TRUE
##   192   107
```

Note how most of the observations are in the second group, as shown in Figure 13.1. The response to be used with INLA is created as follows:

```
# Empty response
yy <- matrix(NA, ncol = 2, nrow = nrow(geyser))

#Add data
yy[idx1, 1] <- geyser$duration[idx1]
yy[!idx1, 2] <- geyser$duration[!idx1]
```

Because we want each group to have a different mean, the intercept must be split in two using a similar structure to that of the observed data. In this case a 2-column matrix will be used with entries 1 and NA.

```
#Create two different intercepts
II <- yy
II[II > 0] <- 1
```

Next, the model can be fit by using values yy and I in the data (which are named duration and Intercept, respectively, in the call to inla()) and two likelihoods:

```
#Fit model with INLA
geyser.inla <- inla(duration ~ -1 + Intercept,
  data = list(duration = yy, Intercept = II),
  family = c("gaussian", "gaussian"))
summary(geyser.inla)
```

```
##
## Call:
##    c("inla(formula = duration ~ -1 + Intercept, family =
##    c(\"gaussian\", ", " \"gaussian\"), data = list(duration = yy,
##    Intercept = II))" )
## Time used:
##     Pre = 1.08, Running = 0.177, Post = 0.132, Total = 1.39
## Fixed effects:
##              mean    sd 0.025quant 0.5quant 0.975quant  mode kld
## Intercept1 1.999 0.030      1.941    1.999      2.058 1.999   0
## Intercept2 4.275 0.027      4.222    4.275      4.328 4.275   0
```

```
##
## Model hyperparameters:
##                                              mean     sd 0.025quant 0.5quant
## Precision for the Gaussian observations     10.71 1.458       8.08    10.63
## Precision for the Gaussian observations[2]   7.22 0.736       5.87     7.20
##                                           0.975quant  mode
## Precision for the Gaussian observations        13.80 10.50
## Precision for the Gaussian observations[2]      8.76  7.15
##
## Expected number of effective parameters(stdev): 2.02(0.001)
## Number of equivalent replicates : 148.35
##
## Marginal log-Likelihood:  -140.45
```

The summary of the model shows that the means of the two groups have estimates 1.9994 and 4.2753, respectively. In addition, the first group has an estimated precision of 10.7114, while the second has an estimated precision of 7.2251, which makes the eruptions times in the second group slightly more variable.

Although this approach leads to reasonable estimates of the eruptions times between the two groups it has two problems. The first one is that we have already used the data once to determine that there are two groups and how these two groups are defined. Secondly, this approach ignores the inherent uncertainty about from which group each observation comes. This is an important issue when classifying observations into groups and a simple cutoff point is seldom a good idea.

From a modeling point a few, what we have just done is fitting a model conditional on the auxiliary variable $\mathbf{z}$, i.e., we have set $\mathbf{z}$ to a given classification. Although this may be useful in practice (see Gómez-Rubio and Palmí-Perales, 2019, for some examples on fitting conditional models with INLA), in a full Bayesian analysis we should also be interested in the posterior distribution of $\mathbf{z}$.

13.3   Fitting mixture models with INLA

Mixture models are hard to fit in general (Celeux et al., 2000) and they do not fall into the class of models that INLA can fit as they cannot be expressed as a latent GMRF. However, as noted in Gómez-Rubio and Rue (2018) and Gómez-Rubio (2017) conditional on $\mathbf{z}$ a mixture model becomes a model that can be fit with INLA.

Gómez-Rubio (2017) note that the posterior marginal of the model parameter of a mixture model can be written down as

$$\pi(\theta_t \mid \mathbf{y}) = \sum_{z \in \mathcal{Z}} \pi(\theta_t \mid \mathbf{y}, \mathbf{z} = z) \pi(\mathbf{z} = z \mid \mathbf{y}), \; t = 1, \ldots, \dim(\boldsymbol{\theta})$$

Note that this requires the posterior distribution of $\mathbf{z}$ that is usually not known. However, this can be easily estimated using INLA within MCMC, as shown in Gómez-Rubio and Rue (2018).

In this example, the Metropolis Hastings algorithm will be used to estimate the posterior distribution of $\mathbf{z}$. Hence, a proposal distribution is required to propose new values of $\mathbf{z}$ and all of the assignments will be accepted or rejected as a single block (i.e., there is not individual acceptance or rejection for each $z_i, i = 1, \ldots, n$).

The proposal distribution $q(\mathbf{z}' \mid \mathbf{z})$ defines the probability of a new value $\mathbf{z}'$ given the current value $\mathbf{z}$. This is taken so that the probability of each individual z_i being 1 is (Marin et al., 2005)

$$P(z_i' = 1 \mid \mathbf{z}) = \frac{w_1 f_1(y_i \mid \mu_1, \tau_1)}{w_1 f_1(y_i \mid \mu_1, \tau_1) + w_2 f_2(y_i \mid \mu_2, \tau_2)}$$

$$P(z_i' = 2 \mid \mathbf{z}) = 1 - P(z_i' = 1 \mid \mathbf{z})$$

Here, $f_1(\cdot \mid \mu_1, \tau_1)$ is Normal distribution with mean μ_1 and precision τ_2, which are the ones for group 1 obtained from fitting the model conditional to $\mathbf{z}$. $f_2(\cdot \mid \mu_2, \tau_2)$ is defined analogously. Note that the values of the means and precisions here depend on $\mathbf{z}$.

The example developed here is taken from Gómez-Rubio and Rue (2018) as the associated code available from `https://github.com/becarioprecario/INLAMCMC_examples`, which relies on function `INLAMH()` from package `INLABMA`. See Chapter 11 for details on how to fit new models with INLA by using the Metropolis-Hastings algorithm.

The different functions required to fit a mixture model using INLA within MCMC are described below. In order to have an overview of the overall picture, the different functions needed to implement this algorithm are:

- `get.probs()`: compute the weights of the different components given an observed value of the latent variable $\mathbf{z}$.

- `dq.z()`: density probability function of the proposal distribution.

- `rq.z()`: random number generator function from the proposal distribution.

- `fit.inla.internal()`: fits the required INLA model given the value of $\mathbf{z}$. This is used to compute the conditional marginal likelihood $\pi(\mathbf{y} \mid \mathbf{z}$ required to compute the acceptance probability.

- `prior.z()` computes the prior of $\mathbf{z}$.

Also, note that the variable that stores the classification of the observations in the functions below is not simply a vector with the groups to which the observation belongs, but a more complex data structure. In particular, it is a list with the following elements:

- z: Vector that indicates to which observation belongs.

- m: Model fit with `INLA` conditional on the value of $\mathbf{z}$. It is a list of two components: `model` with the INLA model fit and `mlik` with the marginal likelihood of the model fit.

Note that this type of object is returned, for example, by function `rq.z()`. This is the data structure used to represent variable $\mathbf{z}$ and it is passed to several functions for the computations. The reason to include the model fit is to avoid fitting it more than once in the implementation of the Metropolis-Hastings algorithm.

Before describing the required functions, the number of groups to be used is 2, which is set in variable `n.grp` to be used by some of the functions defined below. Also, variable `grp` is defined as a vector to store the initial groups to which observations belong:

```
# Number of groups
n.grp <- 2

# Initial classification
grp <- rep(1, length(geyser$duration))
grp[!idx1] <- 2
```

Function `fit.inla.internal()` is used to actually fit the required model given `z` and it is used inside `rq.z()` below. Note that another similar function `inla.fit()` is defined below for a similar purpose. The main difference between these two functions is that `fit.inla.internal()` is the one that calls `inla()` to fit the conditional model on `z` and that `fit.inla()` simply takes the fit model from the complex data structure that represents the value of `z` and the model fit.

```
#y: Vector of values with the response.
#grp: Vector of integers with the allocation variable.
fit.inla.internal <- function(y, grp) {

  #Data in two-column format
  yy <- matrix(NA, ncol = n.grp, nrow = length(y))
  for(i in 1:n.grp) {
    idx <- which(grp == i)
    yy[idx, i] <- y[idx]
  }

  #X stores the intercept in the model
  x <- yy
  x[!is.na(x)] <- 1

  d <- list(y = yy, x = x)

  #Model fit (conditional on z)
  m1 <- inla(y ~ -1 + x, data = d,
    family = rep("gaussian", n.grp),
    #control.fixed = list(mean = list(x1 = 2, x2 = 4.5), prec = 1)
    control.fixed = list(mean = prior.means, prec = 1)
  )

  res<- list(model = m1, mlik = m1$mlik[1, 1])
  return(res)
}
```

The initial data structure to represent the assignment to groups and the associated model fit (as described above) is defined next in variable `grp.init`. Note that given that this includes the model fit the prior means of the Gaussian prior distributions on the group means are defined through variables `prior.means`. Also, variable `scale.sigma` is set to be used in the proposal distribution.

```
y <- geyser$duration

prior.means <- list(x1 = 2, x2 = 4.5)
scale.sigma <- 1.25
grp.init <- list(z = grp, m = fit.inla.internal(y, grp))
```

Below, the functions required for the implementation of the Metropolis-Hastings algorithm are shown. Some information about their respective parameters is given as R comments.

Function `get.probs()` will compute the weights for each component given the current value of z, which is passed as a vector of integers from 1 to K.

```
#Probabilities of belonging to each group
#z: Vector of integers with values from 1 to the number of groups
get.probs <- function(z) {
  probs <- rep(0, n.grp)
  tab <- table(z)
  probs[as.integer(names(tab))] <- tab / sum(tab)
  return(probs)
}
```

Next, we define function `dq.z()` to compute the density of a new value (z.new) of z given the current one (z.old). Note that these values are a data structure as described above and not simply a vector of integers.

```
#Using means of conditional marginals
#FIXME: We do not consider possble label switching here
#z.old: Current value of z.
#z.new: Proposed value of z.
#log: Compute density in the log-scale.
dq.z <- function(z.old, z.new, log = TRUE) {
  m.aux <- z.old$m$model
  means <- m.aux$summary.fixed[, "mean"]
  precs <- m.aux$summary.hyperpar[, "mean"]

  ww <- get.probs(z.old$z)

  z.probs <- sapply(1:length(y), function (X) {
    aux <- ww * dnorm(y[X], means, scale.sigma * sqrt(1 / precs))
    (aux / sum(aux))[z.new$z[X]]
  })

  if(log) {
    return(sum(log(z.probs)))
  } else {
    return(prod(z.probs))
  }
}
```

The function to sample random observations of z using the proposal distribution given the current value of **z**, z, is rq.z(). Note that **z** is a complex data structure that includes the vector of indicators and the model fit, as described above.

```
#FIXME: We do not consider possible label switching here
#z: Current value of z.
rq.z <- function(z) {
  m.aux <- z$m$model
  means <- m.aux$summary.fixed[, "mean"]
  precs <- m.aux$summary.hyperpar[, "mean"]

  ws <- get.probs(z$z)

  z.sim <- sapply(1:length(z$z), function (X) {
    aux <- ws * dnorm(y[X], means, scale.sigma * sqrt(1 / precs))
    sample(1:n.grp, 1, prob = aux / sum(aux))
  })

  #Fit model
  z.model <- fit.inla.internal(y, z.sim)

  #New value
  z.new <- list(z = z.sim, m = z.model)

  return(z.new)
}
```

The prior distribution on **z** is simply the product of Bernoullis with probability 0.5 to provide a vague prior:

```
#z: Vector of integer values from 1 to K.
prior.z <- function(z, log = TRUE) {

  res <- log(1 / n.grp) * length(z$z)
  if(log) {
    return(res)
  }
  else {
    return(exp(res))
  }
}
```

Function `fit.inla()` is the function used by `INLAMH()` to fit the model given the value pf z. In this particular implementation, the actual model fitting is done inside function `rq.z()` using function `fit.inla.internal()`, so that `fit.inla()` simply retrieves element m from the data structure:

```
fit.inla <- function(y, grp) {
  return(grp$m)
}
```

Next, we need to call function `INLAMH()` to fit the model. Given that the starting point is close to the optimal partition of the data (but note that this is not usual), it is not necessary to have a large number of burn-in iterations. Furthermore, the number of iterations is kept low to 100 (after thinning one in five) because in this particular example there are only a few observations that may have a posterior probability which is not close to zero or one. In more complex examples the number of simulations is probably required to be higher.

```
#Run simulations
library("INLABMA")
inlamh.res <- INLAMH(geiser$duration, fit.inla, grp.init, rq.z, dq.z,
   prior.z, n.sim = 100, n.burnin = 20, n.thin = 5, verbose = TRUE)
```

Once the model has been fit, it will return a list with the fitted models and the values of **z** (that includes many auxiliary variables that are not actually needed). The sampled values of **z** are obtained as

```
zz <- do.call(rbind, lapply(inlamh.res$b.sim, function(X){X$z}))
```

From this sample from the posterior distribution $\pi(\mathbf{z} \mid \mathbf{y})$ we can compute the posterior probabilities of belonging to each group:

```
zz.probs <- apply(zz, 2, get.probs)
```

Note that probabilities for most observations are 0 and 1, i.e., classification is quite clear, and only a few observations will show some uncertainty in the classification. Figure 13.2 shows the observed values against the posterior probabilities of belonging to the group of eruptions with the lower durations (i.e., $z_i = 1$).

The conditional marginal likelihoods of all the models associated with the sampled values of **z** can also be obtained to gain some insight on the simulation process:

```
mliks <- do.call(rbind, lapply(inlamh.res$model.sim, function(X){X$mlik}))
```

These are also shown in Figure 13.2 (right plot) and they show how the sampling algorithm produces an increase of the conditional marginal likelihoods as compared to the initial model fit above in Section 13.2 (which had a marginal likelihood of -140.16). This also means that the short burn-in period is enough.

Furthermore, the chain shows that only a few classifications are explored. This behavior can be easily changed by increasing the number of iterations for thinning or choosing a different proposal distribution, for example, one that takes higher values of the standard deviations (e.g., twice their values). However, in this particular case most of the observations have high posterior probabilities of belonging to one of the two groups, which means that they are always classified in the same group. Hence, the posterior probabilities are accumulated in a few classifications where only the observations with a duration time of about 3 minutes are classified in either of the two groups.

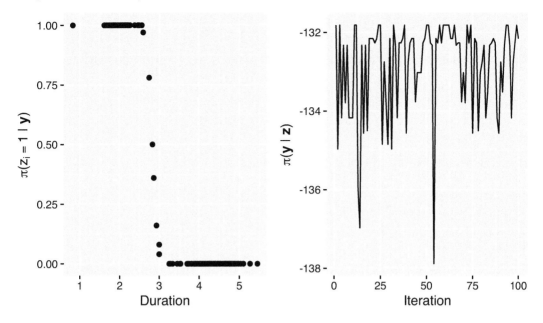

FIGURE 13.2 Posterior probabilities of the observed data (left) and conditional marginal likelihood (right) of the model fit to the duration of geyser eruptions (in minutes).

13.4 Model selection for mixture models

Determining the number of components in a model is often difficult and a number of proposals have been made so far. Here we will simply approach the estimation of the marginal likelihood of the mixture model with a known number of groups by noting that it can be computed as (Gómez-Rubio, 2017):

$$\pi(\mathbf{y}) = \sum_{z \in \mathcal{Z}} \pi(\mathbf{y} \mid \mathbf{z} = z)\pi(\mathbf{z} = z)$$

Note that $\pi(\mathbf{y} \mid \mathbf{z} = z)$ can be approximated with accuracy by the marginal likelihood returned by fitting a model with INLA given $\mathbf{z}$. Furthermore, $\pi(\mathbf{z})$ is the prior distribution which is always known.

Alternatively, the marginal likelihood of a mixture model can be computed by noting that (Chib, 1995):

$$\pi(\mathbf{y}) = \frac{\pi(\mathbf{y} \mid \mathbf{z} = z^*)\pi(\mathbf{z} = z^*)}{\pi(\mathbf{z} = z^*) \mid \mathbf{y})}, \; z^* \in \mathcal{Z}$$

Note that in order to make the previous computation stable the posterior probability of z^* must be bounded away from zero. A good choice would be the posterior mode of $\mathbf{z}$.

For example, we can take the value of $\mathbf{z}$ with the highest marginal likelihood (note that all values of $\mathbf{z}$ have the same value of the prior), which is the one obtained at iteration 60:

```
z.idx <- 60
```

Then, the estimate of the conditional marginal likelihood $\pi(\mathbf{y} \mid \mathbf{z} = z^*)$ provided by INLA is

```
#Marginal likelihood (log-scale)
mliks[z.idx]
```

```
## [1] -131.8
```

Next, the prior at the z^*, $\pi(\mathbf{z} = z^*)$, is computed as

```
#Prior (log-scale)
prior.z(inlamh.res$b.sim[[z.idx]])
```

```
## [1] -207.3
```

Finally, the posterior probability of z^* is obtained from the sample from the posterior distribution of $\mathbf{z}$ obtained from the MCMC algorithm. This is done by simply checking the proportion of times z^* appears in the sample from the posterior distribution of $\mathbf{z}$:

```
#Posterior probabilities
z.post <- table(apply(zz, 1, function(x) {paste(x, collapse = "")})) / 100

# Get post. prob. of z^* in the log-scale
log.pprob <- unname(
  log(z.post[names(z.post) ==
    paste(inlamh.res$b.sim[[z.idx]]$z, collapse = "")])
)
log.pprob
```

```
## [1] -1.561
```

Note that the `paste()` function has been used above in order to create an unique label for each value of $\mathbf{z}$ by appending all its values together. The resulting label has the same length of the number of observations and it can be very long. In any case, this is a simple way to identify each value of the latent variable with a label, although shorter options should be preferred in practice (such as hash tables). Having an unique label for each value of $\mathbf{z}$ allows us to use the `table()` function on the sample values directly to compute the number of times each value of the latent variable appears in the MCMC sample.

Hence, the estimate of the marginal likelihood (in the log-scale) is

```
mlik.mix <- mliks[z.idx] + prior.z(inlamh.res$b.sim[[z.idx]]) - log.pprob
mlik.mix
```

```
## [1] -337.5
```

Note that this estimate of the marginal likelihood relies on the approximations to $\pi(\mathbf{y} \mid \mathbf{z} = z^*)$ (which is provided by INLA) and $\pi(\mathbf{z} = z^* \mid \mathbf{y})$ (which is obtained from the MCMC samples). Hence, in order to obtain reliable estimates it may be required to run the MCMC algorithm for a longer number of iterations.

This value of the marginal likelihood obtained can be compared to the one reported by `INLA` when a Gaussian model with a single likelihood is fit to the whole dataset:

```
inla(duration ~ 1, data = geyser)$mlik[1,1]
```

```
## log marginal-likelihood (integration)
##                                    -478.6
```

Finally, the same approach can be used to fit a model with three components to the data. This will require setting the number of groups to three and generating a suitable starting point (which in this case is splitting the data into three groups of equal size):

```
#Number of groups
n.grp <- 3

#Initial classification
grp3 <- as.numeric(cut(geyser$duration, 3))
grp.init3 <- list(z = grp3, m = fit.inla.internal(y, grp3))
```

Next, the prior means and scale of the standard deviation of the proposal distribution are set:

```
#Priors for  the means
prior.means <- list(x1 = 2, x2 = 3.5, x3 = 5)
#Scale st. dev. of proposal distribution
scale.sigma <- 1
```

Once all parameters have been defined to fit a mixture model with three components, model fitting is carried out with the `INLAMH()` function:

```
inlamh.res3 <- INLAMH(geiser$duration, fit.inla, grp.init3, rq.z, dq.z,
   prior.z, n.sim = 100, n.burnin = 20, n.thin = 5, verbose = TRUE)
```

Then, the marginal likelihood of this mixture model with three components can be computed similarly as before. First, the value of **z** with the largest conditional marginal likelihood (z^*) is obtained:

```
##Conditional (on z) marg. lik.
mliks3 <- do.call(rbind, lapply(inlamh.res3$model.sim, function(X){X$mlik}))
#z^* with maximum cond. marg. lik.
z.idx3 <- which.max(mliks3)
```

Next, the log-posterior probability of z^* is estimated from the MCMC sample:

```
#Get all values of z in the sample
zz3 <- do.call(rbind, lapply(inlamh.res3$b.sim, function(X){X$z}))
#Table of posterior probabilities
z.post3 <- table(apply(zz3, 1, function(x) {paste(x, collapse = "")})) / 100
```

```
#Log-posterior probability of z^*
log.pprob3 <- unname(
  log(z.post3[names(z.post3) == paste(inlamh.res3$b.sim[[z.idx3]]$z,
    collapse = "")])
)
```

Finally, the marginal likelihood is estimated by combining these two values with the prior probability of z^*:

```
#Marginal likelihood
mlik.mix3 <- mliks3[z.idx3] + prior.z(inlamh.res3$b.sim[[z.idx3]]) -
  log.pprob3
mlik.mix3
```

```
## [1] -291.4
```

Note how the estimate of the marginal likelihood obtained now is larger than for the models with 1 and 2 components. This means that there are probably (at least) three groups in the data and not two, as discussed in Zucchini et al. (2016).

In order to summarize the fit model using the model with 2 and 3 components, Figure 13.3 shows the mixture using the posterior means of the model parameter. Function `inla.merge()` will be used to merge all the models obtained in the Metropolis-Hastings algorithms. This will provide the posterior means of the means and precisions in the model. The posterior means of weights **w** will be obtained from the posterior mean of the proportions of observations in each group (which assumes a very vague flat prior).

```
#Merge models
models <- lapply(inlamh.res$model.sim, function(X) {X$model})
mix.model <- inla.merge(models)

#Post. means
mix.means <- mix.model$summary.fixed[, "mean"]
mix.precs <- mix.model$summary.hyperpar[, "mean"]

#Post. means of weights
n.grp <- 2
mix.w <- apply(apply(zz, 1, get.probs), 1, mean)
```

Similarly, for the model with 3 components:

```
#Merge models
models3 <- lapply(inlamh.res3$model.sim, function(X) {X$model})
mix.model3 <- inla.merge(models3)

#Post. means
mix.means3 <- mix.model3$summary.fixed[, "mean"]
mix.precs3 <- mix.model3$summary.hyperpar[, "mean"]
```

```
#Post. means of weights
n.grp <- 3
mix.w3 <- apply(apply(zz3, 1, get.probs), 1, mean)
```

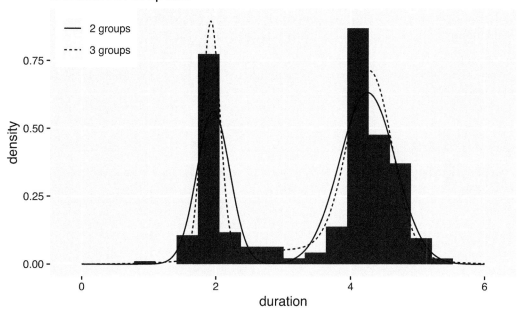

FIGURE 13.3 Mixtures estimated at the posterior mode of z using the posterior means of the parameters for the models with 2 and 3 groups.

13.5 Cure rate models

Survival models described in Chapter 10 assume that all subjects will eventually experience the event of interest. However, in some situations subjects may get cured and, hence, will not be susceptible to experience this event. A typical situation is a patient who is cured from a disease after receiving proper treatment.

This situation can be conveniently represented by a mixture model with two groups: a group of cured subjects and a group of non-cured that have experienced the event or that will eventually. This is a particular type of mixture model with only two classes. Furthermore, some of the subjects will automatically be assigned to the second group as they have already experienced the event. This makes cure rate models easier to identify as these subjects will help to identify the second group, which in turn will help to identify the first group.

In INLA, cure rate models are represented by a constant density (equal to 1) for the first group and a Weibull density for the second group. See inla.doc("weibullcure") for details.

This model can be described as follows:

$$y_i \mid w, \boldsymbol{\theta} \sim w \cdot 1 + (1 - w) f(y_i \mid \boldsymbol{\theta}), \ i = 1, \ldots, n$$

Here, $f(\cdot \mid \theta)$ represents a Weibull distribution and its parameterization in `INLA` is:

$$f(y_i \mid \alpha) = \alpha y_i^{\alpha - 1} \lambda \exp\{-\lambda y_i^{\alpha}\}.$$

Note that this parameterization of the Weibull distribution is similar to the `variant=0` of the Weibull family available in likelihood `weibull`. See `inla.doc("weibullcure")` for details.

In the equation above, y_i represent survival times and it is a non-negative variable, α is a positive shape parameter and λ is a parameter that is linked to the linear predictor. This link is as follows:

$$\lambda = \exp(\eta)$$

where η is the linear predictor.

Priors for this model are defined on the internal representation of parameters α and w. In particular, the internal parameterization is

$$\theta_1 = \log(\alpha)$$

$$\theta_2 = \log(\frac{w}{1 - w})$$

This parameterization makes sure that θ_1 and θ_2 are not in a bounded interval, which simplifies optimization and model fitting. The default prior on θ_1 is a log-gamma with parameters 25 and 25, while the prior on θ_2 is Gaussian with mean -1 and precision 0.2. These priors can be changed as described in Chapter 5.

Package `smcure` (Cai et al., 2012a,b) provides dataset `e1684` from the Eastern Cooperative Oncology Group (ECOG) phase III clinical trial e1684 (see, Kirkwood et al., 1996, for details). The clinical trial was conducted to test whether Interferon alpha-2b (IFN alpha-2b) exhibits antitumor activity in metastatic melanoma. Table 13.2 describes the variables in the dataset.

TABLE 13.2: Variables in the `e1684` dataset.

Variable	Description
TRT	Treatment (0=control, 1=IFN treatment)
FAILTIME	Observed relapse-free time.
FAILCENS	Censoring indicator (1=event happens, 0=event not observed)
AGE	Age of patient (centered to the mean).
SEX	Sex (1 for female and 0 for male).

The original dataset can be loaded as follows:

```
library("smcure")
data(e1684)
summary(e1684)
```

```
##        TRT              FAILTIME          FAILCENS           AGE
## Min.    :0.000    Min.    :0.033    Min.    :0.000    Min.    :-29.99
## 1st Qu.:0.000    1st Qu.:0.356    1st Qu.:0.000    1st Qu.:-11.32
## Median :1.000    Median :1.238    Median :1.000    Median :  0.58
## Mean    :0.509    Mean    :2.763    Mean    :0.691    Mean    :  0.00
## 3rd Qu.:1.000    3rd Qu.:4.956    3rd Qu.:1.000    3rd Qu.: 11.03
## Max.    :1.000    Max.    :9.644    Max.    :1.000    Max.    : 31.70
##                                                        NA's    :1
##        SEX
## Min.    :0.000
## 1st Qu.:0.000
## Median :0.000
## Mean    :0.398
## 3rd Qu.:1.000
## Max.    :1.000
## NA's    :1
```

In order to make summary results more informative, factors in the dataset will be assigned these labels:

```
#Assign labels to factors
e1684$TRT <- as.factor(e1684$TRT)
levels(e1684$TRT) <- c("Control", "IFN")

e1684$SEX <- as.factor(e1684$SEX)
levels(e1684$SEX) <- c("Female", "Male")
```

Finally, observation number 37 will be removed because of missing observations:

```
# Remove observation 37 because it has missing values
d <- na.omit(e1684)
```

Now, the data can be summarized as follows:

```
summary(d)
```

```
##        TRT              FAILTIME          FAILCENS           AGE
## Control:140    Min.    :0.033    Min.    :0.00    Min.    :-29.99
## IFN     :144    1st Qu.:0.354    1st Qu.:0.00    1st Qu.:-11.32
##                 Median :1.215    Median :1.00    Median :  0.58
##                 Mean    :2.754    Mean    :0.69    Mean    :  0.00
##                 3rd Qu.:4.950    3rd Qu.:1.00    3rd Qu.: 11.03
##                 Max.    :9.644    Max.    :1.00    Max.    : 31.70
##        SEX
## Female:171
## Male  :113
##
##
##
##
```

Next, a Kaplan-Meier estimate of the survival times is obtained using function `survfit()` from package `survival` (see Chapter 10 for details):

```
library("survival")

km <- survfit(Surv(d$FAILTIME, d$FAILCENS) ~ 1)
```

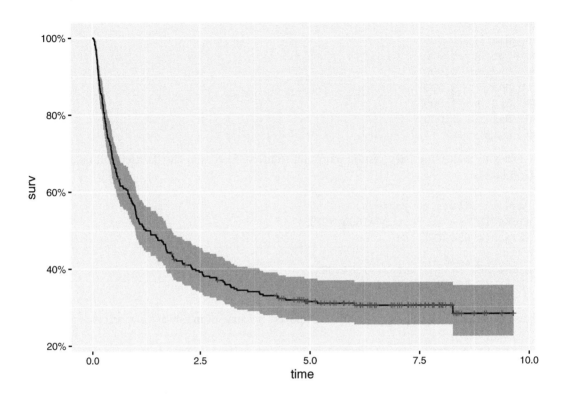

FIGURE 13.4 Kaplan-Meier estimate of the survival times in the `e1684` dataset.

This has been plotted in Figure 13.4. Next, the model is fit. Note that first the response variable needs to be created by using function `inla.surv()`. See Chapter 10 for details.

```
d.inla <- list(y = inla.surv(d$FAILTIME, d$FAILCENS),
  Treatment = d$TRT, Age = d$AGE, Female = d$SEX)

cure.inla <- inla(y ~ Treatment + Age + Female, family = "weibullcure",
  data = d.inla)
summary(cure.inla)
```

```
##
## Call:
##    c("inla(formula = y ~ Treatment + Age + Female, family =
##    \"weibullcure\", ", " data = d.inla)")
## Time used:
##    Pre = 0.976, Running = 0.299, Post = 0.0619, Total = 1.34
```

```
## Fixed effects:
##                mean     sd 0.025quant 0.5quant 0.975quant    mode kld
## (Intercept)  -0.070 0.120     -0.314   -0.068      0.158 -0.063   0
## TreatmentIFN -0.134 0.160     -0.454   -0.132      0.176 -0.129   0
## Age          -0.007 0.006     -0.017   -0.007      0.004 -0.006   0
## FemaleMale    0.142 0.161     -0.178    0.143      0.454  0.145   0
##
## Model hyperparameters:
##                          mean     sd 0.025quant 0.5quant 0.975quant  mode
## alpha parameter for ps  0.928 0.050      0.829    0.929      1.026 0.933
## p parameter for ps      0.297 0.028      0.244    0.296      0.354 0.295
##
## Expected number of effective parameters(stdev): 4.00(0.00)
## Number of equivalent replicates : 70.98
##
## Marginal log-Likelihood:  -401.64
```

The estimates are similar to those reported in Lázaro et al. (2020), which compare MCMC and a different model fitting approach similar to Gibbs sampling with INLA.

Note that the cure rate model estimates that the posterior mean of the proportion of cured patients is 0.2969. A typical analysis using a Weibull survival model (i.e., ignoring the possibility of being cured) will yield the following results:

```
weibull.inla <- inla(y ~ Treatment + Age + Female, family = "weibullsurv",
  data = d.inla, control.family = list(list(variant = 0)))
summary(weibull.inla)
```

```
##
## Call:
##    c("inla(formula = y ~ Treatment + Age + Female, family =
##    \"weibullsurv\", ", " data = d.inla, control.family =
##    list(list(variant = 0)))" )
## Time used:
##     Pre = 0.97, Running = 0.138, Post = 0.0594, Total = 1.17
## Fixed effects:
##                mean     sd 0.025quant 0.5quant 0.975quant    mode kld
## (Intercept)  -0.641 0.122     -0.885   -0.639     -0.407 -0.635   0
## TreatmentIFN -0.379 0.144     -0.662   -0.379     -0.098 -0.379   0
## Age           0.007 0.005     -0.004    0.007      0.017  0.007   0
## FemaleMale    0.001 0.147     -0.290    0.002      0.286  0.003   0
##
## Model hyperparameters:
##                               mean     sd 0.025quant 0.5quant 0.975quant
## alpha parameter for weibullsurv 0.606 0.035       0.54    0.606      0.677
##                               mode
## alpha parameter for weibullsurv 0.605
##
## Expected number of effective parameters(stdev): 4.00(0.00)
## Number of equivalent replicates : 70.98
##
## Marginal log-Likelihood:  -433.14
```

Notice how the effect of the treatment is significant now. Hence, making the assumption that patients can be cured can have an important effect on the estimation of the main effects in the model. Furthermore, the marginal likelihood of the cure rate model is larger than the one of the Weibull model, which suggests a better fit of the cure rate model. However, bear in mind that the marginal likelihood does not penalize for the complexity of the model. Overfit models tend to have higher values of the marginal likelihood.

13.5.1   Joint cure rate models

When studying cure rate models also of interest is the probability of being cured for each patient. Note that a survival model will look at survival times (that may be affected by receiving a treatment) and that a cure rate model will look at the proportions of cured subjects. This probability can also be modeled on the covariates. However, the `weibullcure` latent effect does not allow for the inclusion of the covariates to model cure rate proportion w.

Lázaro et al. (2020) propose a joint model that includes a cure rate model and a logistic regression to model w. Modeling relies on introducing a latent variable $\mathbf{z}$ to assign each subject to the cured or uncured groups. The model is fit using an algorithm similar to Gibbs sampling and at each step the survival model is fit on the uncured population and a logistic regression using the complete dataset to model $\mathbf{z}$ on the explanatory covariates. Hence, this joint model can estimate survival times as well as the probability of being cured.

13.6   Final remarks

Here we have provided an introduction on how to use INLA to fit mixture models. This approach is based on fitting conditional models on $\mathbf{z}$ and seems to provide good results for the examples presented herein. However, fitting mixture models is difficult in general. Furthermore, this approach relies on having good approximations to the marginal likelihoods of the conditional models, which may not always be the case (see Gómez-Rubio and Rue, 2018, for a discussion on this).

On the other hand, the computational approach described here to fit mixture models with INLA has the advantage of providing a toolbox for building different types of mixture models, with different types of likelihoods and priors on the hyperparameters not restricted to conjugate priors. These are probably the two major advantages of this approach.

Packages used in the book

The list of packages used when compiling this book is listed below. This can be very useful when reproducing the examples in this book as results may vary when different versions of R and installed packages are used.

```
## [1] "2020-01-09 14:37:10 CET"
```

```
## R version 3.6.1 (2019-07-05)
## Platform: x86_64-apple-darwin15.6.0 (64-bit)
## Running under: macOS Catalina 10.15.1
##
## Matrix products: default
## BLAS:   R_HOME/Versions/3.6/Resources/lib/libRblas.0.dylib
## LAPACK: R_HOME/Versions/3.6/Resources/lib/libRlapack.dylib
##
## attached base packages:
## [1] splines    parallel   stats      graphics   grDevices utils
## [7] datasets   methods    base
##
## other attached packages:
##  [1] viridis_0.5.1         viridisLite_0.3.0
##  [3] USAboundaries_0.3.1   tmap_2.3-1
##  [5] spelling_2.1          spatstat_1.62-2
##  [7] rpart_4.1-15          spatstat.data_1.4-0
##  [9] smcure_2.0            SemiPar_1.0-4.2
## [11] SDraw_2.1.8           rmarkdown_2.0
## [13] rgeos_0.5-2           rgdal_1.4-8
## [15] RColorBrewer_1.1-2    mice_3.7.0
## [17] lattice_0.20-38       maptools_0.9-9
## [19] MixtureInf_1.1        logitnorm_0.8.37
## [21] lme4_1.1-21           leaflet_2.0.3
## [23] knitr_1.26            KFAS_1.3.7
## [25] JMbayes_0.8-83        rstan_2.19.2
## [27] StanHeaders_2.19.0    doParallel_1.0.15
## [29] iterators_1.0.12      foreach_1.4.7
## [31] survival_3.1-8        nlme_3.1-143
## [33] inlabru_2.1.12        INLABMA_0.1-11
## [35] INLA_19.09.03         Matrix_1.2-18
## [37] gridExtra_2.3         ggfortify_0.4.8
## [39] ggplot2_3.2.1         faraway_1.0.7
## [41] drc_3.0-1             dlm_1.1-5
## [43] deldir_0.1-23         DClusterm_1.0-0
## [45] DCluster_0.2-7        MASS_7.3-51.5
## [47] spdep_1.1-3           sf_0.8-0
## [49] spData_0.3.2          boot_1.3-24
## [51] spacetime_1.2-2       sp_1.3-2
## [53] bookdown_0.16.5
```

```
##
## loaded via a namespace (and not attached):
##    [1] tidyselect_0.2.5       htmlwidgets_1.5.1
##    [3] grid_3.6.1             munsell_0.5.0
##    [5] codetools_0.2-16       units_0.6-5
##    [7] withr_2.1.2            colorspace_1.4-1
##    [9] AlgDesign_1.2.0        rstudioapi_0.10
##   [11] stats4_3.6.1           pscl_1.5.2
##   [13] tensor_1.5             polyclip_1.10-0
##   [15] coda_0.19-3            LearnBayes_2.15.1
##   [17] vctrs_0.2.1            generics_0.0.2
##   [19] TH.data_1.0-10         xfun_0.11
##   [21] R6_2.4.1               jagsUI_1.5.1
##   [23] spatstat.utils_1.15-0  assertthat_0.2.1
##   [25] promises_1.1.0         scales_1.1.0
##   [27] multcomp_1.4-11        nnet_7.3-12
##   [29] gtable_0.3.0           lwgeom_0.1-7
##   [31] processx_3.4.1         goftest_1.2-2
##   [33] sandwich_2.5-1         rlang_0.4.2
##   [35] zeallot_0.1.0          lazyeval_0.2.2
##   [37] acepack_1.4.1          dichromat_2.0-0
##   [39] rjags_4-10             broom_0.5.3
##   [41] checkmate_1.9.4        inline_0.3.15
##   [43] yaml_2.2.0             abind_1.4-5
##   [45] crosstalk_1.0.0        backports_1.1.5
##   [47] httpuv_1.5.2           spsurvey_4.1.1
##   [49] Hmisc_4.3-0            tools_3.6.1
##   [51] raster_3.0-7           Rcpp_1.0.3
##   [53] base64enc_0.1-3        classInt_0.4-2
##   [55] purrr_0.3.3            ps_1.3.0
##   [57] prettyunits_1.0.2      tmaptools_2.0-2
##   [59] zoo_1.8-6              haven_2.2.0
##   [61] cluster_2.1.0          magrittr_1.5
##   [63] data.table_1.12.8      openxlsx_4.1.4
##   [65] gmodels_2.18.1         crossdes_1.1-1
##   [67] mvtnorm_1.0-11         mitml_0.3-7
##   [69] matrixStats_0.55.0     hms_0.5.2
##   [71] mime_0.8               evaluate_0.14
##   [73] xtable_1.8-4           XML_3.98-1.20
##   [75] rio_0.5.16             jpeg_0.1-8.1
##   [77] readxl_1.3.1           compiler_3.6.1
##   [79] tibble_2.1.3           KernSmooth_2.23-16
##   [81] crayon_1.3.4           minqa_1.2.4
##   [83] htmltools_0.4.0        mgcv_1.8-31
##   [85] later_1.0.0            Formula_1.2-3
##   [87] tidyr_1.0.0            expm_0.999-4
##   [89] DBI_1.1.0              car_3.0-6
##   [91] cli_2.0.0              quadprog_1.5-8
##   [93] gdata_2.18.0           pan_1.6
##   [95] forcats_0.4.0          pkgconfig_2.0.3
##   [97] foreign_0.8-74         stringr_1.4.0
```

```
##   [99] callr_3.4.0             digest_0.6.23
## [101] cellranger_1.1.0        leafsync_0.1.0
## [103] intervals_0.15.1        htmlTable_1.13.3
## [105] curl_4.3                shiny_1.4.0
## [107] gtools_3.8.1            jomo_2.6-10
## [109] nloptr_1.2.1            lifecycle_0.1.0
## [111] carData_3.0-3           fansi_0.4.0
## [113] pillar_1.4.3            loo_2.2.0
## [115] fastmap_1.0.1           plotrix_3.7-7
## [117] pkgbuild_1.0.6          glue_1.3.1
## [119] xts_0.11-2              zip_2.0.4
## [121] png_0.1-7               class_7.3-15
## [123] stringi_1.4.3           latticeExtra_0.6-29
## [125] dplyr_0.8.3             e1071_1.7-3
```

Bibliography

Andersen, P. K., O. Borgan, R. D. Gill, and N. Keiding (1993). *Statistical Models Based on Counting Processes*. New York: Springer.

Auguie, B. (2017). *gridExtra: Miscellaneous Functions for "Grid" Graphics*. R package version 2.3.

Azzalini, A. and A. W. Bowman (1990). A look at some data on the old faithful geyser. *Applied Statistics 39*, 357–365.

Bachl, F. E., F. Lindgren, D. L. Borchers, and J. B. Illian (2019). inlabru: an R package for Bayesian spatial modelling from ecological survey data. *Methods in Ecology and Evolution 10*, 760–766.

Baddeley, A., E. Rubak, and R. Turner (2015). *Spatial Point Patterns: Methodology and Applications with R*. London: Chapman and Hall/CRC Press.

Bakka, H. (2019). Small tutorials on INLA. `https://haakonbakka.bitbucket.io/organisedtopics.html`.

Banerjee, S., B. P. Carlin, and A. E. Gelfand (2014). *Hierarchical Modeling and Analysis for Spatial Data* (2nd ed.). Boca Raton, FL: Chapman & Hall/CRC.

Bates, D., M. Mächler, B. Bolker, and S. Walker (2015). Fitting linear mixed-effects models using lme4. *Journal of Statistical Software 67*(1), 1–48.

Bates, D. and M. Maechler (2019). *Matrix: Sparse and Dense Matrix Classes and Methods*. R package version 1.2-17.

Belenky, G., N. J. Wesensten, D. R. Thorne, M. L. Thomas, H. C. Sing, D. P. Redmond, M. B. Russo, and T. J. Balkin (2003). Patterns of performance degradation and restoration during sleep restriction and subsequent recovery: a sleep dose-response study. *Journal of Sleep Research 12*(1), 1–12.

Bivand, R., T. Keitt, and B. Rowlingson (2019). *rgdal: Bindings for the 'Geospatial' Data Abstraction Library*. R package version 1.4-8.

Bivand, R. and N. Lewin-Koh (2019). *maptools: Tools for Handling Spatial Objects*. R package version 0.9-9.

Bivand, R., J. Nowosad, and R. Lovelace (2019). *spData: Datasets for Spatial Analysis*. R package version 0.3.2.

Bivand, R. and C. Rundel (2019). *rgeos: Interface to Geometry Engine - Open Source ('GEOS')*. R package version 0.5-2.

Bivand, R. and D. W. S. Wong (2018). Comparing implementations of global and local indicators of spatial association. *TEST 27*(3), 716–748.

Bivand, R. S. (2017). Revisiting the Boston data set - changing the units of observation affects estimated willingness to pay for clean air. *REGION 1*(4), 109–127.

Bivand, R. S., V. Gómez-Rubio, and H. Rue (2014). Approximate Bayesian inference for spatial econometrics models. *Spatial Statistics 9*, 146–165.

Bivand, R. S., V. Gómez-Rubio, and H. Rue (2015). Spatial data analysis with R-INLA with some extensions. *Journal of Statistical Software 63*(20), 1–31.

Bivand, R. S., E. Pebesma, and V. Gómez-Rubio (2013). *Applied Spatial Data Analysis with R* (2nd ed.). New York: Springer.

Blair, A. L., D. R. Hadden, J. A. Weaver, D. B. Archer, P. B. Johnston, and C. J. Maguire (1976). The 5-year prognosis for vision in diabetes. *American Journal of Ophthalmology 81*, 383–396.

Blangiardo, M. and M. Cameletti (2015). *Spatial and Spatio-temporal Bayesian models with R-INLA*. Chichester, UK: John Wiley & Sons Ltd.

Blatchford, P., H. Goldstein, M. C., and W. Browne (2002). A study of class size effects in English school reception year classes. *British Educational Research Journal 28*, 169–185.

Bliese, P. (2016). *multilevel: Multilevel Functions*. R package version 2.6.

Bliss, C. I. (1967). *Statistics in Biology*. McGraw Hill, New York.

Box, G., W. Hunter, and J. Hunter (1978). *Statistics for Experimenters*. Wiley, New York.

Box, G. E. P. and N. R. Draper (1987). *Empirical Model Building and Response Surfaces*. New York, NY: John Wiley & Sons.

Box, G. E. P., G. M. Jenkins, and G. C. Reinsel (1976). *Time Series Analysis, Forecasting and Control* (3rd ed.). Holden-Day.

Brooks, S., A. Gelman, G. L. Jones, and X.-L. Meng (2011). *Handbook of Markov Chain Monte Carlo*. Boca Raton, FL: Chapman & Hall/CRC Press.

Brooks, S. P. and A. Gelman (1998). General methods for monitoring convergence of iterative simulations. *Journal of Computational and Graphical Statistics 7*, 434–455.

Cai, C., Y. Zou, Y. Peng, and J. Zhang (2012a). smcure: An R-package for estimating semi-parametric mixture cure models. *Computer Methods and Programs in Biomedicine 108*(3), 1255–1260.

Cai, C., Y. Zou, Y. Peng, and J. Zhang (2012b). *smcure: Fit Semiparametric Mixture Cure Models*. R package version 2.0.

Cameletti, M., V. Gómez-Rubio, and M. Blangiardo (2019). Bayesian modelling for spatially misaligned health and air pollution data through the INLA-SPDE approach. *Spatial Statistics 31*, 100353.

Carlin, B. P. and S. Chib (1995). Bayesian model choice via Markov chain Monte Carlo methods. *Journal of the Royal Statistical Society, Series B 57*(3), 473 – 484.

Carlin, B. P. and T. A. Louis (2008). *Bayesian Methods for Data Analysis* (3rd ed.). Boca Raton, FL: Chapman & Hall/CRC Press.

Carpenter, J., H. Goldstein, and M. Kenward (2011). Realcom-impute software for multilevel multiple imputation with mixed response types. *Journal of Statistical Software, Articles 45*(5), 1–14.

Celeux, G., Merrilee, and C. P. Robert (2000). Computational and inferential difficulties with mixture posterior distributions. *Journal of the American Statistical Association 95* (451), 957–970.

Cheng, J., B. Karambelkar, and Y. Xie (2019). *leaflet: Create Interactive Web Maps with the JavaScript 'Leaflet' Library.* R package version 2.0.3.

Chib, S. (1995). Marginal likelihood from the Gibbs output. *Journal of the American Statistical Association 90* (432), 1313–1321.

Chib, S. and I. Jeliazkov (2001). Marginal likelihoods from the Metropolis-Hastings output. *Journal of the American Statistical Association 96*, 270–281.

Condit, R. (1998). *Tropical Forest Census Plots.* Springer-Verlag Berlin Heidelberg.

Condit, R., S. P. Hubbell, and R. B. Foster (1996). Changes in tree species abundance in a neotropical forest: impact of climate change. *Journal of Tropical Ecology 12*, 231–256.

Cox, D. R. (1972). Regression models and life-tables. *Journal of the Royal Statistical Society. Series B 34* (2), 187–220.

Cressie, N. (2015). *Statistics for Spatial Data* (Revised ed.). Hoboken, New Jersey: John Wiley & Sons, Inc.

Cressie, N. and N. H. Chan (1989). Spatial modelling of regional variables. *Journal of the American Statistical Association 84*, 393–401.

Cressie, N. and T. R. C. Read (1985). Do sudden infant deaths come in clusters? *Statistics and Decisions , Supplement Issue 2*, 333–349.

Cressie, N. and C. K. Wikle (2011). *Statistics for Spatio-Temporal Data.* Hoboken, New Jersey: John Wiley & Sons, Inc.

Davies, O. L. (1954). *The Design and Analysis of Industrial Experiments.* Wiley.

Dempster, A. P., N. M. Laird, and D. B. Rubin (1977). Maximum likelihood from incomplete data via the EM algorithm (with discussion). *Journal of the Royal Statistical Society: Series B 39*, 1–38.

Diebolt, J. and C. P. Robert (1994). Estimation of finite mixture distributions through Bayesian sampling. *Journal of the Royal Statistical Society, Series B 56* (2), 363–375.

Diggle, P. J. (2013). *Statistical Analysis of Spatial and Spatio-Temporal Point Patterns* (3rd ed.). Chapman and Hall/CRC Press.

Diggle, P. J., V. Gómez-Rubio, P. E. Brown, A. G. Chetwynd, and S. Gooding (2007). Second-order analysis of inhomogeneous spatial point processes using case–control data. *Biometrics 2* (63), 550—-557.

Fahrmeir, L. and T. Kneib (2011). *Bayesian Smoothing Regression for Longitudinal, Spatial and Event History Data.* New York: Oxford University Press.

Faraway, J. (2006). *Extending the Linear Model with R.* Chapman; Hall, London.

Faraway, J. (2016). *faraway: Functions and Datasets for Books by Julian Faraway.* R package version 1.0.7.

Faraway, J. J. (2019a). Inferential methods for linear mixed models. `http://www.maths.bath.ac.uk/~jjf23/mixchange/index.html#worked-examples`.

Faraway, J. J. (2019b). INLA for linear mixed models. `http://www.maths.bath.ac.uk/~jjf23/inla/`.

Frühwirth-Schnatter, S., G. Celeux, and C. P. Robert (Eds.) (2018). *Handbook of Mixture Analysis*. Boca Raton, FL: Chapman & Hall/CRC Press.

Fuentes, M., L. Chen, and J. M. Davis (2007). A class of nonseparable and nonstationary spatial temporal covariance functions. *Environmetrics 19*(5), 487–507.

Garnier, S. (2018a). *viridis: Default Color Maps from 'matplotlib'*. R package version 0.5.1.

Garnier, S. (2018b). *viridisLite: Default Color Maps from 'matplotlib' (Lite Version)*. R package version 0.3.0.

Gelman, A. (2006). Prior distributions for variance parameters in hierarchical models. *Bayesian Analysis 1*(3), 515–534.

Gelman, A., J. B. Carlin, H. S. Stern, D. B. Dunson, A. Vehtari, and D. B. Rubin (2013). *Bayesian Data Analysis* (3rd ed.). Boca Raton, FL: Chapman & Hall/CRC Press.

Gelman, A., J. Fagan, and A. Kiss (2007). An analysis of the New York City police department's "stop-and-frisk" policy in the context of claims of racial bias. *Journal of the American Statistical Association 102*(479), 813–823.

Gelman, A. and J. Hill (2006). *Data Analysis Using Regression and Multilevel/Hierarchical Models*. Cambridge University Press.

Gelman, A., J. Hwang, and A. Vehtari (2014, Nov). Understanding predictive information criteria for bayesian models. *Statistics and Computing 24*(6), 997–1016.

Gelman, A. and T. C. Little (1997). Poststratification into many categories using hierarchical logistic regression. *Survey Methodology 23*, 127–135.

Gelman, A., X.-L. Meng, and H. Stern (1996). Posterior predictive assessment of model fitness via realized discrepancies. *Statistica Sinica 6*, 733–807.

Gelman, A. and D. B. Rubin (1992). Inference from iterative simulation using multiple sequences. *Statistical Science 7*, 457–511.

Geman, S. and D. Geman (1984). Stochastic relaxation, Gibbs distributions, and the Bayesian restoration of images. *IEEE Transactions on Pattern Analysis and Machine Intelligence 6*(6), 721–741.

Gilks, W., W. Gilks, S. Richardson, and D. Spiegelhalter (1996). *Markov Chain Monte Carlo in Practice*. Boca Raton, Florida: Chapman & Hall.

Gilley, O. W. and R. K. Pace (1996). On the Harrison and Rubinfeld data. *Journal of Environmental Economics and Management 31*, 403–405.

Goicoa, T., A. Adin, M. D. Ugarte, and J. S. Hodges (2018). In spatio-temporal disease mapping models, identifiability constraints affect PQL and INLA results. *Stochastic Environmental Research and Risk Assessment 3*(32), 749–770.

Goldstein, H. (2003). *Multilevel Statistical Models* (3rd ed.). Kendall's Library of Statistics. Arnold, London.

Gómez-Rubio, V. (2017, December). Mixture model fitting using conditional models and modal Gibbs sampling. *arXiv e-prints*, arXiv:1712.09566.

Gómez-Rubio, V. and H. Rue (2018). Markov chain Monte Carlo with the integrated nested Laplace approximation. *Statistics and Computing 28*(5), 1033–1051.

Gómez-Rubio, V., R. S. Bivand, and H. Rue (2017, Mar). Estimating Spatial Econometrics Models with Integrated Nested Laplace Approximation. *arXiv e-prints*, arXiv:1703.01273.

Gómez-Rubio, V., R. S. Bivand, and H. Rue (2019, Nov). Bayesian model averaging with the integrated nested Laplace approximation. *arXiv e-prints*, arXiv:1911.00797.

Gómez-Rubio, V., M. Cameletti, and M. Blangiardo (2019, Dec). Missing data analysis and imputation via latent Gaussian Markov random fields. *arXiv e-prints*, arXiv:1912.10981.

Gómez-Rubio, V., M. Cameletti, and F. Finazzi (2015). Analysis of massive marked point patterns with stochastic partial differential equations. *Spatial Statistics 14*, 179 – 196. Spatio-Temporal Stochastic Modelling of Environmental Hazards.

Gómez-Rubio, V., P. Moraga, J. Molitor, and B. Rowlingson (2019). DClusterm: Model-based detection of disease clusters. *Journal of Statistical Software, Articles 90*(14), 1–26.

Gómez-Rubio, V. and F. Palmí-Perales (2019). Multivariate posterior inference for spatial models with the integrated nested Laplace approximation. *Journal of the Royal Statistical Society: Series C (Applied Statistics) 68*(1), 199–215.

Gómez-Rubio, V., F. Palmí-Perales, G. López-Abente, R. Ramis-Prieto, and P. Fernández-Navarro (2019). Bayesian joint spatio-temporal analysis of multiple diseases. *SORT 43*(1), 51–74.

Haining, R. (2003). *Spatial Data Analysis: Theory and Practice*. Cambridge University Press.

Harrison, D. and D. L. Rubinfeld (1978). Hedonic housing prices and the demand for clean air. *Journal of Environmental Economics and Management 5*, 81–102.

Hastie, T., R. Tibshirani, and J. Friedman (2009). *The Elements of Statistical Learning* (2nd ed.). New York: Springer.

Held, L., B. Schrödle, and H. Rue (2010). Posterior and cross-validatory predictive checks: A comparison of MCMC and INLA. In T. Kneib and G. Tutz (Eds.), *Statistical Modelling and Regression Structures – Festschrift in Honour of Ludwig Fahrmeir*, pp. 91–110. Berlin: Springer Verlag.

Helske, J. (2017). KFAS: Exponential family state space models in R. *Journal of Statistical Software 78*(10), 1–39.

Hoeting, J., D. Madigan, A. Raftery, and C. Volinsky (1999). Bayesian model averaging: A tutorial. *Statistical Science 14*, 382–401.

Holst, U., O. Hössjer, C. Björklund, P. Ragnarson, and H. Edner (1996, 7). Locally weighted least squares kernel regression and statistical evaluation of LIDAR measurements. *Environmetrics 7*(4), 401–416.

Horikoshi, M. and Y. Tang (2018). *ggfortify: Data Visualization Tools for Statistical Analysis Results*.

Hubbell, S. P. and R. B. Foster (1983). Diversity of canopy trees in a neotropical forest and implications for conservation. In S. L. Sutton, T. C. Whitmore, and A. C. Chadwick (Eds.), *Tropical Rain Forest: Ecology and Management*, pp. 25–41. Oxford: Blackwell Scientific Publications.

Hubin, A. and G. Storvik (2016, Nov). Estimating the marginal likelihood with integrated nested Laplace approximation (INLA). *arXiv e-prints*, arXiv:1611.01450.

Huster, W. J., R. Brookmeyer, and S. G. Self (1989). Modelling paired survival data with covariates. *Biometrics 45*, 145–156.

Ibrahim, J. G., M.-H. Chen, and D. Sinha (2001). *Bayesian Survival Analysis.* Springer.

James, G., D. Witten, T. Hastie, and R. Tibshirani (2013). *An Introduction to Statistical Learning.* New York: Springer.

Jovanovic, M. (2015). R playbook: Introduction to mixed-models. multilevel models playbook. `http://complementarytraining.net/r-playbook-introduction-to-multilevelhierarchical-models/`.

Juan, P., J. Mateu, and C. Díaz-Avalos (2010). Characterizing spatial-temporal forest fire patterns. In *METMA V: International Workshop on Spatio-Temporal Modelling*, Santiago de Compostela, Spain.

Kalbfleisch, D. and R. L. Prentice (1980). *The Statistical Analysis of Failure Time Data.* New York: Wiley.

Kirkwood, J. M., M. H. Strawderman, M. S. Ernstoff, T. J. Smith, E. C. Borden, and R. H. Blum (1996). Interferon alfa-2b adjuvant therapy of high-risk resected cutaneous melanoma: the eastern cooperative oncology group trial est 1684. *Journal of Clinical Oncology 14*(1), 7–17. PMID: 8558223.

Knorr-Held, L. (2000). Bayesian modelling of inseparable space-time variation in disease risk. *Statistics in Medicine 19*(17-18), 2555–2567.

Koop, G. and M. F. J. Steel (1994). A decision-theoretic analysis of the unit-root hypothesis using mixtures of elliptical models. *Journal of Business and Economic Statistics 12*, 95–107.

Krainski, E. T., V. Gómez-Rubio, H. Bakka, A. Lenzi, D. Castro-Camilo, D. Simpson, F. Lindgren, and H. Rue (2018). *Advanced Spatial Modeling with Stochastic Partial Differential Equations Using R and INLA.* Boca Raton, FL: Chapman & Hall/CRC.

Kruschke, J. K. (2015). *Doing Bayesian Data Analysis, Second Edition: A Tutorial with R, JAGS, and Stan* (2nd ed.). Amsterdam: Academic Press.

Kulldorff, M., W. F. Athas, E. J. Feurer, B. A. Miller, and C. R. Key (1998). Evaluating cluster alarms: a space-time scan statistic and brain cancer in Los Alamos, New Mexico. *American Journal of Public Health 88*, 1377–1380.

Leroux, B., X. Lei, and N. Breslow (1999). Estimation of disease rates in small areas: A new mixed model for spatial dependence. In M. Halloran and D. Berry (Eds.), *Statistical Models in Epidemiology, the Environment and Clinical Trials*, pp. 135–178. New York: Springer-Verlag.

Li, S., J. Chen, and P. Li (2016). *MixtureInf: Inference for Finite Mixture Models.* R package version 1.1.

Lindgren, F., H. Rue, and J. Lindström (2011). An explicit link between Gaussian fields and Gaussian Markov random fields: the stochastic partial differential equation approach (with discussion). *Journal of the Royal Statistical Society, Series B 73*(4), 423–498.

Link, W. A. and M. J. Eaton (2012). On thinning of chains in MCMC. *Methods in Ecology and Evolution 3*(1), 112–115.

Little, R. J. A. and D. B. Rubin (2002). *Statistical Analysis with Missing Data* (2nd ed.). New York: Wiley & Sonc, Inc.

Lovelace, R., J. Nowosad, and J. Muenchow (2019). *Geocomputation with R*. Boca Raton, FL: Chapman & Hall/CRC.

Lázaro, E., C. Armero, and V. Gómez-Rubio (2020). Approximate Bayesian inference for mixture cure models. *TEST , to appear*.

MacKay, D. J. C. (2003). *Information Theory, Inference, and Learning Algorithms*. Cambridge University Press.

Marin, J.-M., K. Mengersen, and C. P. Robert (2005). Bayesian modelling and inference on mixtures of distributions. In D. K. Dey and C. R. Rao (Eds.), *Handbook of Statistics*, Volume 25. Elsevier.

Marshall, E. C. and D. J. Spiegelhalter (2003). Approximate cross-validatory predictive checks in disease mapping models. *Statistics in Medicine 22*(10), 1649–1660.

Martins, T. G., D. Simpson, F. Lindgren, and H. Rue (2013). Bayesian computing with INLA: New features. *Computational Statistics & Data Analysis 67*, 68–83.

McDonald, T. and A. McDonald (2019). *SDraw: Spatially Balanced Samples of Spatial Objects*. R package version 2.1.8.

McElreath, R. (2016). *Statistical Rethinking: A Bayesian Course with Examples in R and Stan*. Boca Raton, FL: Chapman & Hall/CRC Press.

Moberg, A., D. M. Sonechkin, K. Holmgren, N. M. Datsenko, and W. Karlén (2005). Highly variable northern hemisphere temperatures reconstructed from low- and high-resolution proxy data. *Nature 443*, 613–617.

Moore, D. F. (2016). *Applied Survival Analysis Using R*. Springer.

Morrison, K. (2017). A gentle INLA tutorial. `https://www.precision-analytics.ca/blog/a-gentle-inla-tutorial/`.

Mullen, L. A. and J. Bratt (2018). USAboundaries: Historical and contemporary boundaries of the United States of America. *Journal of Open Source Software 3*, 314.

Møller, J. and R. Waagepetersen (2007). Modern spatial point process modelling and inference (with discussion). *Scandinavian Journal of Statistics 34*, 643–711.

Neuwirth, E. (2014). *RColorBrewer: ColorBrewer Palettes*. R package version 1.1-2.

New York Attorney General (1999). The New York police department's "stop and frisk" practices. `https://ag.ny.gov/sites/default/files/pdfs/bureaus/civil_rights/stp_frsk.pdf`.

Ooms, J. and J. Hester (2019). *spelling: Tools for Spell Checking in R*. R package version 2.1.

Palmí-Perales, F., V. Gómez-Rubio, and M. A. Martínez-Beneito (2019, Sep). Bayesian Multivariate Spatial Models for Lattice Data with INLA. *arXiv e-prints*, arXiv:1909.10804.

Pebesma, E. (2012). spacetime: Spatio-temporal data in R. *Journal of Statistical Software 51*(7), 1–30.

Pebesma, E. (2018). Simple Features for R: Standardized Support for Spatial Vector Data. *The R Journal 10*(1), 439–446.

Pebesma, E. J. (2004). Multivariable geostatistics in S: the gstat package. *Computers & Geosciences 30*, 683–691.

Petris, G. (2010). An R package for dynamic linear models. *Journal of Statistical Software 36*(12), 1–16.

Petris, G., S. Petrone, and P. Campagnoli (2009). *Dynamic Linear Models with R.* useR! Springer-Verlag, New York.

Pettit, L. I. (1990). The conditional predictive ordinate for the normal distribution. *Journal of the Royal Statistical Society. Series B (Methodological) 52*(1), pp. 175–184.

Pinheiro, J., D. Bates, S. DebRoy, D. Sarkar, and R Core Team (2018). *nlme: Linear and Nonlinear Mixed Effects Models.* R package version 3.1-137.

Pinheiro, J. C. and D. M. Bates (2000). *Mixed-Effects Models in S and S-PLUS.* Springer, New York.

R Core Team (2019a). *R: A Language and Environment for Statistical Computing.* Vienna, Austria: R Foundation for Statistical Computing.

R Core Team (2019b). *Writing R Extensions.*

Richardson, S. and P. J. Green (1997). On Bayesian analysis of mixtures with an unknown number of components (with discussion). *Journal of the Royal Statistical Society: Series B (Statistical Methodology) 59*(4), 731–792.

Ritz, C., F. Baty, J. C. Streibig, and D. Gerhard (2015). Dose-response analysis using R. *PLOS ONE 10*(e0146021).

Rizopoulos, D. (2016). The R package JMbayes for fitting joint models for longitudinal and time-to-event data using mcmc. *Journal of Statistical Software 72*(7), 1–45.

Rue, H. (2009). INLA: An introduction. INLA users workshop May 2009.

Rue, H. and L. Held (2005). *Gaussian Markov Random Fields: Theory and Applications.* Chapman and Hall/CRC Press.

Rue, H., S. Martino, and N. Chopin (2009). Approximate Bayesian inference for latent Gaussian models by using integrated nested Laplace approximations. *Journal of the Royal Statistical Society, Series B 71*(2), 319–392.

Rue, H., A. Riebler, S. H. Sørbye, J. B. Illian, D. P. Simpson, and F. K. Lindgren (2017). Bayesian computing with INLA: A review. *Annual Review of Statistics and Its Application 4*(1), 395–421.

Ruiz-Cárdenas, R., E. T. Krainski, and H. Rue (2012). Direct fitting of dynamic models using integrated nested Laplace approximations — INLA. *Computational Statistics & Data Analysis 56*(6), 1808 – 1828.

Ruppert, D., M. P. Wand, and R. J. Carroll (2003). *Semiparametric Regression.* New York: Cambridge University Press.

Schafer, J. (1997). *Analysis of Incomplete Multivariate Data.* London: Chapman & Hall.

Schonbeck, Y., H. Talma, P. van Dommelen, B. Bakker, S. E. Buitendijk, R. A. Hirasing, and S. van Buuren (2011). Increase in prevalence of overweight in Dutch children and adolescents: A comparison of nationwide growth studies in 1980, 1997 and 2009. *PLoS ONE 6*(11), e27608.

Schonbeck, Y., H. Talma, P. van Dommelen, B. Bakker, S. E. Buitendijk, R. A. Hirasing, and S. van Buuren (2013). The world's tallest nation has stopped growing taller: the height of Dutch children from 1955 to 2009. *Pediatric Research 73*(3), 371–377.

Simpson, D. (2016). INLA for spatial statistics. Grouped models. http://faculty.washington.edu/jonno/SISMIDmaterial/8-Groupedmodels.pdf.

Simpson, D., J. B. Illian, S. H. Sørbye, and H. Rue (2016). Going off grid: computationally efficient inference for log-Gaussian Cox processes. *Biometrika 1*(103), 49–70.

Simpson, D. P., H. Rue, A. Riebler, T. G. Martins, and S. H. Sørbye (2017). Penalising model component complexity: A principled, practical approach to constructing priors. *Statistical Science 32*(1), 1–28.

Sørbye, S. H. (2013). *Tutorial: Scaling IGMRF-models in R-INLA*. Availabe from https://www.math.ntnu.no/inla/r-inla.org/tutorials/inla/scale.model/scale-model-tutorial.pdf.

Sørbye, S. H., J. B. Illian, D. P. Simpson, D. Burslem, and H. Rue (2019). Careful prior specification avoids incautious inference for log-Gaussian Cox point processes. *Journal of the Royal Statistical Society: Series C (Applied Statistics) 68*(3), 543–564.

Sørbye, S. H. and H. Rue (2014). Scaling intrinsic gaussian markov random field priors in spatial modelling. *Spatial Statistics 8*, 39 – 51. Spatial Statistics Miami.

Spiegelhalter, D. J., N. G. Best, B. P. Carlin, and A. Van der Linde (2002). Bayesian measures of model complexity and fit (with discussion). *Journal of the Royal Statistical Society, Series B 64*(4), 583–616.

Stephens, M. (2000). Dealing with label switching in mixture models. *Journal of the Royal Statistical Society: Series B (Statistical Methodology) 62*(4), 795–809.

Tennekes, M. (2018). tmap: Thematic maps in R. *Journal of Statistical Software 84*(6), 1–39.

Terry M. Therneau and Patricia M. Grambsch (2000). *Modeling Survival Data: Extending the Cox Model*. New York: Springer.

Therneau, T. M. (2015). *A Package for Survival Analysis in S*. version 2.38.

Tierney, L. and J. B. Kadane (1986). Accurate approximation for posterior moments and marginal densities. *Journal of the Americal Statistical Association 81*(393), 82–86.

Turner, R. (2019). *deldir: Delaunay Triangulation and Dirichlet (Voronoi) Tessellation*. R package version 0.1-23.

Ugarte, M., A. Adin, T. Goicoa, and A. Militino (2014). On fitting spatio-temporal disease mapping models using approximate Bayesian inference. *Statistical Methods in Medical Research 23*, 507–530.

Ugarte, M. D., A. Adin, and T. Goicoa (2016). Two-level spatially structured models in spatio-temporal disease mapping. *Statistical Methods in Medical Research 25*(4), 1080–1100. PMID: 27566767.

van Buuren, S. (2018). *Flexible Imputation of Missing Data* (2nd ed.). Boca Raton, FL: CRC Press.

van Buuren, S. and K. Groothuis-Oudshoorn (2011). mice: Multivariate imputation by chained equations in R. *Journal of Statistical Software 45*(3), 1–67.

Venables, W. N. and B. D. Ripley (2002). *Modern Applied Statistics with S* (fourth ed.). New York. Springer.

Wand, M. (2018). *SemiPar: Semiparametic Regression*. R package version 1.0-4.2.

Wang, X., Y. Y. Ryan, and J. J. Faraway (2018). *Bayesian Regression Modeling with INLA.* Boca Raton, FL: Chapman & Hall/CRC.

Watanabe, S. (2013). A widely applicable Bayesian information criterion. *Journal of Machine Learning Research 14,* 867–897.

Wickham, H. (2016). *ggplot2: Elegant Graphics for Data Analysis.* Springer-Verlag New York.

Wikle, C. K., L. M. Berliner, and N. Cressie (1998). Hierarchical Bayesian space-time models. *Environmental and Ecological Statistics 5,* 117–154.

Wutzler, T. (2018). *logitnorm: Functions for the Logitnormal Distribution.* R package version 0.8.37.

Xie, Y. (2015). *Dynamic Documents with R and knitr* (2nd ed.). Boca Raton, Florida: Chapman and Hall/CRC. ISBN 978-1498716963.

Xie, Y. (2016). *bookdown: Authoring Books and Technical Documents with R Markdown.* Boca Raton, Florida: Chapman and Hall/CRC. ISBN 978-1138700109.

Xie, Y., J. Allaire, and G. Grolemund (2018). *R Markdown: The Definitive Guide.* Boca Raton, Florida: Chapman and Hall/CRC. ISBN 9781138359338.

Zucchini, W., I. MacDonald, and R. Langrock (2016). *Hidden Markov Models for Time Series: An Introduction Using R* (2nd ed.). CRC Press.

Index

Bayesian inference, 1
Bayesian model averaging, 243
BMA, 243

CCD strategy, 16
central composite design strategy, 16
conjugate prior, 2
control options, 28
    control.compute, 24, 27, 28, 35, 136
    control.expert, 28
    control.family, 28, 103, 136, 179, 191,
        229
    control.fixed, 19, 28, 39, 40
    control.hazard, 28
    control.inla, 28, 29, 122, 252
    control.lincomb, 28, 121
    control.mode, 28
    control.predictor, 28, 96, 119, 162, 262
    control.results, 28
    control.update, 28
cumulative hazard, 219
cure rate model, 293

dataset
    1988 US presidential election, 93
    bei, 142
    Boston housing data, 149
    cement, 18
    class size, 87
    clmfires, 167
    diabetic retinopathy, 230
    e1684, 294
    ECOG phase III clinical trial e1684, 294
    eggs, 82
    fdgs, 260
    Fifth Dutch growth study 2009, 260
    forest fires, 167
    geyser, 280
    H.virescens, 214
    heavy metals, 156
    lidar, 201
    liver cirrhosis, 234, 235
    meuse, 156

Meuse river, 156
National Health and Nutrition
    Examination Survey (NHANES),
    272
nc.sids, 21
nhanes2, 272
North Carolina SIDS, 21, 41, 243
NYC stop and frisk, 97
Old Faithful dataset, 280
penicillin, 75
prothro, 235
prothros, 234
reaction time, 90
retinopathy, 230
tropical rain forest, 142
veteran, 220
Veteran's administration lung cancer
    trial, 220

empirical Bayes, 17

forecasting, 187
function
    inla, 19
    inla.dmarginal, 30
    inla.doc, 50, 59, 63, 73, 106, 107, 112,
        138, 245, 293
    inla.emarginal, 30, 152
    inla.group, 209
    inla.hpdmarginal, 30
    inla.hyperpar, 30, 123
    inla.hyperpar.sample, 37
    inla.make.lincomb, 121
    inla.make.lincombs, 121
    inla.merge, 253, 254, 270, 276, 292
    inla.mesh.2d, 159
    inla.mmarginal, 30
    inla.models, 63, 104
    inla.pc.dprec, 112
    inla.pc.pprec, 112
    inla.pc.qprec, 112
    inla.pc.rprec, 112
    inla.pmarginal, 30, 228

`inla.posterior.sample`, 35–37, 270
`inla.posterior.sample.eval`, 37
`inla.qmarginal`, 30
`inla.rgeneric.define`, 247, 249
`inla.rmarginal`, 30
`inla.smarginal`, 30
`inla.spde.make.A`, 160, 161
`inla.spde.make.index`, 160, 162
`inla.spde2.matern`, 160
`inla.spde2.pcmatern`, 170
`inla.spde2.result`, 163
`inla.stack`, 161, 213
`inla.stack.A`, 162
`inla.stack.data`, 162
`inla.stack.index`, 163
`inla.surv`, 222, 296
`inla.tmarginal`, 10, 30, 152, 223
`inla.zmarginal`, 10, 30, 163, 223, 250
`kn.models`, 198

Gaussian approximation, 15
Gibbs sampling, 4
grid strategy, 16

hazard function, 219

imputation, 267, 272
INLA
    CCD strategy, 16
    central composite design strategy, 16
    empirical Bayes strategy, 17
    Gaussian approximation, 15
    grid strategy, 16
    `inla` object, 19
    Laplace approximation, 16
    simplified Laplace approximation, 16
`inla` object, 19
INLA within MCMC, 243, 272

joint model, 233

Laplace approximation, 16
latent effect, 39
    `ar`, 58
    `ar1`, 58
    `ar1c`, 58
    `besag`, 149, 153
    `besagproper`, 149, 153
    `bym`, 149, 153
    `clinear`, 40
    `copy`, 131
    `crw2`, 52

`generic0`, 46
`generic1`, 47
`generic2`, 48
`generic3`, 48
`iid`, 43
`iid1d`, 49
`iid2d`, 49
`iid3d`, 49
`iid4d`, 49
`iid5d`, 49
`linear`, 40
linear combination, 121
linear constraints, 121, 138
`matern2d`, 142, 147
`replicate`, 134
`rgeneric`, 117, 245
`rw1`, 52, 207
`rw2`, 52, 208
`rw2d`, 142, 146
scaling, 114
smoothing, 201
space-state, 188
spatial, 141
spatio-temporal, 192
`spde`, 155, 158, 173, 212
spline, 201
time series, 177
`weibullcure`, 293
`weibullsurv`, 297
`z`, 45
likelihood, 1
linear combination, 121
linear constraints, 138
longitudinal model, 235

MAP, 6
marginal likelihood, 1, 289
Markov chain Monte Carlo, 3
maximum a posteriori, 6
MCMC, 3
Metropolis-Hastings, 3
missing covariates, 267
missing values, 259
missingness mechanism, 259
mixture model, 279
model
    CAR, 149, 243
    cure rate model, 293
    joint, 233
    joint cure model, 298
    longitudinal, 235

mixture model, 279, 293
multilevel, 75
point pattern, 166
random effects, 75
spatial, 141
survival, 219
multilevel model, 75
multiple imputation, 267, 272
multiple likelihoods, 128
multivariate prior, 117

point pattern, 166
posterior marginal, 30
predictive distribution, 259, 260, 277
predictor matrix, 119
prior
    `expression`, 108
    half-Cauchy, 110
    half-normal, 109
    half-t, 110
    multivariate, 117
    new, 107, 116
    scaling, 114
    sensitivity analysis, 113
    `table`, 107
    uniform, 111
    uninplemented, 107, 116
prior distribution, 1

scaling, 114
sensitivity analysis, 113
simplified Laplace approximation, 16
smoothing, 201
space-state model, 188
spatial model, 141
spatio-temporal model, 192
SPDE, *see* Stochastic Partial Differential
        Equation
spline, 201
Stochastic Partial Differential Equation, 158
survival
    analysis, 219
    cumulative hazard, 219
    density function, 219
    distribution function, 219
    function, 219
    hazard function, 219
    models, 219
survival function, 219

time series, 177
    forecasting, 187

Printed and bound by CPI Group (UK) Ltd, Croydon, CR0 4YY

18/10/2024

01776247-0001